Surgeons, Smallpox, and the Poor

Surgeons, Smallpox, and the Poor

A History of Medicine and Social Conditions in Nova Scotia, 1749–1799

ALLAN EVERETT MARBLE

McGill-Queen's University Press

Montreal & Kingston • London • Buffalo

Legal deposit third quarter 1993
Bibliothèque nationale du Québec

Printed in Canada on acid-free paper

This book has been published with the help of
grants from the Social Science Federation of Canada,
using funds provided by the Social Sciences and
Humanities Research Council of Canada, the Hannah
Institute for the History of Medicine, and the
Dalhousie Medical Alumni Association.

Canadian Cataloguing in Publication Data

Marble, Allan Everett
    Surgeons, smallpox and the poor: a history of medicine
    and social conditions in Nova Scotia, 1749–1799
    Includes bibliographical references and index.
    ISBN 0-7735-0988-7
    1. Medical care – Nova Scotia – History – 18th century.
    2. Medicine – Nova Scotia – History – 18th century.
    3. Nova Scotia – Social conditions. I. Title.
    R463.N68M37 1993   362.1'09716'09033
    C93-090263-7

This book was typeset by Typo Litho composition inc.
in 10/12 Baskerville.

Dedicated to the memory of
Drs James Boggs and John Fraser,
ancestors of the author

Contents

Portraits   12, 36, 72, 100

Acknowledgments   ix

Figures and Tables   xi

Preface   xv

Introduction   3

1   Arrival, Settlement, and an Initial Concern for Health Care, 1749 (o.s.)–1753 (n.s.) / 13

2   A Decade of Military and Naval Surgeons, 1753–1763 / 37

3   Poor Relief Takes Precedence over Health Care, 1763–1775 / 73

4   A New Order of Medical Men: The Loyalists, 1775–1784 / 101

5   Health Care and Poor Relief at the End of the Century, 1784–1799 / 145

Appendices

1   Passengers in the Cornwallis Mess Lists with Health-Care Occupations / 193

2   An Explanation of Medications and Treatments Administered by Surgeons in Halifax during the Period 1750–53 / 195

3 An Act to Prevent the Spreading of
Contagious Distempers, 1761 / 200

4 An Act to Prevent Importing Impotent,
Lame, and Infirm Persons into this
Province / 202

5 Loyalist Physicians and Surgeons Who
Settled in Nova Scotia during 1783 / 204

6 Summary of Claims for Property and Loss
of Income Made by Loyalist Doctors Who
Came to Nova Scotia, Compared with the
Sums Allowed and the Pensions Awarded
by the Loyalist Claims Commissioners / 209

7 The Indenture of Apprenticeship of
William James Allmon / 212

8 Physicians and Surgeons in Charge of
Hospitals in Halifax and Environs,
1749–99 / 214

9 Causes of Death of Nova Scotians
between 1749 and 1799 / 217

Notes   219

Bibliography   319

Index   331

Acknowledgments

During the last fourteen years, I have accumulated a debt of gratitude to archivists and librarians at Trinity College Library in Dublin, the Royal College of Surgeons of England Library, The Wellcome Institute for the History of Medicine, the British Museum, the Public Records Office, and the medical archives at each of Guy's Hospital, St George's Hospital, St Thomas' Hospital, and St Bartholomew's Hospital, in London. In Scotland, I was provided with the very able and friendly assistance of librarians and archivists at the universities of Edinburgh, Glasgow, and St Andrews, as well as at the Royal Colleges of Surgeons in Edinburgh and Glasgow and the Royal College of Physicians in Edinburgh.

In the United States, I was fortunate to be able to study records at the Countway Library at Harvard University, the University of Pennsylvania Archives, the Massachusetts Historical Society, the Boston Public Library, the New England Historic Genealogical Society, the Museum of Fine Arts in Boston, the Medical Society of New Jersey, the American Antiquarian Society of Worcester, Massachusetts, and the New York Public Library. In Canada, I found the staff at the Osler Library at McGill University very helpful, as were the staff at the Centre d'Études Acadiennes, Université de Moncton, and the New Brunswick Museum. I also received useful advice and permission to study and copy valuable maps and paintings from both the National Archives and the National Gallery of Canada. Within Nova Scotia, the staff at the Public Archives of Nova Scotia (PANS) have been particularly helpful over the last fourteen years, identifying source material which has greatly enriched this book. Other archives and museums in Nova Scotia that have assisted me are the Nova Scotia Museum, Parks Canada, the Legislative Library, the Kellogg and Killam libraries at Dalhousie University, the Acadia

University Archives, the Colchester Historical Society Museum, the Yarmouth County Museum and Historical Research Library, the Beaton Institute at the University College of Cape Breton, the Simeon Perkins Museum, and the Art Gallery of Nova Scotia.

Two of my colleagues have spent many hours helping me prepare and edit this book. I refer here to Donald F. Maclean and Terrence Punch, both of Halifax. Mr Maclean read the entire manuscript and made several suggestions regarding style and presentation that have enhanced the literary quality of the book. Mr Punch has very generously provided me with information of both an historical and biographical nature and has also offered valuable suggestions that were implemented in the final version of the manuscript. Others who assisted me by providing items of information included Mary Archibald of Shelburne, Dr George Bate of Saint John, Robert Bond of Toronto, Leone Cousins of Kingston, Laleah Cunningham of Toronto, John Duncanson of Falmouth, Brenda Dunn of Parks Canada, Marie Elwood of the Nova Scotia Museum, Olga Grant of Rothesay, Andrew Gunter of Kentville, Gary Hartlen of Liverpool, Roy Kennedy of Tatamagouche, L.S. Loomer of Windsor, Dr Ron McDonald of Parks Canada, Ronald Angus MacDonald of Antigonish, Shirley McCormick of Middleton, Bev Miller of Halifax, Marion Robertson of Shelburne, Scott Robson of the Nova Scotia Museum, Vernon Spurr of Dartmouth, David States of Halifax, Jim St Clair of Mull River, Dr Brenton Stewart of Moncton, Ira Sutherland of Ottawa, John Swift of Maine, Margaret Wagner of Annapolis Royal, Ellen Webster of Halifax, Robert Webster of Toronto, and Stephen White of the Centre D'Études Acadiennes, Moncton. From PANS, I was assisted by the late Dr Phyllis Blakeley, Darlene Brine, Barry Cahill, Margaret Campbell, Allan Dunlop, Philip Hartling, Sandra Haycock, John MacLeod, Gary Shutlak, and Lois Yorke.

Finally, I am grateful to Mr Peter Blaney of McGill-Queen's Press for the advice and direction he gave me during the review and publication process, and to the staff at the Audio Visual Division, Faculty of Medicine, Dalhousie University, who prepared the many figures which appear in the book.

Figures and Tables

FIGURES

1 A plan for fortifying the town of Halifax by John Bruce / 20

2 A map of the south part of Nova Scotia, including the plan of Halifax surveyed by Moses Harris, and a view of Halifax drawn from a top mast by Harris / 21

3 Evidence of an epidemic at Halifax, 1750–51 / 28

4 Civilian, naval, and military surgeons, apothecaries, chymists, and druggists in Halifax, 1749–53 / 35

5 Text of the first newspaper advertisement by a medical practitioner in Canada / 39

6 Civilian deaths in Halifax from January 1755 to August 1756 / 49

7 Plan of Halifax showing line of forts, batteries, and all buildings in the town, *circa* June 1755 / 50

8 "A View of Hallifax [*sic*] in Nova Scotia from Cornwallis Island, with a Squadron going off to Louisbourgh [*sic*] in the year 1757," by Thomas Davies / 53

9 Patients in the naval hospital at Halifax, 1757–61 / 54

10 Deaths in Halifax during the period June 1757 to May 1758 / 56

11 "Part of the Town and harbour of Halifax in Nova Scotia looking down George Street to the opposite shore called Dartmouth," by Richard Short / 60

12 Annual grant (in British pounds) from Whitehall for the province of Nova Scotia and for the civilian hospital, the orphan house, and all medical services, 1753–63 / 63

13 Number of children in the orphan house at Halifax, 1752–62, and the yearly mortality / 69

14 Civilian, naval, and military surgeons in Nova Scotia, 1753–63 / 71

15 Location of the civilian hospital, military hospital, orphan house, and workhouse in Halifax / 77

16 "A Plan representing Part of the Town of Halifax in Nova Scotia looking down Prince Street to the opposite Shore," by Richard Short / 78

17 Civilian, naval, and military surgeons in Nova Scotia, 1763–74 / 97

18 Description of Nova Scotia as a healthy place to live by an anonymous author / 99

19 Total number of deaths in Nova Scotia during the period 1775–76 / 104

20 "The Hospital and Entrance of Bedford Basin," by James S. Meres / 132

21 Plan of the Naval Yard, Halifax, drawn from the original prepared by Captain Charles Blaskowitz in 1784 / 134

22 Civilian, naval, and military surgeons in Nova Scotia, 1775–83 / 143

23 Plan of Sydney drawn by James Miller in 1795 / 166

24 Civilian, naval, and military surgeons, physicians, apothecaries, chymists, and druggists in Nova Scotia, 1750–1800 / 173

25 Deaths in Nova Scotia, 1749–99 / 186

26 Mean age of civilian Nova Scotians at time of death during the period 1780–99, as compared to life expectancy at birth of Canadians in 1981 / 187

27 Death rate of civilians in Nova Scotia during the period 1749–84, as compared to 1984 / 188

28 The shingle of Dr Isaac Webster, physician and surgeon at Cornwallis from 1791 to 1851 / 189

TABLES

1 Treatment for William Kneeland by William Merry, Surgeon, 1750–53 / 40

2 Treatments for Joseph Kent, John Buttler, and John Winston by John Grant, Surgeon, 1752–53 / 41

3 Number of Families and Inhabitants in Nova Scotian Settlements, and Medical Practitioners Serving Them, 1755–61 / 70

4 Civilian Surgeons Who Came to Nova Scotia in 1775–82 / 142

5 Regimental Surgeons who Came to Halifax during the American Revolution / 142

6 Academic Qualifications of Civilian Doctors in Nova Scotia, 1784–99 / 170

7   Members of Nova Scotian Families Who
Studied Medicine/Surgery Abroad / 172

Preface

The history of eighteenth-century medicine and surgery in Nova Scotia has, to date, received very little attention from either amateur or professional historians. Nor has much been written on the history of the poor, the workhouse, or social conditions in general in Nova Scotia during the last half of the eighteenth century. The purpose of this book, therefore, is to address these topics and to present an accurate account of the type of health care available to Nova Scotians during the period, as well as the nature of the charitable and humanitarian attitudes and treatment that confronted the poor, the insane, and the criminal element of society in the province from 1749 to 1799.

On 5 March 1937, Miss Relief Williams read a paper[1] before the Nova Scotia Historical Society entitled, "Poor Relief and Medicine in Nova Scotia, 1749–1783." This paper, which dealt specifically with the poor, the orphan house, and smallpox and inoculation in Halifax during the pre-Loyalist period, represented the first scholarly paper on these topics. Earlier, in 1904, Dr D.A. Campbell wrote an article on the history of medicine in Nova Scotia for the *Maritime Medical News*.[2] This article, entitled "Pioneers of Medicine in Nova Scotia," described the major groups of people who settled in Nova Scotia and gave short biographical sketches of over seventy eighteenth- and early nineteenth-century physicians and surgeons who practised there. Unfortunately, Dr Campbell's paper was of limited use since he did not identify the sources for much of the information he presented.

During the fifty or so years since Miss Williams's paper was published, only two papers, both of which I wrote myself, have appeared on the history of eighteenth-century medicine in Nova Scotia. In 1980, I read "The History of Medicine in Nova Scotia, 1783–1854"[3] before the Nova Scotia Historical Society. This paper, which was later published in the Society's *Collections*, began with the year in which Miss Williams's study ended and extended the story up to 1854, when the Medical Society of Nova Scotia was established. It dealt mainly with the education of doctors who practised in Nova Scotia, the enactment of legislation to regulate the profession, and the difficulties associated with the establishment of civilian hospitals. The second paper,[4] entitled "He Successfully Exercised the Medical Profession: the Career of Michael Head in Eighteenth-Century Nova Scotia," was published in the *Nova Scotia Historical Review* in 1988. It gave a detailed account of the life and experience of a surgeon who practised in Nova Scotia from 1755 to 1805, in both the town of Halifax and in rural Nova Scotia. To my knowledge, this is the only extensive biography of an eighteenth-century Nova Scotian surgeon that has been published, though several short biographies of eighteenth-century Nova Scotian surgeons can be found in the *Dictionary of Canadian Biography*.

In this book, I have purposely presented the history of medicine and social conditions within the context of general Nova Scotian history. In taking this approach, I am following the advice of William Bynum, who has written[5] that a more comprehensive picture of the history of medicine would result if writers would consider such matters as the role of the state in providing for medical care, the structure of the total medical community, and the physical conditions which people had to endure, and study individual patients through wills, diaries, and personal letters. Another author, Thomas McKeown, has recommended[6] that writers of medical history should examine the conditions under which men and women have developed, along with the major factors that have affected their level of health care: "It is imperative that there should be a critical evaluation of the influences on which human health depends." Over the past fourteen years, I have researched the conditions under which the health-care system developed in Nova Scotia and the influences that the many government, military, and religious bodies had on its development, in every primary source I have been able to identify in archives in Nova Scotia, Canada, United States, Great Britain, and Ireland. The result is this book, which I believe represents the first definitive history of medicine and social conditions in Nova Scotia during the eighteenth century.

Surgeons, Smallpox, and the Poor

Introduction

In the last half of the eighteenth century, a large number of surgeons were sent to Nova Scotia because the colony, particularily Halifax, was the rendezvous for many military regiments and naval ships preparing to attack Louisbourg and Quebec. Halifax was also, during the American Revolution, Britain's major naval base in North America.[1]

Although the surgeons were welcomed by the local residents, two concomitants of the regiments and ships decidedly were not: the smallpox and the poor. All the major smallpox epidemics in Nova Scotia during the last half of the eighteenth century occurred soon after the arrival of Royal Navy ships and regiments from Europe. The regiments also brought to Halifax many camp followers who frequently were left destitute when the regiments either departed for battle or returned to Europe. These abandoned people added to the large number of transient poor and represented a crippling financial burden for the small town.

Of the 366 medical personnel who arrived in Nova Scotia during the period 1749 to 1799, 340 were surgeons, twenty-one were described as physicians, and five were referred to as apothecaries, chymists, or druggists. This meant that during the last half of the eighteenth century in Nova Scotia, the surgeon was often called upon to perform the duties of physician and apothecary, as well as practise surgery. The disease that the surgeons were most frequently asked to treat was the smallpox. Their patients, in addition to soldiers and seamen, were for the most part the poor, many of whom were inmates of the workhouse and the poor house.

This role was quite different from that of the eighteenth-century surgeon in Great Britain, where the division of responsibilities among physician, surgeon, and apothecary had been delineated clearly since the sixteenth century; the physician diagnosed illness and administered medication, the surgeon performed surgical operations, and the apothecary prepared and compounded drugs.[2] Each of the three disciplines had a strong college or society to protect its own area of responsibility[3], and, in the eighteenth century, the British army recognized all three by having on staff a physician general, a surgeon general, and an apothecary general.

On 1 July 1745, the Company of Surgeons of London was created when the surgeon members, led by William Cheselden (1688–1752), separated from the barbers. The new company continued the barber-surgeons' established practice of having students examined by a court of examiners at the end of a seven-year apprenticeship.[4] The court was also responsible for examining surgeons for the navy and the army. Although there was no compulsory professional curriculum, it was customary for surgery students to spend some time at one or more of the medical schools and hospitals in London, Edinburgh, or Glasgow.[5] Each student was required, afterwards, to write an examination in anatomy and surgery. If successful, he would receive qualification as a surgeon, assistant surgeon, or hospital mate and be given a specific rating. The surgeon could apply to write, at a later date, an examination to improve his level of qualification.[6]

Surgery in the eighteenth century was a very crude art. Antiseptics and sterile techniques[7] were unknown, and patients usually were not anaesthetized during surgical procedures.[8] It is not surprising, therefore, that eighteenth-century surgeons did not open the thorax at all, and that the only abdominal procedures were the management of external ruptures, and lithotomy (perineal incision to remove stones in the bladder). The two principal surgical procedures were amputation and blood-letting. On the battlefield, wounds to the arms and legs were treated by simple amputation; because of almost certain infection at the incision site, there was a high degree of mortality. Blood-letting, or phlebotomy,[9] had been practised since ancient times, for early physicians noticed that febrile patients who haemorrhaged frequently recovered, while those who did not bleed naturally succumbed to the fever. The use of blood-letting was supported by physicians and surgeons in the eighteenth century. Even Dr Hermann Boerhaave (1668–1738), considered to be the century's most influential physician, prescribed moderate blood-letting to relieve fevers.

As the eighteenth century progressed, three additional subjects were added to the surgeon's curriculum. These were physiology, pathology, and chemistry. John Hunter (1728–93), the most highly esteemed surgeon of his day in Great Britain, raised surgery to the level of a definite branch of science with his research into comparative anatomy and physiology. A student of William Cheselden's in London, Hunter is considered by some to have been the founder of surgical pathology, and his *Treatise on the Blood, Inflammation, and Gunshot Wounds* (1794) is a classic. However, Giovanni-Battista Morgagni (1682–1771) of the University of Padua, Italy, is more generally considered to be the founder of modern pathology. His book *On the Seats and Causes of Diseases Investigated by Anatomy* (1761) became a classic reference. The third subject, chemistry, was introduced in 1747 into the medical curriculum at the University of Glasgow by Dr William Cullen (1710–90), who, from 1755 to 1778, taught chemistry and later medicine at the University of Edinburgh. His book, entitled *First Lines of the Practice of Physic for the Use of Students in the University of Edinburgh*, published in 1776 and reprinted in many editions, was read by surgeons and physicians alike.[10]

The eighteenth-century hospital was a place to heal the sick, a benevolent institution established primarily for the treatment of the poor and helpless. However, while it was not intended to house the criminal element of society, it did, as Porter put it, "function as a social balm as well."[11] William LeFanu has written that although hospitals in the eighteenth century were intended to care for the poor, in the first half of the century they functioned "more like Dickensian work-houses than like hospitals as we know them today."[12] The concept that a hospital was to be solely a medical institution is of relatively recent origin. Specialty medical treatment such as for the insane was totally disregarded in the eighteenth century; Arnold Chaplin has estimated that there were "thirty-seven mad-houses in London" during the century. Prisons were hotbeds of disease, and very little, if anything, was done to provide medical treatment for the prisoners. The general condition of hospitals and infirmaries during the eighteenth century has been described as unpleasant. James Gregory (1753–1821), who succeeded William Cullen as professor of medicine at Edinburgh in 1790, wrote of the Edinburgh Infirmary, when he was first appointed there in 1779, that "both the deficiency of good air and the great abundance of noxious effluvia contribute to make the air in hospitals bad, and almost poisonous." In the same year he initiated a program to ensure hospital and personal hygiene and to ventilate and cleanse the Infirmary. A daily fumigation using tar water and muriatic acid was used to clean the air, the tile floors were mopped daily, and the walls of the rooms were whitewashed on a regular basis.[13]

The majority of London hospitals were established or rebuilt between 1719 and 1745. The medieval hospitals of St Bartholomew and St Thomas were rebuilt during that period, and they were supplemented by the establishment of the Westminister Hospital in 1719, Guy's in 1725, St George's in 1733, the London in 1740, and the Middlesex in 1745. By 1755 there were twelve hospitals in London housing upwards of a thousand beds.[14] It is important to understand, however, that this development was not brought about by the medical profession or by governments, but was the result of humanitarian and philanthropic motives. Porter, in his study of the underlying ideology of the eighteenth-century hospital in England and Scotland, has pointed out that the hospitals and infirmaries founded during the eighteenth century owed their birth not so much to the great landowners as to the prosperous manufacturers and merchants.[15] The voluntary hospitals, such as St George's and the Edinburgh Infirmary (founded in 1741), were financed by subscriptions, collections following charity sermons, proceeds from theatre performances, donations from societies, and donations of materials and labour by the general public,[16] as part of what Porter has described as a popular movement rather than an aristocratic one. The hospitals so established were intended as places were the sick would be healed, as opposed to workhouses where discipline was of primary importance. Patients with chronic, terminal, and infectious diseases were barred from the hospital, whereas those with curable illnesses such as scurvy, abscesses, burns, broken limbs, etc., were treated. No patient who could pay for a cure was admitted to the hospital, since this would interfere with the private practice of local physicians, apothecaries, and surgeons.

THROUGHOUT ITS HISTORY, SMALLPOX has been confused with measles, probably because of the small size of the skin eruptions. Syphilis, or *la grosse vérole*, caused major skin eruptions and was therefore called the great pox. Smallpox has three forms: *variola major*, or true virulent smallpox; *variola minor*, a mild form; and *variola vaccinae*, the disease, primarily of cattle, known as cowpox.[17]

The origin of smallpox is obscure, but it was described in China as early as the third century. Smallpox probably first appeared in western Europe during the early Middle Ages.[18] By the eleventh century, it was a well-known disease in England but was thought, prior to the seventeenth century, to be mainly an affliction of children. During the last half of the seventeenth century, smallpox appears to have become more virulent: the number of deaths from the disease among both children and adults increased so considerably that it became included as one of the principal causes of death. Peter Razzell compared the number of smallpox deaths to the number of all deaths in London between 1574 and 1730 and found that the percentage of deaths from smallpox rose from 1.6 to 8.2 percent during that period.[19] And in Europe, smallpox is said to have destroyed more young people throughout the eighteenth century than any other disease.[20] Major smallpox epidemics were recorded in London on numerous occasions during the last half of the seventeenth century, but unlike most fevers, smallpox disregarded class lines and attacked the upper class and royalty with the same ruthlessness as it did the poor.[21]

Thomas Sydenham, the leading British physician of the seventeenth century, proposed a treatment for smallpox involving a cold regimen that included light bed coverings, an abundance of fresh air, and cool beverages. This was contrary to the treatment that was prevalent at the time based on heat, sweating, bleeding, and purging. Hermann Boerhaave followed Sydenham's method, but there was no universally accepted treatment or cure for smallpox identified during the eighteenth century.

The procedure of using inoculation as a preventative measure against smallpox was introduced into Constantinople around 1672 and appears to have arrived there from Persia or China. It involved removing some of the thick liquid from a pustule borne by a person with smallpox and rubbing it into a small scratch on the recipient's skin. Inoculation soon became generally accepted in Turkey. In March 1718, the British ambassador to Turkey and his wife, Lady Mary Wortley Montague, instructed the embassy surgeon, Charles Maitland, to inoculate their son. The inoculation proved successful and, upon their return to England, they had Maitland inoculate their daughter in London. In April 1722, Maitland inoculated the two daughters of the Prince of Wales. However, the success of these inoculations did not ensure immediate acceptance of the practice.[22] All during the eighteenth century in England, there was a measure of reluctance to inoculate, due, mainly, to the expense of the procedure; the belief by some religious groups that it was against the teachings of their church; the absence of major smallpox epidemics in Great Britain from 1725–46; and the fear of contagion. A significant number of those who had been inoculated developed the virulent smallpox, rather than the expected mild attack. It also became clear that the inoculated were capable of spreading the disease. On the other hand, people vaccinated with *variola vaccinae*, or matter from a cowpox pustule, were protected against smallpox and incapable of transmitting it. This observation was made later, in 1797, by Dr Edward Jenner,[23] and by 1801, over 100,000 people in England had been vaccinated.

In North America the first inoculation for smallpox took place in Boston on 26 June 1721, when the physician Zabdiel Boylston inoculated his son Thomas during a smallpox epidemic that has been described as the worst in Boston's history. Of a total population of 10,700, more than half, 5,789 contracted smallpox naturally, and of these, 842 died. In contrast to the general but cautious acceptance of inoculation in Britain, Boylston and the Reverend Cotton Mather, the person who had urged that inoculation be adopted by Boston physicians, found themselves embroiled in a vicious controversy. Leading citizens in Boston were outraged and horrified that Boylston had deliberately infected someone with smallpox and for a brief period his life was in danger. This fracas delayed the general acceptance of inoculation, which only came into use in Philadelphia and New York in 1731. The fear of contracting smallpox from inoculation persisted, however, and in the 1740s, the colonial governments in New York, Connecticut, Maryland, and Virginia issued proclamations prohibiting its use. It was many years before the general public recognized that, while some persons died from inoculation, most were made immune by the procedure. There were still some who believed that inoculation could spread the disease to other members of the community, but the experience gained from a smallpox epidemic in Boston in 1752 caused many people to change their minds: a total of 5,545 Bostonians caught smallpox naturally, during the epidemic, and 539 of them died. However, of the 2,214 who were inoculated, only thirty died.[24]

In England, the London Smallpox Hospital was established in 1746, and the College of Physicians declared its strong approval of inoculation in 1754. Whereas inoculation had hitherto been a procedure carried out for a fee, it was now available gratis to the poor and the general public. In North America, the first inoculation hospital was established within the city of Boston in 1764, and in Russia, Empress Catherine summoned the English physician, Thomas Dimsdale, to St Petersburg in 1768 to inoculate herself and her family. In the same year, William Buchan published the first edition of his very popular *Domestic Medicine*, in which he recommended that parents should inoculate their own children and outlined clearly how the procedure should be executed. He also advocated that clergymen inoculate their parishioners.[25]

In Canada, Quebec suffered a terrible epidemic of smallpox in 1702-03 when, according to J.J. Heagerty, nearly one-quarter of the town's nine thousand residents died.[26] In 1732–33, over 1,700 Quebecers died from smallpox, while from 1755–57, the disease is said to have decimated the native Indian population in the vicinity of the town of Quebec, as well as about five hundred residents of the town itself. Heagerty writes, "The worst sufferers at this time were the Acadians [expelled from Nova Scotia in 1755] who had endeavoured to recoup their fortunes by settling in and around Quebec."

Meanwhile, in seventeenth-century England, widespread poverty and dislocation arose from the unemployment created by the necessity of modernizing industry and agriculture. Craft guilds and manorial feudal systems were undermined by expanding industries such as clothweaving and mining; wood burning gave way to coal and large factories were established. Drifting men and women gathered in the cities, especially London, where they constituted a large mass of casual workers, criminals, and the poor. It has been estimated that, at the turn of the eighteenth century, more than half of the population of England were earning less than they spent. This meant that many had to be supported from the poor rates which represented, at one time, half of the revenue of the Crown.[27] It is not surprising that in the eighteenth century there was significant emigration to the new world, both voluntary and forced, from London and all parts of England, Scotland, and Ireland.[28] As described by Hofstadter,

The great Immigrations of the eighteenth century were a motley compound of the white and the black, the free, the semi-free, and the enslaved ... The eighteenth century settlers of America were men and women who had seen ... the ravages of war and social conflict, and whether they came as freemen with some capital, as indentured servants, or as transported convicts, they were the off-scourings and the victims of the wars and economic dislocations, the exploitation and religious persecution, that racked Europe at the end of the seventeenth and the beginning of the eighteenth century.

THIS BOOK DESCRIBES HOW MEDICINE AND SURGERY were practised in Nova Scotia during the province's period of early settlement, while it was serving as a major military and naval base, and after it became a refuge for the Loyalists. At the time of the settlement of Halifax, as chapter 1 shows, the Lords of Trade and Plantations, under the leadership of Lord Halifax, took great care to provide proper food and health care during the settlers' passage across the Atlantic in May and June 1749. Upon arrival in Halifax, settlers were provided with a hospital ship, the services of surgeons and a midwife and, within the first year, a general-hospital building. In this period, the colony also saw its first major epidemic, which raged in Halifax during the fall and winter of 1750–51.

Chapter 2 describes the rendezvous of many regiments and ships in Halifax during the period 1755 to 1763, and the two smallpox epidemics they brought with them. Many temporary hospitals for soldiers and seamen were established at this time in Halifax and Louisbourg, along with Halifax's first civilian hospital, the operation of which caused a dispute among the civilian surgeons. The latter part of the chapter is concerned with the demise of the civilian hospital, and London's severe reduction of financial support for the services of surgeons and a midwife for the civilian population. The court records of the period indicate the type of medication and treatment which, during the 1750s, Halifax civilians received from surgeons. Appendix 2 explains these medications and the disease or illness that each was expected to treat.

Chapter 3 is concerned primarily with the treatment of the poor in Nova Scotia between the Seven Years' War and the American Revolution. Many were camp followers who had been abandoned by regiments that had left Halifax either for war or to return to Great Britain. Surgeons were involved in the operation of the workhouse (Bridewell) and, later, the poor house set up to cope with the multitude of idle, helpless, and indigent people. Financial resources directed previously towards providing medical services for civilians were used, because of the destitute condition in which much of the province's population lived, to feed, clothe, and shelter poor people. The chapter also indicates the degree to which surgeons in Nova Scotia, prior to the American Revolution, participated in the deliberations of the recently established House of Assembly.

The American Revolution dominated every aspect of life in Nova Scotia during the period 1775–83, not the least because of the arrival in the province of thirty thousand Loyalists, including fifty-five civilian surgeons, who increased the number of medical personnel in the province from seventeen in 1775 to sixty-five in 1785. These events are described in chapter 4, along with the smallpox epidemic experienced during the fall and winter of 1775–76. Ironically, this epidemic was a major factor in the American decision to cancel a planned attack on Halifax.

The concluding chapter describes the provincial government's renewed attempts to provide for the poor, once again by diverting money that could have been spent on medical services to the workhouse, the poor house, and the indigent poor. Halifax and Dartmouth had also to provide medical services for 530 Maroons from

Jamaica during the period 1796 to 1800, as well as for a large number of prisoners taken in 1793 from the French islands of St Pierre and Miquelon and from French warships during the Napoleonic Wars. The chapter also looks at the initial, unsuccessful attempt to regulate the practice of medicine in Nova Scotia and the reasons why the province lagged behind Lower Canada and the American colonies in this respect. Finally, statistics are provided on the number of deaths in Nova Scotia during the period 1749–99, the mean age at time of death, infant and child mortality, the death rate, and leading causes of death during the last half of the eighteenth century.

A WORD IS REQUIRED ABOUT THE METHOD of dating used in this book. The Gregorian calendar was not adopted by Great Britain until 2 September 1752, and the day following was declared to be 14 September 1752. To bring "old style" dates into line with modern reckoning for the eighteenth century, add eleven days. I distinguish old style (o.s.) from "new style" (n.s.) dates in chapter 1, but in later chapters the reader should understand that all dates are modern or new style, unless otherwise indicated. At the time that the calendar was adjusted as described above, the date of the new year was also changed. Whereas hitherto the year had begun on 25 March, the years following 1752 were declared to begin on 1 January. Because different countries in Europe did not all use the same calendar before 1752, it was common until then to designate the dates between 1 January and 25 Marsh using two years. Thus, 1 February 1749/50 meant 1 February 1750 according to the Gregorian calendar, but 1 February 1749 according to the Julian calendar. At a meeting of Council held on 31 August 1752 (o.s.),[30] it was resolved "that an advertisement be printed and dispersed thro' the Province for the better information and regulation of all persons in regard to the alteration of the chronological stile [sic], for regulating commencement of the year, and for correcting the Calendar now in use."

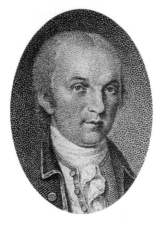

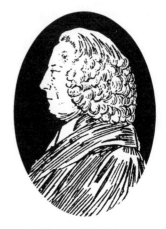

Dr John Cochran (1730–1807) came to
Halifax with the 1st Regiment of Foot
in 1758 and was in Halifax in 1761. He
was director general of the medical
department of the American army in 1781
and died in New York State.
Miniature in oil on canvas, artist
unknown. (Medical Society of New
Jersey)

Rev. Dr Thomas Wood (ca.1711–1778)
arrived in Halifax from New Jersey in
1752. He ministered and practised in
Halifax and Annapolis Royal until his
death at Annapolis.
Silhouette by unknown artist.

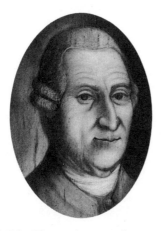

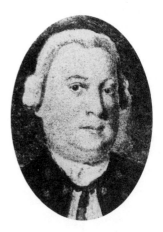

Dr John Thomas (1724–1776) came to
Nova Scotia with New England troops
in May 1755 and was present at the siege
of Fort Beausejour. He returned to
Boston in April 1756 and died of smallpox
near Quebec City in June 1776.
Pastel on paper by Benjamin Blyth.
(Massachusetts Historical Society)

Dr John Day (–1775) arrived in Nova
Scotia in 1758, the year he was
appointed an assistant surgeon at the
naval hospital in Halifax. He died in a
fire in Boston Harbour.
Portrait by unknown artist.

Arrival, Settlement, and an Initial Concern for Health Care, 1749 (o.s.) − 1753 (n.s.)

At the beginning of 1749, the land mass known today as Nova Scotia held approximately 14,000 people: about 10,800 persons of French origin[1], 1,000 native Indians,[2] and 2,300 civilian and military personnel of English origin.[3] Between the ceding of mainland Nova Scotia to the English by the Treaty of Utrecht in 1713 and the arrival of the Cornwallis settlers in June 1749, Britain made no attempt to colonize Nova Scotia. The only major influx of English-speaking people into the colony during this thirty-six year period was from June 1745 to July 1749, when New England troops and their British army replacements occupied the fortress of Louisbourg.[4] Meanwhile, the Acadian French population quadrupled in this period from 2,500 in 1713[5] to 10,800 in 1749.

In March 1749, an advertisement[6] appeared in the *London Gazette* regarding a proposal to establish a permanent settlement in Nova Scotia. This advertisement was directed mainly to officers and private men discharged from His Majesty's land and sea services following the War of the Austrian Succession, which had ended in late 1748. In part, it read: "That all such persons as are desirous of engaging in the above settlement, do transmit by letter, or personally give in their names, signifying, in what regiment or company, or on board what ship they last served, and if they have families they intended to carry with them, distinguishing the age and quality of such persons to any of the following officers appointed to receive and enter the same in the Books opened for that purpose." The advertisement stated further that the books[7] would be closed "as soon as the intended number shall be completed, or at least on the 7th day of April 1749." The transports would be made ready to receive such persons on 10 April (o.s.), and be ready to sail on the twentieth.

The same terms proposed to private soldiers and seamen would be granted to carpenters, shipwrights, masons, joiners, brickmakers, bricklayers, and all other artificers necessary in building or husbandry. The concluding paragraph read: "That the same conditions as are proposed to those who have served in the capacity of Ensign shall extend to all surgeons, whether thay have been in His Majesty's service or not, upon their producing proper certificates of their being duly qualified." Edward Cornwallis[8] was appointed captain general and governor-in-chief in and over the province of Nova Scotia on 6 May 1749 (o.s.). On 15 May 1749 (o.s.), thirteen transports under his command sailed from Spithead, England, for Chebucto Harbour.[9] Cornwallis arrived in Chebucto aboard the sloop of war *Sphinx* on 21 June 1749 (o.s.), and by 1 July 1749 (o.s.), all thirteen of the transports, carrying a total of 2,547 passengers, had safely arrived. The passengers included 1,174 families,[10] 665 single men, 440 children, and 420 servants. Because of the large number of single men, the average size of family was only 2.2 persons. A total of 137 heads of family were recently released army personnel and 435 were retired recently from the Royal Navy. Thus, about one-half of the families arriving in Chebucto in June 1749 were recently retired servicemen, and the other half were artificers with various civilian occupations.

Thirty-eight of the passengers[11] gave their occupations as one of the following: apothecary (two); apothecary's mate (two); assistant surgeon (one); chymist and druggist (one); chymist and surgeon (one); doctor and surgeon (one); lieutenant and surgeon (one); midwife (two); pupil surgeon (one); surgeon (sixteen); and surgeon's mate (ten). The names of these thirty-eight persons, and the additional information provided on them in the passengers lists, appear in Appendix 1.

The fifty years preceding the founding of Halifax have been described as "the lost half-century" and the "barren age" in English medicine.[12] Patients in 1750 were treated in the same way that their grandparents had been in 1700. Between the age of Thomas Sydenham and Isaac Newton, which ended *circa* 1700, and the age of Albrecht von Haller and Antoine-Laurent Lavoisier, which covered the last half of the eighteenth century, surgeons in England developed few new operations, and no attempt was made to address the health problems of cities, the army, or the fleets. There was almost no advance in the understanding of disease and its treatment, and there seems to have been no ethical objection to secret remedies, personal nostrums being often a part of the prestige of the successful practitioner of physic. In England, eighteenth-century medicine was "pluralist through and through. An enormous range of healers practised freely and lucratively."[13] The period has been described as the "golden age of quackery."[14]

Dr Thomas Sydenham (1624–89) attempted to direct mens' minds away from speculation and back to the bedside, and toward practise of the straightforward clinical observation originally espoused by Hippocrates. In the early eighteenth century, however, Sydenham's methods were largely ignored by the majority of English physicians and surgeons. The eighteenth century represented "the adolescence of modern medicine," a period when "the wisdom of antiquity was still part of the physician's intellectual background."[15] Diagnostic devices such as the thermometer and the microscope were being used by a few physicians in France and Germany, but were not used in England until the later years of the century, when they were introduced primarily through the efforts of the eminent surgeon John Hunter. These measurement devices were not in general use by physicians and surgeons, however, until the mid-nineteenth century.

In Scotland, a reawakening in medicine took place twenty-five years earlier than in England. Medical education had been reorganized in Scotland mainly due to the influence of Hermann Boerhaave of Leyden. His student, Alexander Monro, *primus*, (1697–1767) at Edinburgh, and Monro's student William Cullen (1712–90) at Glasgow created a growing spirit of enquiry at those two universities. In 1731, the Philosophical Society of Edinburgh began to publish its *Medical Essays and Observations*, some twenty-five years before a similar publication appeared in England. During the period 1700–50, medical teaching was sadly wanting in England. The only two universities, Cambridge and Oxford, were restricted to members of the established church and required twelve years of study before the MD was granted. Also, the degree was largely based on the theoretical since Oxford did not have a hospital until 1758 and no regular instruction in anatomy until 1750. As William LeFanu has pointed out, these two universities were dormant in medicine during the period. Formal education of apothecaries in England did not begin until the 1760s, and surgeons' training was very informal prior to 1745, the year the surgeons separated from the barbers and formed the Company of Surgeons of London.

It is not surprising, therefore, that most of the thirty-eight medical personnel with Cornwallis were surgeons or assistant surgeons. It is surprising, however, considering the stagnation in medicine in England, that those making the plans for the new settlement of Halifax would make the detailed efforts described below to ensure that the passengers had a high level of medical and surgical attendance, both during the crossing and for the first few years after the founding of Halifax. This was, indeed, in marked contrast to the relative neglect which the Lords of Trade had displayed towards the English garrison at Annapolis Royal during the period 1713–49.

On 30 March 1749 (o.s.), Mr Bevan, an apothecary and chymist, made proposals to the Lords of Trade and Plantations[16] for supplying medicines for the settlers destined for Nova Scotia. On that same date, Major Lockman, who had been recommended for employment as surgeon and physician to the intended settlement in Nova Scotia, acquainted their lordships that he was a surgeon to HM Guards at Hanover, had been surgeon at the hospital in Mecklenburgh, and also inspector general of health at Barbados in 1723 and 1724. Their lordships directed Major Lockman to bring forth such persons as might give them further satisfaction of being duly qualified, which he promised to do.

The Lords of Trade met next on 3 April 1749 (o.s.). Presented to them was a paper, prepared by the celebrated physiologist Stephen Hales,[17] relating to the importance of having ventilators on the ships bound for Nova Scotia. The Lords ordered "that Mr Kilby do enquire of Mr Sutton as to what number of ships can be furnished with air pipes before the 20th" of April.[18] At the same meeting were Mr Middleton, surgeon general to the army abroad, and the apothecary general, Mr Garnier, whose opinions had been sought concerning proper measures to be taken for preserving the settlers' health in Nova Scotia. They told their lordships that they had met with the physician general, Dr Wilmot, and were of the opinion "that the best choice of medicines to be sent with the new settlers would be those used in the Hospitals in Flanders, which might be prepared according to the Pharmacopoeia printed for them there, that two chief surgeons and two apothecaries should be sent with them to reside at the head settlement, and a mate at each of the other settlements, who might be appointed out of such as have entered their names to go to Nova Scotia, upon their qualifications being examined at Surgeons' Hall."[19] The Lords ordered further "that the Solicitor and Clerk of the Reports do transmit a list of such surgeons as have entered upon the books of this office for Nova Scotia to Mr Hawkins, Master of Surgeons' Hall, and desire him to make a return of the qualifications of such as have been examined there." Also, "Major Lockman was desired to pass his examinations at Surgeons' Hall, upon return whereof their Lordships would further consider his application."

On 7 April, Mr Middleton, Mr Garnier, and Dr Wilmot related[20] to the board "that the medicines, utensils, etc., be dispensed to the mates of the several divisions from the principal apothecaries, and as we are informed no less than 17 surgeons have entered themselves upon the encouragement offered by the government, [and as] many of whom have served in the Navy and Army, they may be of great service in the several settlements."[21] On 8 April was read the return[22] of surgeons whose qualifications had been examined at Surgeons' Hall: James Handasyde, second mate, third rate, March 1747; Josiah Irwin, second mate, third rate, 4 September 1746; Mark Story, third mate, third rate, April 1747; Edward Turner, second mate, third rate, February 1743; Thomas Wilson, second mate, any rate, July 1744; John Sherman, second mate, third rate, December 1743; John Inman, surgeon, fourth rate, 6 October 1741; Leonard Lockman, surgeon, John Steele, surgeon, Fenton Griffith, John Farquhar, Alexander Abercrombie.

Each of the last five persons listed received certificates of their respective qualifications on the day the return was read. It was ordered further "that the Solicitor and Clerk of the Reports do write to Mr Hawkins to desire a special Court may be held on Thursday next for examining such as have not yet [been] examined, and reexamining those who may be desirous of gaining a higher qualification and make a return thereof to their Lordships. Mr Bevan attending, as desired, and the report and invoice laid before the Board by Dr Wilmot, Mr Garnier, and Mr Middleton, having been communicated to him, he represented to their Lordships that he apprehended the quantity [of medicines] insufficient." He also represented that it would be proper to allow a medicine chest for each ship during the voyage. As a result of this recommendation, medicines were put in twelve chests for the use of the settlers and the *Roehampton* was designated as a hospital ship.[23]

On 14 April, the surgeon general, Mr Middleton, laid before the board a return from the surgeons' company of persons they had examined. The Lords agreed that the following persons should be appointed for the intended settlement of Nova Scotia: William Merry and Thomas Reeves, apothecaries; Robert Carr and Alexander Abercrombie, apothecary's mates; Leonard Lockman, John Steele, and Matthew Jones, surgeons; and Robert Grant, John Grant, and Mr Belchiss, surgeon's mates.[24]

At their last meeting prior to the ships' departure for Nova Scotia, the Lords of Trade authorized Mr Bevan to provide a set of surgical instruments as requested by the surgeons destined for Nova Scotia.

Of the thirty-eight persons who arrived in Nova Scotia with occupations related to medicine and surgery, two were midwives and thirty-six were surgeons, apothecaries, chymists, or druggists. It seems unlikely that these people would have been motivated to emigrate to Nova Scotia to set up practice in a new settlement consisting of only 2,500 settlers. They would have been aware that, as Cornwallis[25] put it, many of the settlers were "poor, idle, worthless vagabonds that embrace the opportunity to get provisions for one year without labour." It would be apparent to anyone, at that time, that a settlement the size of Chebucto[26] would be able to provide employment for no more than three to five practitioners. It seems likely, then, that many of the surgeons who entered their names and who, indeed, came to Chebucto with Cornwallis, did not remain in Halifax, but left, with a large percentage of the passengers, for New England within a month.

There are several reasons why many of the original settlers quit Chebucto (Halifax) and moved to New England during July 1749. To begin with, they could find greater employment opportunities and better agricultural land in and around the established townships of New England. The passenger lists note that 158 heads of family described their occupations as husbandry or related to husbandry; only sixty-nine of these 158 families (forty-four percent) appear in the records of Halifax after the end of July 1749. Settlers were also fearful of attack by the French and Indians. This fear was present also among the New England settlements, but it was more pronounced in the much smaller and more vulnerable town of Chebucto. During the first two weeks after their arrival, the Cornwallis settlers had no military protection. It was only after 25 July that the soldiers in Hopson's 29th and Warburton's 45th regiments were transferred from Louisbourg to Chebucto in order to protect the new settlement.

During the first six to eight weeks after arrival, the majority of settlers continued to live on the transports in Chebucto harbour. The passengers on at least five ships were transferred, however, to George's Island. On 6 July 1749 (o.s.), Cornwallis sent five of the transports to bring Lieutenant Governor Hopson and his garrison from Louisbourg to Halifax.[27] The latter arrived in late July. The Louisbourg garrison consisted of about two thousand persons, military and civilian, but it is difficult to say how many of the civilians or disbanded soldiers[28] took up residence in Chebucto and how many continued on to New England.

Constant fear of attack by the French and the Indians led Cornwallis, on 26 June 1749 (o.s.), to order the transfer to Chebucto, aboard the *Fair Lady*, of a company[29] of the 40th Regiment garrisoned in Annapolis.[30] He requested Paul Mascarene, who had been lieutenant governor of the town and fort at Annapolis Royal, travel with the company of soldiers. All arrived at Chebucto on 12 July 1749 (o.s.). On the following day, aboard the *Beaufort*, Cornwallis held his first council meeting.[31]

Cornwallis mentions[32] in a letter to the Lords of Trade that he is including "A copy of a Plan for the Town with a line of defence offered me by Mr Brewse [Bruce]". Figure 1 is a photograph of this plan.[33] The proposed system of defence fortifications to surround the town was to be built by soldiers of the 29th and 45th regiments. A second plan, which must have been prepared within a month of the Brewse plan, was drawn by Moses Harris,[34] a Cornwallis settler. The Harris plan, which appears in the upper right of the composite map and plan shown in Figure 2, depicts a much more elaborate system of five forts around the town, which was laid out in twenty-nine blocks, each consisting of sixteen lots.[35] Figure 2 also shows the exact location of the town in relation to Chebucto harbour and the site of the military camp of Warburton's Regiment.

Cornwallis's letter to the Lords of Trade gives a first indication of the confusion and chaos which existed in Chebucto during the month of July 1749. The letter begins by informing[36] the board that "the number of settlers, men, women, and children is 1,400." What happened to the remainder of the 2,547 passengers who arrived in Chebucto during the last week of June 1749? in a disgusted tone, Cornwallis stated that many of the settlers were quitting the settlement and that many of the sailors:

only wanted a passage to New England. Many [of the passengers] have come as into a Hospital, to be cured, some of veneral [*sic*] disorders, some even incurables. I do all I can to make them useful, but I shall be obliged, I believe, to send some of them away. I published a proclamation[37] in the terms advised by your Lordships with regard to such as should desert the settlement and made the penalty to whoever should be absent two days together without permission forfeiture of all rights and priviledges of settlers. Eight fellows that had gone off to Canada and were brought back, I punished [them] by striking their names out of the Mess Books, and out of your Lordships Lists, and ordered them to leave the Province.

Cornwallis's penalty proved to be no deterrent whatsoever to the more than one thousand persons who left Chebucto during July. They could obtain easy transportation to New England. A total of eighteen ships are recorded as having cleared Halifax for New England ports during the period 21 July to 31 August 1749 (o.s.).[38] John Salusbury recorded in his diary[39] that "Gates [Horatio Gates,

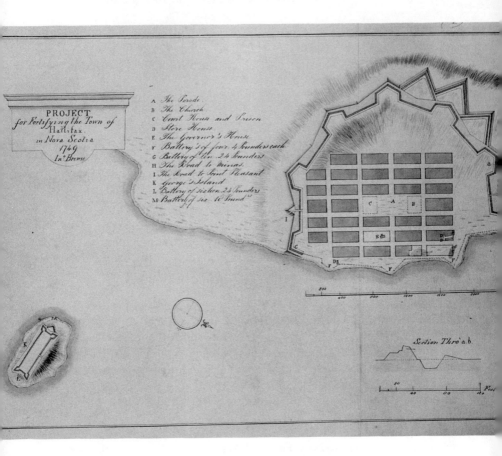

Figure 1
A Plan for Fortifying the town of Halifax by John Bruce, drawn sometime in July 1749. (Public Record Office, Kew, Richmond, Surrey, United Kingdom, SP42/38f224)

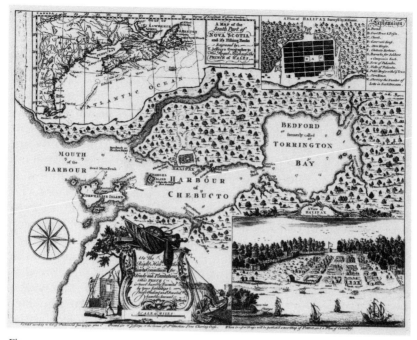

Figure 2

A Map of the south part of Nova Scotia, including the plan of Halifax surveyed by Moses Harris, and a view of Halifax drawn from a top mast by Harris. (National Archives of Canada, NMC 1012)

afterwards a revolutionary general] is ordered to the Harbours mouth after a schooner supposed lurking to take off some of our people [was sighted], we brought [the] four deserts [deserters] from Point Pleasant."

In his third letter[40] to the Lords of Trade, Cornwallis wrote, "The Town has been marked out, lots drawn,[41] and now everyone knows where to build his house. A great many houses are begun, and many huts. Loghouses are already up for about half a mile on each side of the Town." He continued, "A good many people from Louisbourg have settled here and several from New England, and they tell me above 1,000 more desire to come down [to Chebucto] before winter." The Allotment Book,[42] which details the names of those who drew the 464 lots in the five divisions of the town on 8 August 1749 (o.s.), makes clear that, of the total number of 606 heads of family (or single men) who were granted lots or parts of lots in the five divisions, the names of only 419 (69.1 percent) are to be found on the Cornwallis mess or passenger lists. The striking fact is, however, that 419 represents only 35.7 percent of the 1,174 heads of family who made up the Cornwallis passenger lists. The remaining 187 families allotted land on 8 August, whose names are not included on the mess lists, probably arrived in Chebucto as part of the Louisbourg garrison transferred to the new settlement during the period 24-26 July 1749 (o.s.).

Since the Louisbourg garrison did not arrive until after Cornwallis had written his second letter to the Lords of Trade, it can be presumed that the 1,400[43] settlers he referred to had arrived with him. As already noted, only 419 of the 606 families allocated land on 8 August were Cornwallis passengers. If each family that arrived with Cornwallis averaged 2.2 persons, the 419 families represent about 925 people, some 475 fewer than the 1,400 reported by Cornwallis. It is my contention that a significant number of Cornwallis settlers in Chebucto were not allocated lots of land because they were Roman Catholic. Blatant discrimination against Roman Catholics in the new town played a part in the move to New England of many of the original Chebucto settlers. Since the Penal Laws, in effect since 1704, prohibited the granting of land in the colonies to Roman Catholics, it is unclear why officials entering the passengers' names in the books in England would have accepted Roman Catholics. It may have been that prospective passengers were not asked to state their religion, since there was no mention of religious preference in the London Gazette's advertisement of March 1749. It is also possible that many of the 420 anonymous servants, Cornwallis passengers, were Roman Catholic and quit the settlement to escape their servitude.

In any event, a comparison of the names of passengers on the Cornwallis mess lists with a number of eighteenth-century Halifax records indicates that 191 Cornwallis families not allotted land on 8 August 1749 (o.s.) were residing in Chebucto after that date. Why 191 families (representing about 420 persons) were not allotted land is not known.[44] Statements by Cornwallis,[45] Salusbury,[46] and others[47] suggest that every settler who was head of a family was, in fact, allotted land. Nonetheless, there is evidence that those Cornwallis passengers who were Roman Catholic were probably not allotted land.[48]

Among the settlers who apparently quit the settlement of Chebucto during July 1749 were at least twelve surgeons.[49] Eighteen of the medical personnel residing in Chebucto on the day of allotment were granted lots in the five divisions of the town, while in 1750,[50] three received grants of land in the town and in the South Suburbs. Although nine of the twelve surgeons who quitted the settlement (seventy-five percent) were single, only fourteen of the twenty-four who remained (fifty-eight percent) after 8 August were unmarried. It is surprising that twenty-four surgeons would decide to remain in a settlement of about two thousand persons. It may be that a number of them actually did not plan to remain very long, and stayed the winter of 1740–50 because of the subsidization that they and their families were guaranteed until 1 July 1750 (o.s.). The surnames of surgeons listed in Appendix 1 suggest that all were of English origin and that they were Anglican, Presbyterian, or Lutheran, but not Roman Catholic.

It is likely that no more than four or five of the surgeons and apothecaries were actually practising their profession during the fall of 1749 and the winter of 1749–50. It is probable also that they would have been in the employ of Cornwallis and housed in the hospital ship *Roehampton*. The majority of surgeons and apothecaries were occupied, however, in building their houses on the lots which they had drawn. In order to hasten the building, Cornwallis advertised in the Boston newspaper[51] for carpenters to come to Chebucto. Cornwallis had also employed, prior to 24 July, all the carpenters he could get from Annapolis and from the ships in Chebucto harbour, in order to build log houses. He offered the French at Minas considerable wages to work in Chebucto and those who responded stayed until the first of October.[52] Cornwallis's concerted effort to bring in carpenters led to rapid construction of the numerous buildings shown in the sketch by Moses Harris that appears in the lower right of Figure 2.

In his letter[53] to the Lords of Trade in August 1749 (o.s.), Cornwallis stated, "In a few days more I should have been able to have discharged most of the rest [of the Transports]." He continued: "The Council has found it absolutely necessary to continue Warburton's Regiment at least for the winter upon the same footing it was upon at Louisbourg." Later, on 11 September, he wrote that "the Troops have been employed in carrying the line," which meant that they were building a barricade of logs and brushwood around the town.[54] This temporary barricade[55] was erected in order to protect the settlers from attacks by the French and Indians[56] during the winter of 1749–50.

Cornwallis also reported[57] that 1,574 settlers were victualled in Chebucto during the first week of September. This included the 116 settlers who came on the ship *Sarah*, which had arrived from Liverpool on 30 August. Prior arrangements[58] had been made for a surgeon and a chest of medicines to accompany the passengers, but I was unable to determine whether a surgeon actually did arrive on the ship. On 17 October, Cornwallis reported that there were three hundred houses covered in at Halifax;[59] on 7 December, he reported[60] that the number of settlers victualled in the town was 1,876, "besides the artificiers and labourers from Boston and Minas." A letter from Halifax, dated 7 December 1749 (o.s.) and published in *Gentleman's Magazine and Historical Chronicle* (February 1750, 7), states that "there are already about 400 habitable houses within the fortifications and not less than 200 without."

In addition to the twenty-four surgeons and apothecaries who arrived with Cornwallis and who are known to have resided in Halifax after 8 August 1749 (o.s.), at least three surgeons[61] arrived before the end of the year. Two of them, George Slocombe[62] and William Catherwood,[63] were surgeon and surgeon's mate with Warburton's 45th Regiment. The third was William Skene,[64] surgeon with Philipps's Fortieth Regiment, a company of which Cornwallis had summoned to Halifax on 12 July 1749 (o.s.). By the end of 1749, therefore, the number of surgeons and apothecaries in Halifax totalled twenty-five. Two of the surgeons who had been Cornwallis passengers, Robert White and Joshua Sacheverell, died[65] during the fall of 1749.

THE FALL OF 1749 AND THE WINTER OF 1749–50 took its human toll in the new settlement. St Paul's Anglican Church burial records[66] indicate that, between 21 September 1749 (o.s.) and 21 April 1750 (o.s.), a total of 237 persons died, 172 civilians and 65 soldiers or mariners. The mortality rate among the civilian population was, therefore, approximately nine percent during the seven-month period, a rather high figure.[67] Nearly a century later, T.B. Akins[68] claimed that "about this time a destructive epidemic made its appearance in the Town, and it is said nearly 1,000 persons fell victim during the autumn and following winter," which probably refers to the autumn and winter of 1749–50. However, if there were 1,876 settlers victualled on 7 December 1749 (o.s.) and 2,367 victualled[69] during the period from 18 May to 4 June 1750 (o.s.), it seems unlikely that as many as a thousand persons could have died from an epidemic during the winter of 1749–50. Moreover, a study of the Boston newspaper[70] of the period reveals numerous references to Halifax but no mention of an epidemic which ravaged half the population. On 19 March 1749/50, Cornwallis wrote[71] to the Lords of Trade that "a frame is put up for a hospital to receive the sick. There has never been above 25 in the hospital ship at one time." In the same letter, he wrote, "The winter has passed without complaints of any kind." These statements suggest that there could not have been an epidemic of the proportions reported by Akins.

The victualling list from which these figures are drawn, updated to the end of June,[72] includes only fifteen of the twenty-one surgeons (seventy-one percent) known to have been in Halifax in May and June of 1750.[73] Inasmuch as the Halifax settlers were guaranteed provisions until the end of June 1750 (o.s.), one would expect that the names of everyone actually residing in the settlement at that time would appear in the list. Thus, one year after the settlement of Halifax was founded, only nineteen of the thirty-six original surgeons, apothecaries, and chymists (fifty-three percent) were still there.

The frame for the hospital mentioned above had been erected by 19 March 1750 (o.s.). It was located on the site of present-day Government House and was probably one of the two buildings designated by the letter к in the Moses Harris plan of Halifax shown in Figure 2. One of the three buildings shown in the left foreground of the "View of Halifax drawn from ye Topmasthead" may also have been the hospital. However, this drawing positions the hospital (assuming that one of the buildings is, indeed, the hospital) nearer to the water's edge than it actually was. The hospital received its first patients sometime between 19 March and 9 July 1750 (o.s.), the day that the hospital ship *Roehampton* cleared Halifax and sailed to New York.[74]

It appears, from correspondence, that Cornwallis had much difficulty in convincing the Lords of Trade of the necessity of continuing the hospital for a period longer than one year. Their attitude towards maintaining a civilian hospital is not surprising. In mid-eighteenth-century England, only the poor were treated at public expense and only sometimes was treatment given in a hospital. More frequently, it was provided in an alms house or poor house. "It is important," as Knowles states, "to emphasize that during the 18th century most of the care given in Hospitals was nursing and the Hospital remained an institution for the sick poor."[75] In Paris, the death rate among patients at the Hôtel-Dieu Hospital in 1788 was nearly twenty-five percent; frequently two to eight patients occupied one bed. Attendants living in the hospital were noted to have a death rate of six to twelve percent year. Unlike France, which built hospitals in its colonies and staffed them with nuns and surgeons who were members of religious orders,[76] England did not appear to believe that it should provide its colonists with hospitals for an extended period. The first hospital in New England was not established until some two hundred years after the *Mayflower's* arrival at Plymouth. The hospital in Halifax pre-dated similar institutions in Philadelphia (1751) and New York (1771). Military hospitals were very common in both French and English colonies, although for the most part, they were only temporary establishments.

The first indication that the Lords of Trade were becoming uneasy about the new settlement at Halifax appears in a letter to Cornwallis dated 16 Febuary 1749/50. They questioned the number and amount of expenditures.[77] Cornwallis replied.[78] "According to your Lordships directions, I this day discharged some of the surgeons and mates that may be spared." According to an earlier letter,[79] the medical personnel being paid during the first year were two surgeons and two apothecaries at ten shillings per day, two surgeon's mates at five shillings per day, and a midwife at fifty pounds per year. Further scepticism about financial matters relating to Nova Scotia was expressed in a letter dated 5 March 1749/50 from Christopher Kilby, Esq., agent for the settlement, complaining of the poorly filed information about matters concerning Halifax. On the same date, a request for medicines for the hospital in Nova Scotia was turned down and the secretary of the board was ordered to write a letter informing Mr Oswald, one of the commissioners for Trade and Plantations, that without the board's direction,[80] he should not respond to the requests of Mr Davidson, treasurer of the colony of Nova Scotia. Hugh Davidson later was called[81] to London to answer questions regarding his accounts and explain why the cost of the settlement had been £76,976 in 1749, rather than the £40,000 granted[82] by Parliament on 23 March 1749 (o.s.) "towards the charge of transporting to His Majesty's Colony of Nova Scotia, and supporting and maintaining there such reduced officers, etc."

THREE EMIGRANT SHIPS, with a total of 795 passengers, arrived during the summer of 1750: the *Alderney*[83] on 23 August, the *Ann*[84] on 2 September, and the *Nancy* on 16 September.[85] This brought to 3,200 the population of the town by 22 September, according to Hugh Davidson.[86] He stated before the Lords of Trade that, owing to ventilation, the people of the *Nancy* and the *Alderney* had arrived in good health, whereas "Mr Dick's ship was somewhat sickly." There are no specific references to the type or extent of the sickness which affected the *Ann* passengers. On 5 October, Cornwallis wrote[87] to Leonard Lockman "that the sick should be removed to the house of Major Lockman where there are chimneys and the persons that are in health that are there, to be removed to the place where the sick now are. You are hereby directed to make such a disposition to them if it appears to you to be necessary for their comfort and to hire such of the persons in health among them to attend the sick as may be necessary, promising them a reasonable allowance for their service." This order may have been precipitated by the death of Matthew Jones, one of the principal surgeons at the hospital, who was buried[88] on 7 October. Quite likely, "the sick" to whom Cornwallis referred were Germans, since on 5 November, a letter[89] was sent to Mr Lewis Hays, Keeper of the Provisions, informing him that the government had contracted with persons to victual the sick Germans at a certain rate per diem per person, and that Hays should stop this allowance for Germans who were returned by Chief Surgeon Lockman as being well. Salusbury noted in his diary (16 November): "It is hoped this weather will clear the air and make the settlement more healthy. We have had more sickness this fall than last." Cornwallis wrote,[90] referring to the *Ann*, that "the Germans were very sickly and many dead." On 11 December, the *Boston Gazette* reported that "the buildings on the opposite side of the Harbour[91] increases daily. The people are very sickly especially the meaner sort [the poorer people], and the Germans, which is probably owing to change of climate, want of necessaries, and bad [medical] attendance." Dick's explanation to the Lords of Trade concerning the lack of ventilators on the *Ann*[92] was that "there was no person in the country [i.e., Holland], that could have fixed it."

Another possible source of the sickness that appears to have taken its toll during the fall and winter of 1750–51 was the transports that brought Lascelles's Regiment from Ireland. It had been noted that

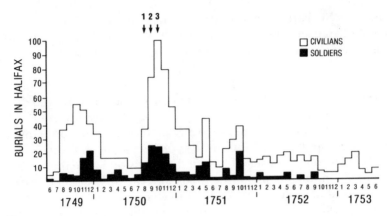

Figure 3
Evidence of an epidemic at Halifax during the winter of 1750–51.

1 Arrival of an Irish regiment, 12 August, 1750
2 Arrival of the *Ann* from Rotterdam, 2 September, 1750
3 Death of Matthew Jones, principal surgeon at the hospital, 5 October, 1750

on at least one of the Irish transports, there was a great deal of sickness. Figure 3, which was constructed from the burials recorded in St Paul's Anglican Church, shows that, during the eight months from August 1750 to March 1751, a total of 333 persons, an average of forty-two per month, had died.[93] In contrast, the average mortality for the twenty-seven months following March 1751 was only twelve per month. It would appear that some form of epidemic ravaged the population during the late summer, fall, and winter of 1750–51.[94] While this epidemic has not been precisely identified from the primary-source literature, it is my belief that it was typhus fever, which, in the middle of the eighteenth century, would have been identified as camp, hospital, jail, or ship fever, or simply under the general category of fever.

Sir John Pringle (1707–82), a student of Boerhaave and later physician to the military hospital at Flanders, began in 1742 to study febrile illnesses prevalent in crowded military camps. He noted that in winter and spring, inflammatory fevers were common, whereas during the summer and fall, the body fibres were more relaxed, fluids more rarefied and disposed to putrefaction. The prevalent disease in the summer and fall was the putrid fever, which he referred to as bilious in his book, *Observations on the Diseases of the Army*, published in 1752. He noted that people with bilious fever became yellow with jaundice. Pringle attempted to investigate fevers by paying special

attention to heat, cold, moisture, and dampness, as well as the putrefaction of the air. He noted that fevers seemed to be endemic in sit-
uations where there were vapours and putrid effluvia from human
excrement lying about the camp during hot weather, as well as from
rotting straw, and from air in crowded places. He enforced sanitary
regulations, attempted to purify the air in military camps, and laid
down guidelines of sanitation and ventilation in military hospitals. It
is likely that Dr Alexander Abercrombie would have known Dr Pringle since they both served in Flanders at the same time. Assuming
that Abercrombie agreed with John Pringle's beliefs concerning the
prevention of fever in military camps and hospitals, it is possible that
Abercrombie applied the same sanitation and ventilation procedures to the civilian hospital that he was in charge of in Halifax from
1750 to 1758.

In his *Synopsis Nosologie Methodicoe*, published in 1769, William
Cullen divided fevers into two general categories: synocha, or inflammatory fever, distinguished by a strong hard pulse; and low
nervous fever or typhus, characterized by prostration, weak pulse,
and delirium.[95] The word typhus means smoke or mist, and was first
used in the medical literature by F.B. de C. Sauvages in his book on
the classification of diseases, published in Leyden in 1759.[96] Cullen
divided typhus fever into typhus *petechialis*, which manifested itself
in a skin rash and haemorrhage spots over the chest and abdomen,
and typhus *icteriodes*, where the patient suffers from a low fever and
jaundice. In typhus *petechialis* the fever is severe and malignant, with
the appearance of gangrene. It is referred to as putrid because of
the dissolution of bodily fluids and solids. This was the type of fever
which Pringle had observed in military barracks or camps, hospitals,
and crowded ships during the summer and fall months, and was
very likely the epidemic which broke out in Halifax in August and
September of 1750, brought there by ships such as the *Ann* and the
Irish transports.

In addition to Matthew Jones, who was one of the chief surgeons
at the hospital, two other surgeons, John Wildman and Robert Kerr,
both Cornwallis passengers, died during the late summer of 1750,
because of the epidemic. This meant that only sixteen of the original
thirty-six surgeons and apothecaries (forty-four percent) who arrived in June 1749 (o.s.) were still in Halifax at the end of 1750. A
total of seven new surgeons appear in the records of Halifax during
1750. William Draper, surgeon, was listed as residing in Halifax
prior to June 1750.[97] Probably he was among the approximately one
thousand persons who are said[98] to have come to the province from
the New England colonies during the winter and spring of 1750.

Each of the three emigrant ships mentioned previously had at least one surgeon on board, John Baxter[99] on the *Alderney*, Johann Ulrich Klett[100] on the *Ann*, and John Duckworth[101] on the *Nancy*. Two additional surgeons were members of regiments stationed in Halifax in 1750. Arthur Price,[102] surgeon with Lascelles's Regiment, arrived in August 1750, and Richard Veale[103] was appointed surgeon with the Forty-fifth Foot on 30 September, replacing George Slocombe who was buried from St Paul's five days earlier. Edward Crafts, "surgeon of the Town of Halifax," sold Lot B4 in Collier's Division on 29 September.[104] Thus, at the end of the year, there were twenty-five surgeons, apothecaries, chymists, and druggists in the town of Halifax.

As already mentioned, the 353 passengers on the *Alderney*, including Doctor John Baxter, were encouraged to establish themselves on "the opposite side of the Harbour over against George's Island"; in other words, to found the settlement which soon became known as Dartmouth. During the first six months of 1751, the settlers residing in Dartmouth were attacked on at least three occasions by Indians. Salusbury records that "the Indians attacked Dartmouth, one poor boy[105] returned scalp'd." On 13 May, he records: "Dartmouth attacked by a large party of Indians. Near 20 killed and taken, men, women, and children." The entry[106] in the *London Magazine or Gentleman's Monthly Intelligencer*, dated Halifax 25 June 1751 (o.s.) probably refers to Salusbury's statement that, "some days ago about 60 Indians attacked the Town of Dartmouth and killed about 8 of the inhabitants. They also carried off about fourteen prisoners." The terror and insecurity which these attacks created was so great that, upon the arrival on 10 July of the *Speedwell* with 212 passengers,[107] the governor and Council decided to employ[108] them to build a picket line of fortification at the back of the settlement of Dartmouth. The *Speedwell* was the first of four transports with foreign Protestants from Germany and Switzerland to arrive in Halifax in 1751. The others were the *Gale*, which arrived on 29 July with 205 passengers;[109] the *Pearl*, which came on 14 September with 232 on board;[110] and the *Murdoch* with 269 passengers,[111] which arrived on 25 September. In all, a total of 918 passengers arrived in Halifax on these ships, having survived a mortality rate during the four crossings from Rotterdam of between 4.2 to 12.1 percent.[112] The intention was to locate the foreign Protestants in a new settlement. However, because of the fear created by repeated Indian attacks, it was decided to have the new settlers remain in Halifax for the winter of 1751–52.

Among the 918 passengers who arrived from Europe in July and

September 1751, eight listed their occupations as surgeon.[113] Only four of these, Johannes Matthew Lutgens, Christopher Adam Nicolai, Johann Berghard Erad, and Alexandre de Rodohan, appear in later eighteenth-century records for Nova Scotia. It is likely that the other four left Halifax shortly after their arrival. In addition to these eight surgeons, at least five new surgeons appeared in Halifax in 1751. One was John Phillipps, who might possibly have been one of the three persons by that name on the Cornwallis passenger lists.[114] He was appointed[115] surgeon for all independent companies of Rangers on 4 June 1751 (o.s.). A second was Jonathan Prescott, who had been a surgeon and captain of a company at Louisbourg in 1745. He addressed a memorial[116] to Council in June of 1751 asking for permission to establish a still in the town. William Urquhart, who could have been in Halifax in 1749 or 1750,[117] was listed[118] as a surgeon in Halifax on 9 September 1751 (o.s.). A fourth, George Francheville, first appeared in Halifax in April 1751, when he bought Lot 14 in Callendar's Division.[119] Dr Francheville remained in the colony until he died[120] in August 1781. A surgeon named George Winslow was recorded[121] as having sold Lot E8 in the North Suburbs on 26 August 1751 (o.s.). Winslow does not appear in either the victualling list of May–June 1750 or in the July 1752 census for Halifax. One of the original surgeons, Alexander Hay, who was surgeon's mate at the hospital, was buried from St Paul's on 2 May 1751 (o.s.). So now only twelve of the original thirty-six surgeons, apothecaries, and chymists on the Cornwallis passenger lists (thirty-three percent) were residing in Halifax at the end of 1751, six having died, and the remaining eighteen having left the settlement.

None of the ships bringing the foreign Protestants to Halifax in 1751 appears to have brought fever into the settlement as the transports had the year before. The *Boston Gazette* of 27 August 1751 (o.s.) reported, "That place [Halifax] is very healthy, and the people in high spirits, and ... they hope soon to see a flourishing settlement." Very little reference to the hospital is made in the records of 1751, except for the memorial[122] of John Grant presented and dismissed at a December meeting of Council. In this memorial, Grant and other (unnamed) persons wrote to Council, "praying that surgeons in Government pay may be prohibited from practicing and dispensing medicines to private persons for money."

A letter[123] from Whitehall to Cornwallis in March 1751/52 stated that the House of Commons had voted £21,069 "to make good the exceedings incurred last year in the services of Nova Scotia, and £40,450 for this year to defray the charges of the current year." The tone of the letter indicated that the Lords of Trade were still disappointed with the magnitude of the cost of the settlement at Halifax. Thus:

Upon considering the establishment of civil officers in the Province, which is very large, we are in hopes that you will be able to reduce it by lessening the profits of such officers as are not held singly, and by striking off some of those officers which were necessary at the very beginning of the settlement, but were never intended to be continued longer. In this particular the people ought to be accustomed to provide for their own convenience and at their own charge, and the public we should imagine might be directly relieved from the charge of [a] midwife, apothecaries, and surgeons, as there must be now many families both used and very well able to bear such expenses. We hope that a reduction may also be made in the expenses of the Hospital.

At this time, Cornwallis had great difficulty in explaining to the Lords of Trade that the settlers were not able to pay for their own medical expenses. Even under constant urging to reduce spending, Cornwallis demonstrated much compassion for the welfare of his people by continuing with construction of the orphan house. That establishment opened on 8 June 1752 (o.s.) with Mrs Ann Wenman as matron at a pay of three pence per day for each orphan housed.[124] The orphan house, probably the second of the two buildings designated by the letter K in the Harris plan (Figure 2), was located on Bishop Street across from the hospital. The first record of the number of children in the orphan house and hospital is for the period August to October 1752, when the two establishments contained fifty-five orphans and forty-nine patients.[125] The minutes of Council[126] for 24 August recorded the direction that "one or more apartments in the Public Hospital in Halifax ... be conveniently fitted up with iron bolts, bars, and locks for the reception, lodging, and detention of sick and infirm prisoners for debt."

The settlement of Halifax increased further with the arrival of five more ships in August and September 1752, carrying a total of 1,007 foreign Protestants.[127] Governor Hopson had been instructed,[128] in April of 1752, "to have all ships or vessels inspected immediately upon arrival before persons on board are landed to enquire into the Health and condition of those on board. If any distemper or infectious disease is found on board, the said persons are to be landed and placed in a Lazaretto or other building erected for that purpose a convenient distance from the settlement." However, none of these five transport ships appears to have brought fever into Halifax, although the mortality rate on the *Pearl* and the *Sally* was 15.5 percent, the highest among any of the eleven ships bringing foreign Protestants to Halifax in 1750, 1751, and 1752. It should be noted that, whereas passengers on the *Ann* were detained aboard in Halifax harbour for only five days, passengers on the *Pearl, Gale,* and *Sally*, which arrived in 1752, were detained for fifteen to twenty-one days.[129] This extended period of detention could be interpreted as a form of quarantine. After the *Pearl* arrived in Halifax harbour on 10 August, it was reported at the Council meeting referred to above that the ship had "been inspected by the surgeon and found to be generally in good health and no appearance of a contagious or infectious disorder" existed. The last ship to arrive in 1752, the *Gale*, experienced twenty-nine deaths during passage and probably had some form of sickness on board. Hopson, who had replaced Cornwallis as governor of Nova Scotia on 3 August 1752 (o.s.), reported to the Lords of Trade on 16 October that on 26 September, "the last of these settlers were landed, when there were about 30 of them that could not stir off the beach, eight of them orphans who immediately had the best care taken of them, notwithstanding which two of them dyed [*sic*] after being carried to the Hospital, within about 12 days time there were 14 orphans belonging to these settlers that were taken into the Orphan House." In addition to the foreign Protestants, Hopson's Regiment (the Twenty-ninth), consisting of 619 personnel,[130] arrived on 3 August 1752 (o.s.). Since the census of Halifax and surrounding area taken in July 1752 listed 906 families and a total of 4,248 persons,[131] the civilian population by the end of 1752 would have totalled about 5,250 persons. The military population consisted of 2,200 soldiers in three regiments: Hopson's 29th; Warburton's 45th; and Lascelles's 47th.

By the end of 1752, there was a total of twenty-five surgeons, apothecaries, and chymists in Halifax, eleven of whom had been Cornwallis passengers. The only new surgeon to arrive in 1752 was the Reverend Thomas Wood, who had been at Louisbourg as surgeon to Shirley's Regiment in 1746. After being ordained a clergyman in the Anglican church in London in 1749 and returning to his home in New Brunswick, New Jersey, he petitioned in late 1751 for a transfer to Nova Scotia.[132] The Reverend Mr Wood was "bred to physick and surgery" and appears to have practised medicine in Halifax while he was vicar of St Paul's Church.[133]

On 16 September 1752 (n.s.), the Shubenacadie Indians signed[134] a peace treaty with Governor Hopson. Soon after, on 22 November, Rev. J.B. Moreau wrote,[135] "Peace having been made with the savages, the Government contemplates establishing a new colony." This alluded, of course, to plans to establish the town of Lunenburg. But the establishment of Lunenburg was delayed for fear of Indian attacks, until, on 12 April 1753 (o.s.), Claude Gisiquash, "an Indian who stiles [sic] himself Governor of LeHeve [sic], appeared this day before Council and having declared his intention of making peace," signed[136] with Governor Hopson a document drawn up for that purpose. This meant that peace treaties had now been signed with most of the Indians in the central and eastern regions of Nova Scotia. In addition to the Indian threat, the governor was also determined that the foreign Protestants destined for the new settlement work off their debts in Halifax before he would allow them to leave the town.[137]

An incident had taken place near Country Harbour, in eastern Nova Scotia, in which Indians had scalped[138] two men and taken captive two others. The latter, John Connor and James Grace, escaped and, bearing six Indian scalps, arrived in Halifax harbour on 15 April 1753 (n.s.), three days after Gisiquash had signed the peace treaty. Governor Hopson must have been perturbed by this untimely incident. His letter[139] reporting the incident concluded, "What turn this may take, I can as yet form no judgement." Apparently, there was no immediate hostile response from the Indians who signed the treaties, and on 10 May, Council "resolved that the settlement intended to be made at Merlegash [sic] be called the Township of Lunenburg and that the District thereof to be hereafter ascertained." On 26 May, Hopson wrote[140] further to the Lords of Trade that, "as everything is now in readiness I propose to send out the Foreigners in three days. They are to go to Merleguash [sic], a harbour about sixteen leagues to the westward from this place where there has been formerly a French settlement by which means there is between three and four hundred acres of cleared land which is to be equally divided amongst the settlers who consist of about sixteen hundred persons." Halifax was the only major English settlement in Nova Scotia during the period 21 June 1749 (o.s.) to 7 June 1753 (n.s.), the day on which the Lunenburg settlers sailed from Halifax for their new home.[141] During that four-year period, the number of medical personnel entering Halifax totalled sixty. While the number of surgeons and assistant surgeons providing medical attention to the settlers was reduced in this time, varying between twenty and thirty (Figure 4), it can be seen that the Lords of Trade ensured that a sufficient level of health-care workers, including a midwife, was provided. Contrary to popular belief, the majority (approximately eighty-seven percent) of the surgeons, apothecaries, and chymists in the new settlement were civilian rather than mili-

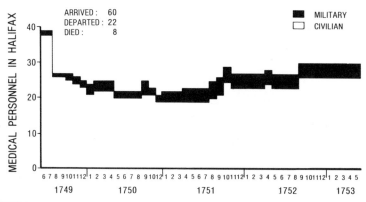

Figure 4
Civilian, naval, and military surgeons, apothecaries, chymists, and druggists in
Halifax, 1749–53.

tary. During the same four-year period, the civilian population of
Halifax had risen from 2,547 on 1 July 1749 (o.s.) to about 5,200 just
prior to 7 June 1753 (n.s.).

THE NEXT CHAPTER concentrates on the transformation of Halifax
from a small civilian town into a military and naval base which, in
1757 and again in 1758, was a temporary home for 22,000 soldiers
and sailors. Although the large number of military and naval personnel in Halifax during the decade brought money to the town,
and created employment there as well, it will be seen that they also
brought smallpox, which led to epidemics in 1755 and 1757. They
also left behind them a great number of camp followers and destitute people to be cared for by the small civilian population. A further result of the presence of this large, transient military and naval
population was the decline and elimination of the civilian hospital.
The Lords of Trade were adamant that the civilian population of
Halifax could be treated in the military hospitals there, but were not
sensitive to the eventuality, recognized by Governor Lawrence, that
when the military left, their hospitals closed.

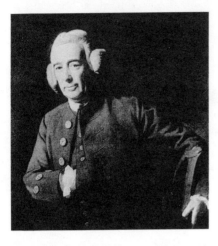

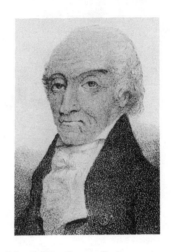

Dr Silvester Gardiner (1707–1786) arrived in Halifax in April 1776 after the evacuation of Boston, having studied with William Cheselden at St Thomas's. He died in Rhode Island.
Oil on canvas by J.S. Copley.

Dr John Jeffries (1745–1819) came to Halifax in April 1776 after the evacuation of Boston. He was surgeon to the military hospital at Halifax from 1776 to 1779. He died in Boston.
Oil on panel by an unknown artist. (Museum of Fine Arts, Boston.)

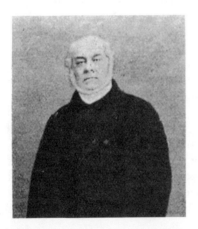

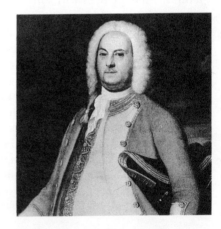

Dr Duncan Clark (ca.1760–1808) arrived in Halifax in 1778 with the 82nd Regiment from Scotland, having studied at Edinburgh University during 1777–78. He practised in Halifax until his death. Painting by an unknown artist.

Dr William Brattle (1706–1776), who had been the attorney general of Massachusetts Bay, arrived in Halifax in April 1776 after the evacuation of Boston. He died in Halifax in October 1776.
Oil on canvas by J.S. Copley.

A Decade of Military and Naval Surgeons, 1753–1763

Four years after the founding of Halifax the British presence in Nova Scotia was still largely confined to that town, apart from a small anglophone population at the old capital, Annapolis Royal. Within a decade, British ownership had been established and an English-speaking population predominated. Beginning with the placing of foreign Protestants at Lunenburg, the trend continued as the bulk of the French Acadian inhabitants were deported and the forts at Beauséjour and Louisbourg were captured by the British. By the time the Treaty of Paris was signed in February 1763, an increasing immigration of New Englanders was opening up a network of townships across western Nova Scotia. During those years of demographic change and great-power conflict, the activities of civilian medical practitioners were overshadowed by those of the military and naval surgeons in attendance upon servicemen and civilians alike.

For almost a decade, Halifax was truly a rendezvous for armies and fleets. During the period 1755–63, the town was transformed from a small, insignificant seaport on the North Atlantic into a major military and naval base. The establishment of numerous regimental hospitals, a general military hospital, and a naval hospital in the town gave the Lords of Trade sufficient leverage to force the governor to close the civilian hospital and to eliminate almost all of the expenditures that had previously been allowed for health care and charitable purposes. Meanwhile, Halifax was visited by two smallpox epidemics during this period, in 1755 and again in 1757. The second epidemic was at least partly responsible for the cancellation of the planned attack on Louisbourg by the combined forces of Lord Loudon and Admiral Holburne.

With the departure of the foreign Protestants for Lunenburg on 7 June 1753, Halifax lost at least eight of its surgeons. Leonard Lockman and Johann B. Erad had been appointed[1] as surgeons to the new settlement, while J. Ulrich Klett, J. Carl Deglen, Christopher A. Nicolai, and Johann C.H. Edmund, were surgeons among the 1,453 original settlers at Lunenburg.[2] John Phillipps, who in early June had been appointed[3] surgeon for all Independent Companies of Rangers, quite likely arrived in Lunenburg with the settlers, or shortly thereafter, for in October 1753, he was married[4] at Lunenburg to Anna de Labertouche. The eighth surgeon who seems to have accompanied the settlers was John Baxter, who remained only a short time before returning to Halifax. Colonel Charles Lawrence, who had been put in charge of transferring the settlers to Lunenburg, recorded in his journal[5] that, while the transports were preparing to leave Halifax harbour in June, he "sent an order to Mr Baxter, one of ye surgeons of the settlement to visit the vessel" to attend a passenger who was sick. Later, in June, Lawrence records in Lunenburg that "Mr Baxter has indicated [that] the settlers are in good health." This exodus of eight surgeons left fifteen surgeons remaining in the town of Halifax, while an additional seven were distributed throughout the province at Annapolis, Grand Pré, and Fort Lawrence.[6]

Halifax in July 1753 appears[7] to have had a civilian population of approximately 3,500. It was protected by one sloop of war[8] and only five hundred soldiers, a fact that concerned both Hopson and Lawrence.[9] The settlement at Dartmouth had all but disappeared and was reported[10] as having "not above five familys ... as there is no trade or fishery to maintain any inhabitants and they apprehend damage from the Indians."

THE EARLIEST ADVERTISEMENTS by medical practitioners in Halifax appeared in the *Halifax Gazette* of 21 July 1753. The first of these (Figure 5), placed by Henry Meriton in July, was also the first such advertisement in Canada. The second, which appeared in the *Gazette* in October, was inserted by Robert Grant, who, among other commodities, was offering medicines for sale. This same Robert Grant, along with two other surgeons, William Merry and John Grant, petitioned[11] Council on 27 December 1753, stating:

that your memorialists having lately met with great difficulties in the recovery of their debts, as surgeons and Apothecaries, which have occasioned great animosities, expense, loss of time and troublesome Lawsuits to your

Notice is hereby given to the Publick that they may be attended during any disorder by a regular bred surgeon and apothecary, with advice gratis, with medicines at the same rate as in England, and without any charge for visits, unless sent for after the nine o'clock gun firing. Likewise all persons under necessity of employing a man midwife, may be served by

Their most humble servant,
Henry Meriton,

Surgeon, Apothecary, and Man Midwife;
Late a Dresser in St Thomas's Hospital, London, and
Pupil to the well known man midwife, Dr Smelley.

Figure 5
Text of the first newspaper advertisement by a medical practitioner in Canada. It appeared in the *Halifax Gazette* of 21 July 1753.

memorialists, and to some of the subjects of this Province from the supposed extravagence of medicine accompts and attendance to them charged.

Your memorialists, in order to prevent disputes of such pernicious tendencies for the future, beg leave to submit the state of their accompts with the price of their visits to the determination of your Honours.

In order to forward such a desirable end, we have transmitted to your Honours, the lowest price of medicines under their different denominations that we believe a living would be procured, under the strictist [*sic*] oeconomy and from the best payments that could be wished for.

If this scheme shall be judged impracticable, or the prices thought too high charged, we pray that your Honours will determine it in such other manner as appears to you more equitable, and more likely to destroy the feuds that are of constant attendants of suits of Law, as they are of great expence and loss of time to the parties concerned, which we shall punctually observe.

Council, of the opinion that to regulate the price of medicine would not only be unprecented but attended with infinitely more inconvenience than that complained of, denied the petition.

The lawsuits mentioned in the petition were, in fact, numerous. John Grant had taken two people to the Supreme Court in 1753, and at least one in 1754, for non-payment of fees for medicines and attendance,[12] while William Merry had taken William Kneeland, a carpenter, to the Inferior Court of Common Pleas in June 1753 for

Table 1
Treatment for William Kneeland by William Merry, Surgeon, 1750–53

Date (o.s.)		Medication or Treatment	Fee (£	s.	d.)
22 May	1750	A large Bottle of Drops	–	2	6
1 June	1750	Glauber Salts	–	1	0
10 June	1750	A Balsamic Bolus	–	2	–
12 June	1750	Four Nervous Powders	–	6	–
12 June	1750	A Cephalic Mixter, 8 oz	–	8	–
20 Aug.	1750	A Coroborating Plaster	–	5	–
21 Oct.	1750	A Comp^d Emetic	–	2	6
10 Feb.	1751	Antie Ietetic Pills, No. 16	–	4	–
26 Mar.	1751	A Rhubarb Bolus	–	2	6
29 May	1751	Scarborough Salts 1½ oz	–	3	–
4 July	1751	A Colic Tincture	2	6	–
21 Aug.	1751	A Cordial Bolus for night	–	2	–
24 Sept.	1751	A Hysteric Mixture, 8 oz	–	8	–
8 Oct.	1751	Elixir Salutes, A Bottle	–	6	–
23 Oct.	1751	Spanish Liquorice	–	–	–
21 Jan.	1753	Ingred^{ts} for an Enema	–	2	6
22 Jan.	1753	Chemical Oyls and two Doses of Pills	–	5	–

Source: Halifax County Inferior Court of Common Pleas, Box 2, file 22, *William Kneeland vs. William Merry*, PANS RG37.

unpaid medical bills.[13] The court records of these cases reveal the types of medical treatment being administered in Halifax at the time, though one can only speculate about the illnesses themselves. A selection of these medications and treatment regimens is shown in Tables 1 and 2. The first listed treatment was administered by William Merry, surgeon, to William Kneeland (Table 1). John Grant administered some of the same medicines as well as those listed in Table 2 to Joseph Kent, attorney at law; John Buttler, distiller; and John Winston, labourer. An explanation of these medicines and the illnesses that they were expected to treat can be found in Appendix 2.

These listings are found in court records because patients had failed to pay for services rendered by their surgeon or doctor of physic. As the petition suggests, medical practitioners found it difficult to make a living. Many were faced with the necessity of pursuing a second occupation; for instance, William Merry and Jonathan Prescott operated stills,[15] while Henry Meriton opened on Sackville Street a school "for the instruction of youth in reading, writing, arithmetic, Latin, French, and dancing."[16] Robert Grant, as his advertisement indicates, operated in Granville Street a store where he

Table 2
Treatments for Joseph Kent, John Buttler, and John Winston by John Grant,
Surgeon, 1752–53

Date (o.s.)		Medication or Treatment	Fee (£	s.	d.)
20 Aug.	1752	An Anodyne Draught	–	2	–
21 Aug.	1752	6 oz of attenuating mixture	–	6	–
25 Aug.	1752	Two Pectoral Boluses	–	3	–
16 Sep.	1752	Two cooling Clysters	–	4	–
23 Sep.	1752	12 Anti Icteric Pills	–	6	–
31 Mar.	1752	A Dose of Purging Pills	–	2	6
31 Mar.	1752	Ingred[ts] for a fermentation	–	1	–
31 Mar.	1752	1 oz. of Disgestive [sic]	–	–	6
3 Apr.	1752	4 oz Camphereted Sp[ts] of Wine	–	4	–
5 Apr.	1752	Blooding	–	2	6
xber 22	1752[14]	Three Asstringent Boluses	–	4	6
xber 22	1752	4 oz of the shavings of hartshorn	–	1	–
xber 22	1752	3 oz of Issinglass	–	1	6
xber 23	1752	Advice and Attendance	1	10	–
21 Jan.	1752	4 ozs of gargarsm	–	4	–
29 Jan.	1752	3 ozs of Asstringent Electuary	–	7	6
5 Jun.	1753	6 oz Detergent Decoction	–	6	–

Source: Halifax County Supreme Court, Box 1, *John Kent vs. John Grant; John Buttler vs. John Grant; Catherine Winston vs. John Grant*, PANS RG39, series C.

sold groceries, medicines, and dry goods, while John Grant engaged in the trading business.[17]

On 1 January 1754, Council issued its first instruction[18] concerning preventive measures to guard against epidemics brought into Halifax by visiting ships. Council instructed Charles Hay, Esq., captain of the Port of Halifax, as follows:

You are to go aboard all ships, snows, brigantines, sloops, schooners coming into the Harbour before they pass George's Island and you are to examine into the Health and condition of the passengers and crew, and know from what Port they last sailed, and if you shall see any causes to suspect the plague or an epidemical disease on board, or if the vessel came from a Port where any sick diseases are supposed to be, you will bring the vessel to an anchor below the Island and forthwith make report thereof to the Governor or Commander-in-Chief.

What prompted this action is unclear. It may be that Lawrence,[19] president of the Council, had decided that in order to reduce the probability of contagious epidemics entering Halifax from immigrant, military, or naval ships, it was time to establish formal quarantine procedures. As dtescribed in chapter 1, at least three ships with contagious epidemics on board (the *Ann*, the *Gale*, and one of the transports for Lascelles's Regiment) had arrived in Halifax during the first few years of settlement.

The civilian hospital at Halifax continued to have the support of Hopson, even though he was constantly being pressured by the Lords of Trade to reduce its staff and expenses. In July 1753, he wrote[20] to the Lords, pleading that

the Orphan House and Hospital are not by any means to be done without at present. Your Lordships may be assured that I shall discontinue these and all other Establishments as soon as they cease to be Indispensably necessary ... As your Lordships seem to be of [the] opinion that some of the surgeons might be spared from the Establishment, I have made the most diligent enquiry into their employment with design if possible to lessen their number, but as I have been obliged to send two to Merlequash [Lunenburg] I find the remaining three barely sufficient to attend the Hospital and take care of the Inhabitants in the Town and Suburbs and at Dartmouth, the greatest part of whom are so extremely necessitous that they are by no means able to pay for the attendance of a surgeon, neither is it worth a surgeon's while to reside amongst them upon his practise only.

Alexander Abercrombie continued to hold the position of surgeon at the hospital, while Thomas Reeve and John Steele were the surgeon's mates. Abercrombie was paid ten shillings per day, and Reeves and Steele received five shillings. In 1754, they were assisted by two nurses;[21] by 1755, the establishment had been reduced to one nurse.[22] Ann Catherwood continued to be paid fifty pounds for her midwifery services to the residents of Halifax.[23] The total expense of medical services provided in the year 1754 was £961, and the number of patients in the hospital during the period July to December 1754 varied from a low of sixteen in September to a maximum of twenty-six in December.[24]

The administration and operation of the hospital was challenged in September of 1754 when the surgeon John Grant, desiring to contract with the government for supplying and attending the hospital, petitioned Council:[25]

That your Memorialist seeing the good intentions of your Honours hath taken the liberty of inclosing you a scheme, proposing a contract for the Hospital of Halifax, also a small allowance for medicines and attendance at the Orphan House, which he hopes will meet with the approbation of your Honours, as a large annual sum would be saved to the Government by such a contract.

That he would engage to supply each patient received into the Hospital with proper and sufficient victuals, drink, medicines, and attendance, necessaries and fire, candles, and nurses at a rate of 1 shilling, 3 pence per day in money and the usual allowance of salt, provisions. The Government to continue the House now occupy'd as an Hospital and to supply Beds and Beddings when wanted for which he would be accountable.

That he would attend and furnish medicines for the Orphan House for 10 pounds per annum.

Council replied, "The Hospital Accounts were called for and inspected, and it appeared therefrom that no advantage would arise from contracting according to the Proposals contained in said Memorial, it appearing also, upon inquiry, that the Hospital was in much better order and better taken care of by Mr Abercrombie, the surgeon thereof, than could be expected from a contractor as well as that it is upon a more certain footing and at as moderate an expence, the Memorial was rejected." It is probably not mere coincidence that a month earlier, on 17 August 1754, there appeared in the *Halifax Gazette* a sarcastic item that cast aspersions on Dr Abercrombie's credibility:

We hear that a certain Northern University justly infamous for Physical Diplomas, hath lately, by Request, transmitted one to this Place, in order to varnish the irregular Education, and to decorate the illegal Promotion of a Person now in a lucrative Station, in a Physical way here. It is therefore necesary, that the Publick may not be imposed upon, to acquaint them with the Nature of Diplomas: They are mostly confined to Theology, Physick, and Surgery, and cannot be obtained from any creditable University, or Corporation, but by Persons of a liberal Education, and that on the strictist Examination, after having defended a Thesis on the subject assigned. Indeed such as lately appeared here, may be obtained without any of the above Requisites, as is verified for the cases of Dr Rock, and Dr A--rc---bie, both which are the merchandise of the same University, and that without having seen, or examined the persons on whom they are conferred. The Practice of such a University, is by all Men of Sense despised, and the Possessors of such Diplomas held in Contempt, in so much that by a late Act of Parliament, and a later Order of his Majesty and Council, no man can be legally admitted into his service without undergoing a public Examination, and bringing a Certificate of his being qualified for the office he is to be employed in. And so greatly absurd it is, to claim Merit from such Diplomas, and producing them as Qualifications, or as a Testimony of a regular Education, will be ridicul'd and gain no credit, but with the Prejudiced, the Ignorant, and the Illiterate, it being well known that such Diplomas can be obtained for a horse, and Ass, or A-be'r.

It seems likely that the author of this statement, possibly John Grant,[26] was attempting to discredit Alexander Abercrombie in order to render available Abercrombie's position as surgeon to the hospital. As indicated in chapter 1, John Grant had petitioned Council in December 1751 (o.s.) to prohibit surgeons in government pay (i.e., at the hospital, or in the military) from practising and dispensing medicines to private persons for money. Council had dismissed the request. In January 1755, Grant wrote to the Lords of Trade[27] that he "was surprised that Mr Abercrombie, an unexperienced youth without qualifications to practise physic and surgery should be appointed" as surgeon to the hospital. Grant continued:

That your memorialist was at the setting out of this Province appointed by your Lordships an Assisting Surgeon to this Colony, in which place, he continued labouring for two years, and being without vanity affirm, was not the least unprofitable of the Professions, having practised the art of midwifery, which was not common to the other surgeons upon the Establishment.

That at the death of Mr Jones, one of the Principal Surgeons, your memorialist apply'd to the then Governor, Colonel Cornwallis to be appointed in his place, humbly hoping that his past service in His Majesty's Navy of Eight years and in this Province, with some assurances of your Lords of having the first vacancy, would have [entitled] your memorialist thereto.

That the sums expended in the support of surgeons and mates attending the Hospital, the victualling, and other contingent expenses thereof, is better known to your Lords then to your memorialist, but the sums that the Public could long ago been served for by putting the Hospital up to offers, and fair contract at but a fifth part, as a contract would have been had for it not exceeding two hundred pounds sterling per annum ...

That the patients of the Hospital are soldiers of the Governor's Regiment, who are supply'd with the provisions, medicines, fire, and other necessaries as well as with the Province surgeons, and the inhabitants that are entertained, or that would accept of the Hospital, are venerals [sic], and miscreants that ought not to be supported or countenanced by the Public.

After receiving an enquiry about Grant's memorial from the Lords of Trade, Council decided to hold a "Public Enquiry ... that all persons might have the opportunity to remark of what the grievances complained of were and of informing Council whether they know them or any of them to be true."[28] In responding to Grant, Council pointed out[29] that, contrary to his assertion regarding patients with venereal disease, only one or two per month were treated at the hospital during the period July 1754 to June 1755.[30] Council also made clear that it was quite happy with the performance of the surgeons at the Hospital. "The surgeon and his mate it is well known have been always ready to attend gratis, out of the Hospital any such poor industrious families as have been recommended to them by persons who have known them unable to pay the exorbitant fees too often demanded by the private practioners here." Lawrence wrote[31] to the Lords of Trade, after the enquiry, that "John Grant is a most audacious impudent fellow whose business it has been for these four years past to breed discontent among the people." The Lords of Trade responded[32] with an apology to Lawrence, stating that they had concluded that Grant's memorial was without the least foundation.

There is a reference to one other hospital in Halifax in 1754. It was called the Hospital for Sick and Hurt Seamen and was mentioned as being in Granville Street.[33] A letter[34] from Robert Grant to the board of this hospital in December 1759 (o.s.) indicates that Major Lockman, surgeon and agent for the sick, had requested that Grant take care of the sick sent ashore on 29 October 1750 (o.s.). Grant explained that Lockman had been appointed surgeon and agent for the hospital by Capt. Rous, but now found that his private business did not permit him to assume these responsibilities. In a second letter,[35] dated 4 October 1752, Robert Grant stated that he had been appointed to act as surgeon and agent for sick seamen at Halifax by Captain Pye, chief commander of the squadron at Halifax, as "Mr Lockman had declined to act since the pay was too low." Richard Veale, who apparently felt that he should have had the position, subsequently wrote that "he should be appointed surgeon of Sick and Wounded in Halifax in place of the person who is now in the position who is not a proper person to undertake the contract."[36] Robert Grant held the appointment on 16 April 1753 and was still in the position in October 1755,[37] when he reported that he had 177 sick sailors from Admiral Edward Boscawen's Fleet and seventy-nine French prisoners under treatment in sick quarters in Halifax. He continued as surgeon and agent to the sick and wounded seamen until at least 10 February 1757, when the question of his pay was referred to in a letter.[38]

The minutes of Council for 27 June 1754 refer[39] to "a stonehouse situated on Hospital Street, built by Richard Wenman." Council resolved that this building be appropriated for use as a workhouse or house of correction. It is likely that Hospital Street was the street leading to the hospital that had been established in March 1750 and was administered, in 1754, by Dr Alexander Abercrombie. The hospital was south of the palisades and just beyond Horseman's Fort.[40] The street was probably an extension of Barrington Street. Just south of the hospital was the orphan house, which was administered by Rev. John Breynton and whose matron was Mrs Ann Wenman, wife of the Richard Wenman mentioned above. It is likely that Richard and Ann Wenman lived in the orphan house and that, adjacent to it, was the stonehouse appropriated for use as a workhouse.

As 1754 drew to a close, the Halifax settlers appear to have been in good health. The average number of patients in the hospital, during the last six months of the year, was a modest twenty. However, Lawrence, president of Council, had reported to the Lords of Trade in June that "there had been a daily decrease in the people in this place [Halifax] occasioned by its inability to support its inhabitants who began to discover that they had too much neglected agriculture.[41] How many persons left Halifax during 1754 is not known, but it appears that none of the surgeons left. However, William Merry, described in the *Gazette* as "a noted surgeon and apothecary of this place,"[42] died during the year.

At the end of its first year of settlement, Lunenburg was reported to have 319 houses and forty huts.[43] The main health concern during this period was the lack of a midwife, so that "many of the inhabitants ... laboured under great disadvantage having lost many of their children from the want of midwifes."[44] This was soon remedied. In November 1754, the Lords of Trade informed Lawrence that ten pounds had been added to the establishment to pay for a midwife for Lunenburg.[45]

One major event which brought at least six new surgeons into Nova Scotia was the successful attack and capture, in June 1755, of Fort Beauséjour, the French stronghold at Chignecto. Ever since the fort had been built in 1750, Governors Cornwallis, Hopson, and Lawrence had agonized about its influence in inciting the Indians and in providing the Acadians with a rallying point so that they did not feel it necessary to take the oath of allegiance. In August 1754, Lawrence had confided Council's concern to the Lords of Trade: "I greatly feel that this evil [attacks by Indians] can never be absolutely and effectively removed while the French possess the north side of the Bay of Fundy."[46]

Governor Shirley of Massachusetts agreed with Lawrence. His thoughts about ridding Nova Scotia of the French were communicated to Lawrence in a letter from the Lords of Trade.[47] Shirley felt that many New Englanders would be interested in settling in Nova Scotia, but only if the French forts at Beauséjour and Baie Verte were destroyed and the French and Indians driven out of Nova Scotia.

To effect the capture of these forts, the Lords of Trade informed.[48] Lawrence "that two Regiments of Foot consisting of 500 men each are to be sent to Virginia, there to be augmented by 700 men each. Orders have also [been] sent to Governor Shirley and Sir William Pepperell to raise two Regiments of 1,000 men each." Lieutenant Governor Lawrence was advised to raise three hundred men for an attack on Fort Beauséjour planned for early summer of 1755. On 15 November 1754, Lt Col Robert Monckton, commander at Fort Lawrence, and Captain George Scott, one of his officers, were sent to New England for a six-month period of preparation for the intended siege.[49]

On 28 May 1755, Col John Winslow, with two battalions of Governor Shirley's Regiment, consisting of approximately two thousand men, arrived at Annapolis Royal on their way to Chignecto.[50] Each battalion had a surgeon (Miles Whitworth in the First Battalion and Philip Geoffrey Cast in the Second) and two surgeon's mates (John Thomas and John Tyler, First Battalion; Jacob March and Cornelius Nye, Second).

The two battalions arrived in Chignecto on 2 June and joined the companies of Warburton's and Lascelles's regiments stationed at Fort Lawrence. Under Colonel Monckton, the combined English troops, encountering very little resistance, captured Fort Beauséjour on 16 June 1755.[51] The New England Provincial Troops, including the six surgeons, remained at Chignecto until early August 1755. On 2 August, Dr Jacob March (who had accompanied a contingent of soldiers to Petitcodiac) was killed,[52] along with twenty-two soldiers, by the French and their Indian allies. Twelve days later, Dr Miles Whitworth left Chignecto with Colonel Winslow for Grand Pré, in order to prepare an evacuation of the Acadians.[53] He appears to have remained at Grand Pré until at least 3 December 1755 and was later paid thirty-seven pounds by the Council of Nova Scotia for fifty days of attendance to the Acadians prior to their departure.[54] Although the Acadians at Grand Pré were notified on 5 September 1755 that they were to be expelled,[55] they did not actually depart until late October.[56] A further 1,664 Acadians from the environs of Annapolis Royal were embarked[57] on 8 December. Records indicate that the only two surgeons available to provide medical attendance for the Acadians in Grand Pré and environs were Doctors Whitworth and de Rodohan.[58]

THE FIRST FLEET OF ROYAL NAVY SHIPS ever to arrive in Halifax dropped anchor during the summer of 1755. This fleet, ordered to intercept all French reinforcements sent to America,[59] had been stricken with illness. So many sailors were incapacitated that the vice-admiral of the fleet, Edward Boscawen, decided to put into Halifax, arriving on 9 July. The sickness could have been the smallpox acquired from French sailors taken prisoner by Boscawen's Fleet. A smallpox epidemic had reportedly broken out in Louisbourg in June 1755.[60] On 12 July, Boscawen wrote[61] that, out of the 6,154 men under his command, 1,624 were sick with "inflamatory fever." Four days later, "Our sick increase dayly. We are now erecting tents and repairing houses for their reception on shore."[62] By September, it was reported[63] that "the people [in Halifax] are very sickly," indicating that the illness brought by the fleet had spread to the local residents. Captain John Rous wrote to Col John Winslow from Halifax[64] that "the Fleet is in high spirits notwithstanding there has been great destruction among them by sickness." The severity of this destruction can be established from the records of the Hospital for Sick and Hurt Seamen, administered by Robert Grant, surgeon. He reports that, between 18 October and 18 November, seventy-six of the 177 who had been captured by Boscawen's Fleet and held in the hospital had died.[65] Although Williams[66] does not mention this outbreak, Figure 6, below, shows that the epidemic did in fact spread to the civilians of Halifax.[67] The average death rate among them, during the six months preceding the arrival of the fleet, was nine per month, whereas the rate increased by a factor of four to thirty-six per month through September, October, and November of 1755. The surgeon William Urquhart died in Halifax in August 1755,[68] possibly from the epidemic.

Two other surgeons are found in the records of Halifax in 1755, John Day and Dr Head. John Day was mentioned briefly in the previous chapter in connection with land allotments. It has not been ascertained whether subsequent references are to the same person, or to two or more persons of the same name who lived in Halifax during the first decade of its settlement. In any case, there is no further mention of the name until 20 October 1755, when a John Day was married at St Paul's to the widow Sarah Mercer. The next mention appears in the report of an autopsy performed by John Day on the body of one Catherine Mackintosh, in Halifax. Day indicates in the autopsy report that he was a surgeon,[69] and on 10 August, Admiral Boscawen appointed him as a surgeon's assistant in Nova Scotia.[70] In the year 1768, John Day was granted[71] two thousand acres of land near Windsor, Hants County, "for service as surgeon in the Naval Hospital."

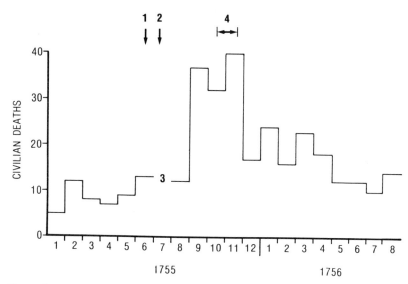

Figure 6
Civilian deaths in Halifax from January 1755 to August 1756. Death totals for each month have been taken from the five sources described in note 67, chapter 2.

1 Smallpox epidemic reported at Louisbourg in June, 1755
2 Arrival of Boscawen's Fleet, 7 July 1755 with prisoners from Louisbourg.
3 No burial records for St Paul's Church for July 1755.
4 Period in which 121 seamen and prisoners died in hospital.

A Dr Head was in Halifax as early as 4 October 1754 and was listed[72] as being of the *Success*, a Royal Navy sloop[73] commanded by Capt. John Rous. It is possible that Dr Head was its surgeon. Apparently, he was resident in Halifax on 30 March 1755, for on that date he was recorded as taking over responsibility for an inmate of the orphan house.[74] It is likely that the Dr Head mentioned in the William Best Account Book was Dr Michael Head, known to have been in Halifax as early as 1759 and to have resided, during the period 1765–1805, in various other towns in Nova Scotia.[75]

After the Acadians had been deported from Nova Scotia in the late fall of 1755, the New England Troops at Grand Pré and Chignecto were transferred to Halifax to provide protection[76] during the winter of 1755–56. Colonel John Winslow arrived with his troops from Grand Pré[77] on 19 November 1755, and Major Jedidiah Prebble brought his men from Chignecto[78] on 9 December 1755. It is likely that John Tyler, Miles Whitworth, Cornelius Nye, Philip Cast, and John Thomas, the surviving surgeons sent with the New England Troops, spent the winter with the men in Halifax. The New

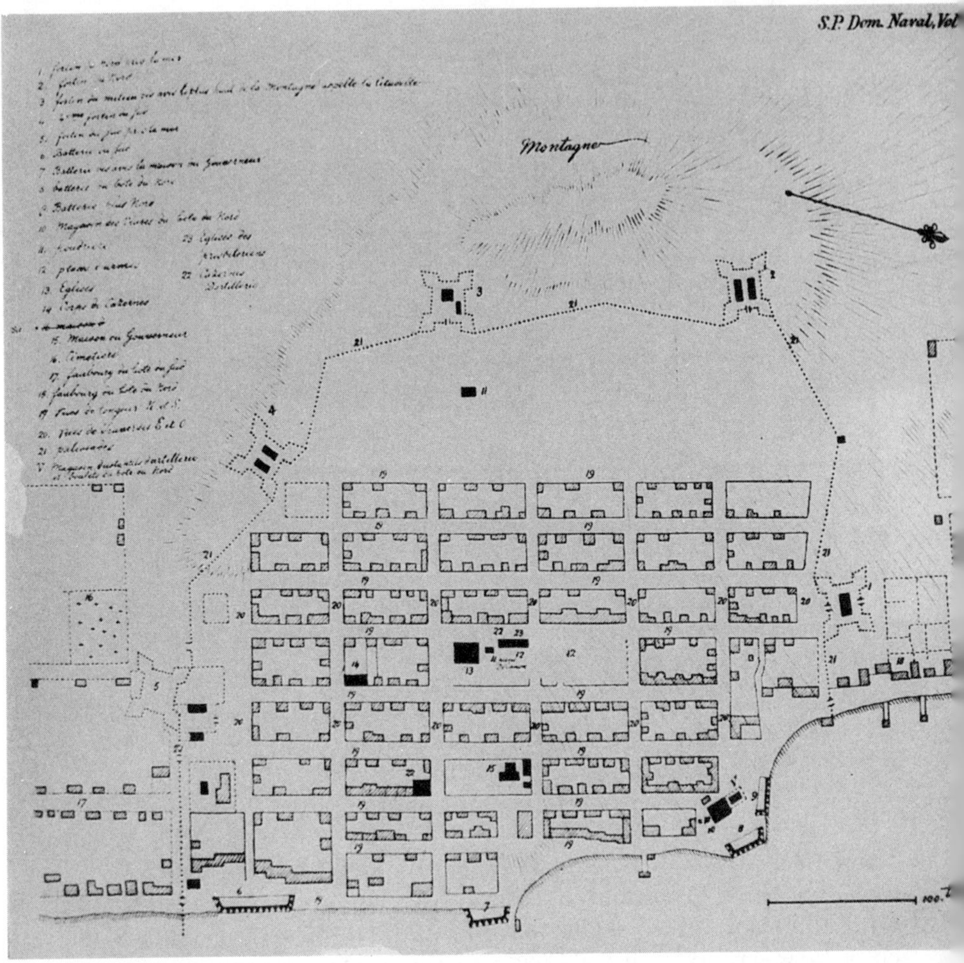

Figure 7
Plan of Halifax showing line of forts, batteries, and all buildings in the town, *circa* June 1755. The story of the acquisition of this plan is given in note 76, chapter 2. (Original in PRO State Papers Domestic, Naval, 1711–1755, vol. 38, folio 224; a reproduction can be found in PANS CO217, 15:256)

England hospital mentioned in William Best's Account Book[79] in February 1756 was probably established for these soldiers and was located in a building on the property of John Solomon whose house was referred to as "the Hospital house."[80]

In March, Governor Shirley of Massachusetts was reported[81] to have hired a number of vessels which "were shortly expected in the Harbour to transport the New England Troops now in the Province to Boston as soon as the term was expired for which they were engaged." Capt. Richard Spry wrote from Halifax that "the Vulture [a sloop], sailed on the 9th April with 12 transports having 900 New England troops on board, which are recalled from this Province."[82] The departure of the New England Provincial Troops from Nova Scotia left the province defended by the regulars of the 40th, 45th, and 47th Regiments, which had been stationed in Nova Scotia since 1750. On 21 June 1756, the army returns[83] gave a total of 2,079 men in the three regiments, with 1,018 rank and file in Halifax and 354 stationed at Chignecto. The remaining soldiers were located at Annapolis Royal (114), Pisiquid (146), Lunenburg (114), Lawrence-town (32), Sackville (31), Dartmouth (45), and George's Island (32). Four military surgeons were in the province: William Skene of the Fortieth at Annapolis Royal; Richard Veale of the 45th at Chignecto; and surgeon and surgeon's mate Arthur Price and John Tyler of the 47th at Halifax.

The sickness that prevailed during the fall of 1755 continued into early 1756. On 18 April of that year, Captain Spry wrote[84] of his seaman, "Numbers of our people are so weak and sickly that they cannot be taken on board" ships on the harbour. There was also a high level of mortality among civilians during the months of January to April 1756, as shown in Figure 6.

In May 1756, Britain declared war on France.[85] By 29 November, the three regiments in Nova Scotia had been increased in strength[86] to a total of 2,702 men. On 4 February 1757, Whitehall wrote to Governor Lawrence that seven regiments, including 5,990 soldiers together with a train of artillery, Ordnance stores, a corps of Engineers, and four companies of Artillery, were to embark from Cork for Halifax at the end of February.[87] These regiments did not sail until 8 May, arriving in Halifax on 9 July.[88] They were carried on forty-five transports and accompanied by a fleet of fifteen ships of war and 7,135 seamen under the command of Admiral Holburne. The hospital ship Alderney sailed as one of this armada of sixty-one vessels. In addition to the more than twelve thousand men brought to Halifax by Holburne, two other smaller bodies of military and naval personnel had arrived in Halifax during the previous two weeks. Sir Charles Hardy had arrived[89] on 30 June with six ships and 951 men, while Lord Loudon arrived from New York on the same day with four regiments totalling about five thousand soldiers.[90] In July 1757, there were in excess of twenty thousand soldiers and seaman in Halifax[91] and a civilian population of about three thousand.

It was probably during late July 1757 that Lieutenant Thomas Davies of the Royal Artillery painted the first view of Halifax. He entitled his painting, "A View of Hallifax [sic] in Nova Scotia taken from Cornwallis [later McNab's] Island with a Squadron going off to Louisbourgh [sic] in the year 1757" (Figure 8). Lieutenant Davies had arrived in Halifax with Admiral Holburne's Fleet on 9 July 1757. Although it is not possible to distinguish in this painting the civilian hospital building (the hospital administered by Dr Abercrombie), it would have been located in one of the large buildings immediately behind the topmast of the vessel in the foreground.

The Hospital for Sick and Hurt Seamen, which, as noted earlier, had been administered by Robert Grant since as early as 1750, was reorganized in 1757, so that:

such sick and wounded seamen as may be set on shore there for cure, will be provided for in much better manner, not only in the articles of Physic and Surgery, but also in that of diet, than can be possibly expected from the method now practiced; for with regard to their cure, we have in our said plan which is herewith enclosed, and which we desire you [the secretary of the Admiralty] to lay before their Lordships, so amply provided for their assistance in that respect, by the proposed number of surgeons [five] and the allowances to be made them, in order to induce fit people to accept those employs, as we hope will not fail of answering the good purposes designed by this alteration: our principal motive for which is, that it cannot reasonably be supposed that in a business so extensive, one man with a few assistants, he may be able to procure in that quarter of the world can be sufficient to properly attend it; and to show their Lordships, we offer this plan to them purely for the good of His Majesty's service, without meaning any reflection upon Mr Grant; we beg leave, if their Lordships should be pleased to suffer it to take place, to recommend him to be Principal Surgeon.

The proposed establishment was to consist of one surgeon at £200 per annum; two assistant surgeons at £150 each; two under assistant surgeons at £80 each; one dispenser at £80; one agent at £200; two clerks to the agent at £50 each; medicines, instruments, "and such necessaries as cannot be well procured at Nova Scotia, to be sent from hence"; five hundred suits of bedding, "and Mr Grant's bed-

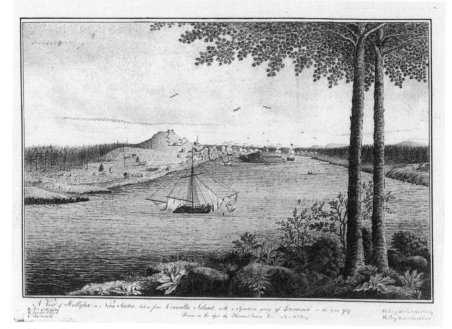

Figure 8
"A View of Hallifax [*sic*] in Nova Scotia from Cornwallis Island, with a Squadron going off to Louisbourgh [*sic*] in the year 1757," by Thomas Davies (1737–1812). Watercolour, pen, and black ink on laid paper. (National Gallery of Canada, No. 6268)

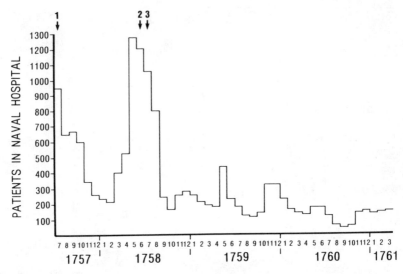

Figure 9
Patients in the naval hospital at Halifax, 1757–61.

1 Arrival of 12,000 soldiers and seamen in Halifax, 9 July, 1757
2 Landing of English troops at Louisbourg, 8 June, 1758
3 Louisbourg surrenders to the English, 26 July, 1758

ding to be taken off his hands at an equitable valuation"; and the houses used by Grant as hospitals, to be hired for the Crown.[92] The location of the houses used by Robert Grant as hospitals is not known. In addition to Grant, surgeon and agent, one of the assistant surgeons is known[93] to have been Godfrey Webb. It is probable that John Baxter was the second assistant surgeon, while the under assistant surgeons could have been John Grant[94] and a Mr McCormick.[95]

On 16 July 1757, Governor Lawrence indicated to Council that "the Earl of Loudon had, this day, represented to him that a fever was beginning to spread amongst the Troops under his Lordships Command, occasioned by the great quantities of rum that are sold to the soldiers by unlicensed retailers, and that ... this if it continues must unavoidably prove of fatal consequences to His Majesty's Service."[96] This was obviously a very contagious fever; it is recorded that in July 1757, up to 949 patients, attended by thirty-two nurses, were victualled in the naval hospital.[97] Figure 9 shows the number of seamen in the naval hospital during the period July 1757 to March 1761. Records of the number in the naval hospital for the months prior to July 1757 have not been found. Robert Grant was dismissed from his position as surgeon and agent at Halifax on 23 September 1757, "for issuing slops to the sick and wounded seamen put under his care." He was replaced on the same day by First Assistant Surgeon Godfrey Webb.[98] It is likely that John Baxter was appointed agent to the Hospital for Sick and Hurt Seamen on or shortly after 23 September;[99] it is recorded that he held that position as early as 28 April 1758.[100]

It is difficult to assess whether the fever among the soldiers and seamen had a significant effect on Lord Loudon and Admiral Holburne's decision, in August 1757, to postpone the invasion of Louisbourg. Their obvious concern over the severity of sickness among their men is indicated in a letter from Holburne to John Cleveland, secretary of the Admiralty. It read, in part, "We had between 900 and 1,000 men put ashore to the Hospital where I must leave 500 sick, besides 200 dead since we sailed."[101] As mentioned earlier, Admiral Holburne had sailed from Spithead on 8 May, approximately three months previously. Almost all of the two hundred deaths are reported to have taken place after Holburne and his men arrived in Halifax on 9 July 1757.[102] Loudon and Holburne had determined, also, that the French at Louisbourg numbered six thousand regular troops, three thousand men resident at Louisbourg, thirteen hundred Indians, and seventeen ships of war.[103] In contrast, the English force at Halifax numbered over twenty thousand soldiers and seamen, with twenty-one ships of war.[104] It would appear that the English had almost twice as many men as the French as well as four more ships of war.

The cancellation of the siege of Louisbourg in 1757 was very unpopular in London and New England. As a letter in *Gentleman's Magazine* put it, "Lord Loudon and Admiral Holburne have been censured for not attempting a descent on Cape Breton."[105] Both Lord Loudon and Admiral Holburne were soon replaced,[106] Loudon after his return from Halifax to New York, and Holburne after his return to England in the fall of 1757.[107]

It is possible, however, that both Loudon and Holburne realized that the fever was so serious among the seamen and troops in Halifax that it would have been unwise to attempt an attack on Louisbourg. Neither Loudon nor Holburne mentions sickness as the main reason for calling off the siege, but it must have been of epidemic proportions. In September 1757, the governor acquainted[108] Council that it was to consider measures that could prevent the spread of the smallpox. Dr Abercrombie reported "that many of the families[109] in the Town were infected and that it would be very difficult to stop [the epidemic]." Further, "The several surgeons should

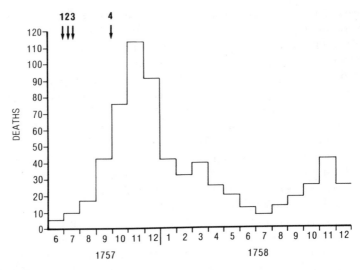

Figure 10
Deaths in Halifax during the period June 1757 to May 1758. The number of
deaths for each month has been taken from the five sources listed in note 67,
chapter 2.

1 Arrival of Lord Loudon's and Sir Charles Hardy's Forces.
2 Arrival of Admiral Holburne's Fleet.
3 Lord Loudon indicates *"fever"* is spreading among the Troops.
4 Dr. Abercrombie indicates smallpox is rampant in the Town.

be desired not to inoculate[110] any person." On 2 August, John Knox,
a military officer in Halifax, wrote,[111] "The Royal [1st] Regiment
with 700 rank and file only have been very sickly," and that "it appears that since this Army last embarked at their respective ports, if
they were then actually complete, have suffered by sickness, etc.,
and perhaps a few deaths, to the amount of 612 men." On 1 September, Knox recorded that "the *Alderney*, the Hospital Ship, one of our
squadron, has landed [at Chignecto] several sick men, and a house is
provided for their reception. Their disorders are spotted fevers and
dysenteries. It is remarkable that 17 men have died on board the
ship in the short passage from Halifax here, which exceeds the number lost by the seven Regiments in their long voyage from Europe."
As was the case in the fall of 1755, the epidemic brought by the fleet
spread to the civilian population. The number of deaths occurring
in Halifax during the fall of 1757 increased rapidly over previous
months (Figure 10). It is clear that the smallpox represented a very
serious epidemic in Halifax during October, November, and December of that year.

J.J. Heagerty, in his writings on the history of medicine in Canada, describes an attempt by the French to introduce smallpox into Halifax in August 1757. Immediately after the French captured Fort William Henry near Lake Champlain, Montcalm is alleged to have ordered that a number of the British prisoners taken at the fort who were ill with smallpox be shipped to Halifax. Heagerty points out that this attempt to transfer the dreaded disease to the enemy backfired, since it is said that all of the prisoners recovered *en route* and than took command of the ship after their French guards contracted smallpox and died almost to a man.

John Grant, mentioned earlier in this chapter in connection with the dispute among surgeons over the administration and operation of the civilian hospital in Halifax, died in September 1757, possibly of the smallpox.[112] He had continued his campaign against what he considered to be the improper operation of the hospital and was one of the committee of freeholders of Halifax who complained in a petition[113] to the Lords of Trade, early in 1757, about Governor Lawrence's inactivity in establishing a House of Representatives, the lack of adequate defences for the town, the use of coercion of get inhabitants to enlist in the various regiments stationed in Halifax, and the use and condition of the hospital.[114]

The Expense of the Government for surgeons and medicines is very great near £1,000 a year besides the great expense of a Hospital such as cooks, nurses, washerwoman, bedding, soap, candles, wood, and provisions that is generally occupied by the soldiers of Hopson's Regiment and a few miscreants of the Town for no sober industrous people will go there for a "cure" to live among soldiers in the greatest riot and confusion as the people who go into this Hospital are of the vilent [*sic*] sort. How much better it would be to have them in a workhouse with a resident apothecary of £20 per annum to exhibit medicines which could be prescribed by the practising surgeons of the Town which they would most readily attend to monthly gratis and as to what may be alleged with respect to the industrous poor being assisted by the means of those surgeons now in Pay. The contrary is pretty well known and that they spend most of their time in attending upon the Governor and place men, with favorite Officers and their families, and leave the poor inhabitants to the mercy of such, as may from necessity be obliged to attend them.

Upon his departure, Lord Loudon left the three regiments formerly in the province (Hopson's 40th, Warburton's 45th, and Lascelles' 47th) and three other regiments (the Royals, or 1st; Bragg's 28th; and Kennedy's 43rd) in Nova Scotia. Colonel Bragg's 28th Regiment was posted to Fort Cumberland, formerly Fort Beauséjour; Colonel Kennedy's 43rd was posted to Annapolis Royal and Pisiquid; and the Royals [the 1st Regiment], was stationed at Halifax for the winter.[115] In addition, Admiral Holburne left eight ships to winter in Halifax for the colony's protection,[116] and Admiral Colville was placed in command at Halifax, in the winter of 1757–58.[117]

During that winter, plans were made in London to send a large military and naval force to Halifax to prepare for an attack on Louisbourg during the late spring or early summer of 1758. The first segment to arrive in Halifax was that of Sir Charles Hardy, who had returned to England from Halifax in September 1757, after the cancellation of the siege of Louisbourg.[118] Now, his six ships of war were anchored in Halifax harbour on 19 March 1758. Hardy wrote to the Secretary of the Admiralty on 22 March: "The *Borias* [a frigate] which arrived here before me brought in a very sickly ships Company."[119] Although the smallpox epidemic of late 1757 had declined significantly in early 1758 (Figure 10) there were still 322 sick seamen in the naval hospital and 171 sick on board the ten ships of war in the harbour on 22 March 1758, representing 13.6 percent of the seamen in Halifax. The report[120] of the state and condition of His Majesty's ten ships in Halifax indicated that 201 seamen belonging to these ships had died since 18 October 1757.

Admiral Boscawen, who had been appointed the naval commander for the forthcoming siege of Louisbourg, arrived[121] in Halifax with twelve ships of war on 8 May 1758. This brought to twenty-two the number of warships in Halifax harbour, manned by a total of 9,525 seamen, of whom 1,070 (11.2 percent) were sick.[122] Boscawen brought not only seamen but also more sickness. Two of his ships, the *Devonshire* and the *Pembroke*, were ultimately left in Halifax during the siege of Louisbourg: "I leave [them] here being sickly."[123]

Major General Jeffery Amherst sailed[124] into Halifax harbour on 28 May on the *Dublin* and transferred immediately to Boscawen's flagship *Namur*, the largest of the twenty-three ships of war. Amherst wrote in his journal that "the *Dublin* went very sickly into Halifax." His brother, Col William Amherst, wrote[125] from Halifax on 28 May, "We went on board the *Namur*, Admiral Boscawen, leaving the *Dublin* to go into the Harbour to water and put her sick on shore, having near two hundred [sick], fourteen died on the voyage."

General Jeffery Amherst was appointed the military commander for the siege of Louisbourg and was to have thirteen regiments,[126] a company of Rangers, a train of Artillery, and a corps of Engineers, totalling 13,463 personnel, under his command. Boscawen and Amherst sailed from Halifax on 29 May for Louisbourg with an armada of 157 sail,[127] transporting 14,215 soldiers and approximately 8,000 seamen, or a combined force of 22,215 men. Halifax was left to be defended by two regiments, the thirty-fifth and the forty-third, consisting of 1,589 army personnel. Many of the soldiers remaining in Halifax were ill, however, and Lieutenant Governor Monckton informed[128] Council, on 2 June 1758, "that the Town was at present, but in a weak state of defence on account of the small number of troops left here, and many of them sick."

John Knox wrote in his journal on 28 May that "the barracks evacuated by the 45th Regiment [is] being prepared as a hospital for the reception of the sick that are unable to proceed on the expedition, every Corps is forthwith to send their sick to that Hospital where the Deputy Director wil receive them."[129] This hospital was probably the realization of the general hospital that Lord Loudon had intended to establish in 1757[130] and was, by November 1758, under the directorship of William Adair, Esquire.[131] It was located on the south side of Blowers Street and opposite the entrance to Argyle Street.[132] This meant that in June 1758, there were at least three hospitals in Halifax: the naval hospital, probably located on Granville Street (since the construction of the King's Naval Yard was not started until the spring of 1759[133]) and administered by Agent John Baxter, with Godfrey Webb as surgeon;[134] the general military hospital, located on Blowers Street and directed by William Adair, surgeon; and the hospital for civilians built in 1750 and administered until October 1750 by Matthew Jones, who was then succeeded by Alexander Abercrombie.

The sickness brought to Halifax by army and navy personnel in May 1758 seems not to have spread to the civilian population as it did in 1757. This can be seen by comparing the number of deaths in Halifax during each month following May 1758 (Figure 10) with the number of deaths during the months following the arrival of Lord Loudon in June 1757. There is no evidence in the primary-source material to suggest that the sickness among the armed forces in Halifax in 1758 was smallpox. It could have been what was frequently referred to during the eighteenth century as "intermittent fever," scurvy, or a combination of these.[135]

Shortly after the English force arrived at Louisbourg on 2 June 1758, it was discovered that smallpox had broken out among the troops. Nathaniel Knap, a carpenter from New England who was a member of the attacking force, wrote[136] on 17 June 1758, "Some of our people was took sick" and, on 18 June, "Building a house for our sick to live in." Between 19 and 30 June, Knap himself was ill with smallpox but recovered and continued building the hospital for

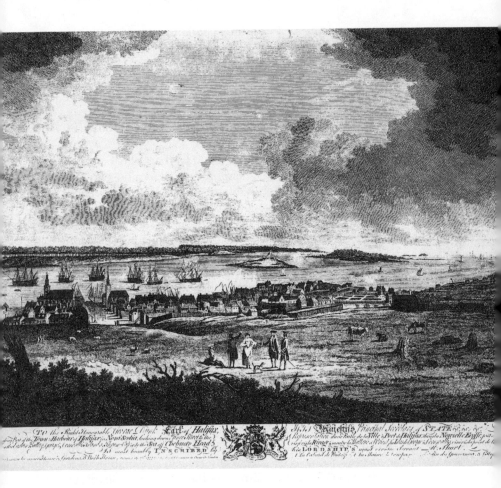

Figure 11
"Part of the Town and harbour of Halifax in Nova Scotia looking down George Street to the opposite shore called Dartmouth," drawn by Richard Short. One of six engravings of different views of Halifax done by Short. See note 133, chapter 2. (Art Gallery of Nova Scotia)

the English troops at Louisbourg. General Amherst wrote[137] on 23 June, "Colonel Messervy and most of his carpenters [have] taken ill of the smallpox." On 28 June, "Col. Messervy and his son both died this day, and of his Company of carpenters of 108 men, all but 16 in the smallpox."

The smallpox was obviously rampant among the French as well, as Boscawen pointed out in a letter on 13 September: "I have sent all the recover'd French soldiers and sailors from the French Hospitals strictly to France as they have an epidemical disorder amongst them which I am afraid will break out again in their passage to Europe. They have buried many since the surrender of the Town."[138] This epidemical fever and other disorders ensured that much sickness was brought to Halifax by the English soldiers returned there. On 2 November, Governor Lawrence wrote[139] to William Adair, director of the general military hospital in Halifax, that he had received a memorial from Colonels Murray, Howe, and Young, of the 15th, 58th, and 60th regiments, indicating that:

the respective corps under their command are, from the fatigues of the compaign, now labouring in extraordinary numbers under epidemical fevers and fluxes and that it is impossible with the Regimental Surgeons and their allowances, to provide for and assist the ailing men ... They have asked that I would order you to establish such a General Hospital as may be sufficient for the relief of those thought fit to direct and you are hereby required and directed to give such assistance to the Regimental Hospitals before your departure from hence as to you shall appear necessary and expedient, and you are to take special care that the same be done with the utmost frugality and oeconomy, and to leave directions with the Principal Surgeon that he make report in writing to me or the Commander-in-Chief when ever the same may, in his opinion, be discontinued with safety to His Majesty's Service.

The year 1758 ended with two noteworthy incidents in Halifax. On 9 December, John Day, mentioned earlier in this chapter, entered an advertisement for drugs and medicines in the *Halifax Gazette*. This is the first advertisement for drugs, and Day's store on Hollis Street could be considered the first drugstore established in Halifax. The second incident was the submission of a petition by Ann Catherwood, the midwife, on 18 December 1758 asking for leave of absence because of ill health.[140] She was granted leave and received a certificate for her "excellent services as Provincial Midwife."[141] Mrs Catherwood was absent for at least the next two or three years. Chief Justice Belcher, appointed[142] early in 1761 to administer the province after Charles Lawrence died[143] in October 1760, reported[144] to the Lords of Trade that "the allowance for midwifery by the absence of Mrs Catherwood beyond the time of her licence being in the disposition of the Government and one person not being sufficient for the duty, I have appointed two persons at the same salary to be divided between them and the rather as one of them Mrs Triggs[145] from her long residence here and skill, fidelity, and charity to the poorer settlers deserved this consideration for her services."

THE NEXT YEAR opened with an announcement[146] by the Lords of Trade to Governor Lawrence that they were omitting the item in the 1759 estimate[147] which listed the projected expenses of the hospital. This reduction was "expressly ordered by His Majesty [George II] to be defrayed by the Commander-in-Chief of the Military and should not therefore be inserted in your estimate." The hospital in question was the civilian hospital established in 1750 and administered by Alexander Abercrombie. As noted in Figure 12, the grant from Whitehall to administer the province of Nova Scotia had decreased from £58,559 in 1753 to £16,753 in 1758, a reduction of 71.4 percent. Their objective, of course, was to reduce the yearly grant to zero and eventually have the province self-supporting. They were also aware, probably, that in 1754, the expenses related to health care in Nova Scotia were only 2.5 percent of the total grant, whereas in 1758, medical expenses had risen to 8.8 percent. The Lords of Trade most likely felt that civilians could be cared for at the many government-supported military and naval hospitals existing in Halifax in 1759. Governor Lawrence was concerned that, if the administration and expenses of the hospital in question were put in the hands of the military, the hospital would disappear after the military left Halifax. This may be why he again included the hospital expenses in the estimates[148] for 1760. Lawrence reminded the Lords of Trade that the hospital had been established for civilians:

The article of the Expenses of the Hospital was inserted in a List of particulars ordered in the year 1757, to be thence forward paid out of the military contingent money, but being at the same time continued amongst the articles for which the Grant for the Colony for 1758 was made it was accordingly paid out of that fund and the Establishment thereof having from the commencement of the settlement been wholly for the benefit of the necessitous Inhabitants exclusive of any of the troops (who have all along had their several Hospitals). It was presumed that it had been designed to be

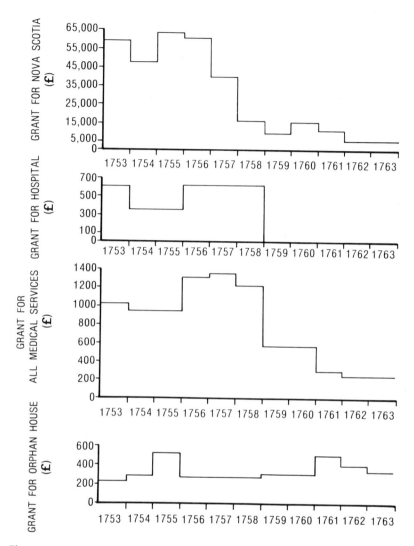

Figure 12
Annual grant (in British pounds) from Whitehall for the province of Nova Scotia
and for the civilian hospital, the orphan house, and all medical services,
1753–63. Information obtained from sources listed in note 146, chapter 2.

continued in the List of the Colony expenses, and was accordingly inserted
in the estimate of the year 1759 of which their Lordships of the Board of
Trade having disapproved and not inserted in that years Grant it would not
have been again inserted in this Estimate but that if the Expenses of it
should not be thought proper to be allowed out of the Military Fund for the

reasons before mentioned, and no provision for it should be made in the Colony Grant, the loss of it would be very distressing. It is therefore again here stated and humbly submitted to their Lordships consideration.

The Lords of Trade responded[149] that "we must now however omit this opportunity of acquainting you that it is not in our power to admit the expenses of the Hospital being put upon the civil establishment. His Majesty having given special directions that it should be considered and defrayed as a military contingent service, and therefore the expense of it must be demanded of the Commander-in-Chief." As shown in Figure 12 the civilian hospital did not receive further yearly grants. In November 1767, Hibbert Newton and others, overseers of the poor, were empowered to use the hospital as an alms house.[150]

The decision by George II to discontinue funding for the civilian hospital is not at all surprising, given that it had never been the policy of the British government to support hospitals. As noted in the Introduction, hospitals that were founded in the eighteenth century usually owed their existence to wealthy manufacturers and merchants rather than to the landed rich or to government. In Halifax, the decline and eventual closing of the civilian hospital does not appear to have been opposed in any way by the few wealthy merchants in the town.

Although the soldiers and seamen had brought so much sickness to Halifax from 1755–58, and the Lords of Trade would not change their policy to allow the civilian hospital to continue as such, Lawrence was convinced that the presence of the army and navy had a positive effect on the continued existence of Halifax. In an address[151] to the House of Assembly in December 1759, he said, "Had it not been for the annual sums graciously granted and the money circulating amongst us from Fleets and Armys, this Town and its environs so much improved, must have sunk in misery."

THE MILITARY AND NAVY were still very numerous in the province in 1759. On 17 March, Admiral Phillip Durell, Commander-in-Chief of the Fleet in America during the winter of 1758–59, reported[152] that he had twelve ships in Halifax carrying a total of 5,419 seamen. Only 271 (or five percent) of these men were sick on that date, with 157 in the hospital on shore and the remaining 114 on their respective ships in the harbour. He lists three ships under his command as being berthed at Louisbourg and manned by 1,148 seamen.

Admiral Charles Saunders, who had arrived in Halifax on 1 May 1759, wrote[153] to the Secretary of the Admiralty on 6 June that he had left Halifax with twelve ships for Louisbourg on 12 May and then left Louisbourg on 4 June for the St Lawrence River with a total of twenty-two ships and 119 other sailing vessels. Saunders lamented the fact that there were so many French prisoners and inhabitants in the hospitals at Louisbourg that there was little room for those of his own men who were sick.

One of the hospitals mentioned in Admiral Saunders's letter was the Grand Battery Hospital.[154] A second hospital known to have been extant at Louisbourg in 1759 was constructed by order of General Jeffery Amherst[155] and referred to by Nathaniel Knap, one of the carpenters who carried out the construction of the hospital during the summer and fall of 1758.[156] The latter hospital was still being maintained by the English in February 1759, when a great quantity of medicines was prepared, presumably in England, for use in the hospitals at Halifax and Louisbourg.[157]

With the fall of Quebec on 18 September 1759, Admiral Saunders returned to England and left Admiral Colville with a strong squadron at Halifax for the winter. On 7 November, Colville reported[158] that he had eight ships and a total of 2,399 men under his command, 320 of whom (13.3 percent) were sick. This force remained in Halifax until 22 April 1760, when Colville sailed for the St Lawrence.[159] In December 1759, the naval hospital at Halifax was reported[160] to have as patients a total of 231 seamen and sixty marines.

On 28 June 1759, Council considered[161] the memorial of Mr John Phillipps, surgeon, to the effect that, since Johann B. Erad's death in March 1757, Phillipps had filled the office of surgeon at Lunenburg and had also acted as man-midwife. He asked to be paid for his services. Council noted that Dr Phillipps had performed the services of a surgeon at Lunenburg from March 1757 to August 1759, for which Dr Leonard Lockman, who was absent from Lunenburg during the period, had been paid. Dr Lockman explained to Council that he had left Lunenburg in March 1757 for health reasons and had resided in Halifax at the time in question. Council decided to cease paying Lockman and installed John Phillipps as surgeon at Lunenburg at a pay of three shillings per day, and also awarded Phillipps £150 for his past services. The only mention[162] of a hospital at Lunenburg during its first decade of its existence was in May 1759, in a return of births and cradles at the settlements, which contains the information: "14 births in the Hospital which has 5 cradles."

The year 1760 saw the arrival of the first settlers belonging to the fourth major group[163] of immigrants to settler in Nova Scotia since 1749. As early as 1754, Governor Shirley had indicated[164] that "a considerable number of people from New England [would] settle [there]," assuming that the French and Indians would be forced from the province. No serious attempt was made to settle New Englanders on the lands vacated by the Acadians or elsewhere in the province until after the capture of Louisbourg, which took place on 26 July 1758.

On 12 October 1758, Lawrence issued a proclamation[165] related to the settling of the vacant lands. The proclamation was revised[166] on 11 January 1759 to conform to concerns raised by the Lords of Trade, to whom Lawrence wrote[167] in December 1758 that he had been informed that hundreds of families in the colonies of Connecticut, Rhode Island, and Massachusetts were preparing to take up land in Nova Scotia. Their reasons for leaving New England were the excellent fertility of the land in Nova Scotia and the burdensome taxation and growing population in the colonies.

In May 1759, the first land grants were made, in the recently established township of Horton,[168] to 197 persons from Connecticut. Lawrence estimated[169] that the thirteen townships surveyed in Nova Scotia would be populated by 650 families (3,250 persons) in 1760; 1300 families (6,000 persons) in 1761; and 600 families (3,000 persons) in 1762. On 11 May 1760, Lawrence wrote[170] that fifty families had arrived in Liverpool, and forty had arrived at Minas and Piziquid. On 16 June, he wrote[171] that there were seventy families at Liverpool and families arriving in Horton, Cornwallis, and Falmouth. On 12 December, Jonathan Belcher, who was administering the government after Lawrence's death in October, sent a record[172] of the state of the new settlements in Nova Scotia, which indicated that the New England settlers who had arrived in eight townships totalled approximately 520 families, comprising some 1,900 persons.

Whereas thirty-six surgeons, mates, and apothecaries, had accompanied the Cornwallis settlers, and thirteen surgeons had arrived with the foreign Protestants, only four persons referred to as doctor and physician (rather that surgeon) were with the New England settlers. Two of these, Samuel Willoughby of Cornwallis Township and Jonathan Woodbury of Yarmouth, later of Granville and Wilmot, continued for many years to practise in the province.[173] Richard Sears, referred to as a physician, came to Horton probably in 1760 and died there in June 1762.[174] The fourth doctor, Samuel Oats, was listed as such in a return of the inhabitants and stock in in the township of Yarmouth at Cape Forchu on 21 June 1762.[175] He was still in Yarmouth Township on 18 October 1762,[176] but his where-abouts after that date are uncertain.[177] Other settlers said to have given medical aid to the New Englanders were Benoni Sweet[178] in Falmouth, and Mrs Elizabeth Doane[179] in Barrington. Mrs Doane was referred to as an "expert midwife ... incomparably well skild [sic] in fisick [sic] and surgery."

In December 1759, the Council prepared a bill[180] entitled an Act to Prevent the spreading of Contagious Distempers, which was then submitted for consideration by the House of Assembly. Surprisingly, as Jonathan Belcher, president of the Council, reported[181] to the Lords of Trade, the House of Assembly rejected the bill. However, in the same month a vessel arrived in Halifax from Louisbourg and landed some people with smallpox. Council reacted by adopting a resolution that all vessels coming into Halifax harbour must be stopped at George's Island.[182] Council sent to the House a new bill concerning contagious diseases, a revision of the former one composed after examination of similar bills that had been enacted in other colonies.[183] It received first reading on 25 July 1761.[184]

There appears to have been, in August 1760, a significant number of sick patients in the Louisbourg hospital. John Baxter, who had reported[185] the state of the Halifax hospital in April 1760, was listed as surgeon at the Louisbourg hospital in August of that year and reported that he had 398 patients sick with fevers, fluxes, and the scurvy.[186] At the same time, there were about 150 patients at the naval hospital in Halifax, where Lord Colville had been ordered to winter with ten ships of war.[187] In April 1761, Lord Colville wrote[188] to the secretary of the Admiralty that he had now spent three winters in Halifax and that "scurvy never fails to pull us down in great numbers, upon our going to sea in the spring." Sickness does not appear, however, to have been too severe during the winter of 1760–61, for on 6 April 1761, Colville reported[189] having 3,563 seamen under his command at Halifax (twelve ships of war), of whom only 161 (4.5 percent) were sick.

The effective demise of the civilian hospital took place in 1761, while the orphan house was reorganized at the request of the Lords of Trade. They instructed[190] Jonathan Belcher that "the salary for a surgeon[191] at Halifax and the allowance for medicine money should cease immediately, as well as the pay of the coroner and his Juries." They continued:

The only article of the estimate [referring to the estimate for 1761] which we have anything to observe is the Orphan House, not that we object to the Establishment itself, but merely to what we think is an abuse of it. It is stated in Gov[r] Lawrence's Account of the conduct of this charity that the children of the poorer sort of people, tho' not orphans, have frequently been admitted by which means a new object is introduced, the expense of the public augmented, and the plan of the charity enlarged, which was meant, in its institution, simply to afford relief to those who by death of their parents would not probably be provided for by others and who were incapable of providing for themselves. We think likewise that a considerable reduction might be made in the salary of the person to whom the inspection of the children is committed, three pence a day for each child appearing to us as a very reasonable demand, especially as there is an additional charge for an allowance to two assistants, by which means the supertending [sic] these children is become a heavier article or expense than the providing for them their labor likewise.

Belcher replied,[192] "Two hundred and seventy-five children, mostly orphans, have been graciously relieved in the course of nine years by this Royal Charity, who might otherwise have perished or been useless to the public ... The last years expense my Lords for the support of 32 children amounted as by the presentation to your Lordships to the sum of £713 exceeding the grant of £580 estimate." Belcher concludes by suggesting that an allowance for twenty-five orphans would answer the purpose of the charity. Figure 13 indicates the number of orphans cared for in the orphan house from its opening in 1752 to the end of 1762,[193] and shows that Belcher was successful in limiting the number of orphans to twenty-five.

More New Englanders emigrated to Nova Scotia in 1761 to the townships mentioned previously, as well as to those of Onslow, Truro, Cumberland, Annapolis, Barrington, Newport, and Yarmouth. The location and size of each of these townships is shown very clearly in a map[194] which depicts the various land grants awarded Colonel Alexander McNutt,[195] who had a grandiose plan to bring to Nova Scotia ten thousand settlers from Northern Ireland.[196] The first contingent of McNutt settlers, about three hundred, arrived in Halifax in October 1761.[197] These settlers were to be transferred to the lands "around Cobequid and the River Chubenacadie [sic]" in the spring of 1762, after spending the winter in Halifax. In addition to the three hundred McNutt settlers, 445 Acadians,[198] 1,617 seamen,[199] and an undetermined number of soldiers[200] wintered in Halifax with the approximately 2,500 civilian residents.[201]

On 9 January 1762, Halifax was described as having seven hundred houses.[202] Considering that John Kingslaugh had reported[203] to the Lords of Trade in December 1749 (o.s.) that Halifax had

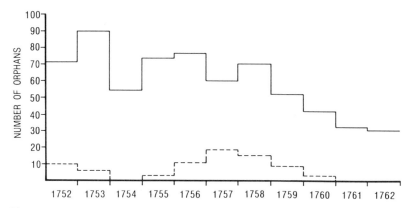

Total Number of Orphans : 243
Deaths in Orphan House : 74
Per Cent Mortality : 30.4 %

——————— NUMBER OF ORPHANS
- - - - - DEATHS OF ORPHANS

Figure 13
Number of children in the orphan house at Halifax, 1752–62, and the yearly
mortality.

seven hundred houses, one might conclude that in the intervening
twelve years, very few new residential houses were built in the town.
This reflects a stagnant civilian population after the departure of the
Lunenburg settlers and during the period 1755 to 1761, when great
numbers of military and naval personnel, in addition to those stationed there, were passing through Halifax.

The names of the other settlements in the province, the number
of families and inhabitants in each, and the names of the doctors of
physic, surgeons, and apothecaries providing medical service in each
settlement is given in Table 3.

THE TOTAL NUMBER OF DOCTORS of physic, surgeons, and apothecaries in Nova Scotia in January 1762 was thirty-one, including the
thirty noted above and Richard Veale, surgeon of Warburton's
Forty-fifth Regiment, by that date stationed at Louisbourg.[205]

By July 1762, Yarmouth had an additional 153 inhabitants,[206]
bringing its population to 253, and Barrington and the district between Yarmouth and Barrington had, by the date, a total of 248 inhabitants. In November 1762, Colonel Alexander McNutt brought
his second group of settlers from Northern Ireland. It numbered
170 persons destined for the township of New Dublin.[207] The total

Table 3
Number of Families and Inhabitants in Nova Scotian Settlements, and Medical
Practitioners Serving Them, 1755–61

Settlement	Families	Inhabitants	Medical Personnel
Halifax	700	2,500	Total of 19[204]
Chester	30	150	
Lunenburg	300	1,400	John Phillipps and Johann Carl Deglen
Liverpool	90	504	
Barrington	20	180	Mrs Elizabeth Doane
Yarmouth	20	100	Jonathan Woodbury and Samuel Oats
Granville	30	140	
Annapolis	60	240	Ebenezer Hartshorn and John Steele
Cornwallis	115	600	Samuel Willoughby
Horton	150	900	Richard Sears
Falmouth	80	350	Benoni Sweet
Newport	60	240	Edward Ellis
Onslow	50	160	
Truro	53	120	
Cumberland	35	100	
Totals	1,793	7,684	

Source: "Description of the State of Nova Scotia, 9 January 1762," PANS CO217, 18:245.

population of Nova Scotia was, by August, about 12,000, including 1,200 men in the army and navy;[208] about 1,200 Acadians, and about 1,500 Indians.[209]

Figure 14 shows the number of civilian and military surgeons in Nova Scotia during the period 1753–63. The number of civilian surgeons remained almost constant at about twenty-three during that eleven-year period. Military surgeons dominated the decade, however, with a total of ninety-three surgeons (thirty-nine naval, fifty-four military) arriving in and departing from Halifax.[210] They represented approximately seventy percent of the surgeons in Nova Scotia during the decade. Halifax was, as the Reverend John Breynton put it,[211] a "rendezvous of Fleets and Armies" during the previous decade.

A recommendation made by Dr Alexander Abercrombie to Council in September 1757 that surgeons in the town of Halifax not be allowed to inoculate is, as far as I could find, the first mention of the procedure in primary-source material related to Nova Scotia. In his letter, Dr Abercrombie stated, "The several surgeons should be de-

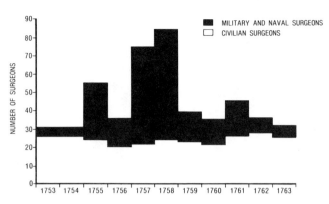

Figure 14
Civilian, naval, and military surgeons in Nova Scotia, 1753–63.

Total number of surgeons in Halifax during period: 132
Number of surgeons who departed from Halifax during period: 90
Number of surgeons who died in Halifax during period: 10

sired not to inoculate," presumably because of his fear that the inoculation had, and would continue to, spread the contagious disease. It
is likely, however, that inoculation was practised in Halifax from the
very beginning of the settlement. In an advertisement placed in the
Nova Scotia Gazette and Weekly Advertiser of 10 April 1787, Christopher Nicolai, surgeon and man-midwife who had come to Halifax in
1751, stated that he had been inoculating for smallpox for over
thirty years. Barbare Tunis, in her article[212] on Dr James Latham,
describes him as the "Pioneer Inoculator in Canada," having been
recorded as carrying out the procedure at Quebec and at Montreal
as early as 1768. It is likely that surgeons in Nova Scotia were carrying out the preventative measure of inoculation a decade earlier,
and might thereby have saved some lives during the two major epidemics of smallpox that were brought to Halifax by the army and
navy, as described in this chapter.

THE NEXT CHAPTER turns from a military to a civilian focus, concen-
trating on factors affecting the health care of Nova Scotians, particularly the numerous poor who sought refuge in the colony, and the
often uneasy attempts to accommodate both the needs of the poor
and the need for adequate medical services.

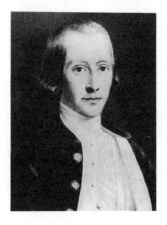

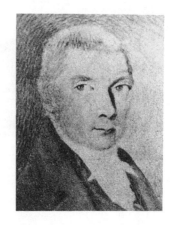

Dr William Paine (1750–1833) arrived in Halifax in October 1782 to take charge of military hospitals and remained in Halifax until 1784. He was a licentiate of the Royal College of Physicians. He eventually returned to Worcester, Massachusetts.
Pastel, artist unknown. (American Antiquarian Society, Worcester, Massachusetts)

Dr Stephen Thomas (n.d.) came to Liverpool, Nova Scotia, in 1782 with the King's Orange Rangers, and remained there until March 1784, when he returned to England to further his studies. Upon his return in 1785 he moved to Grand Manan Island.
Oil on canvas, artist unknown. (New Brunswick Museum)

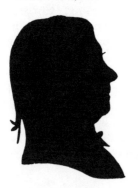
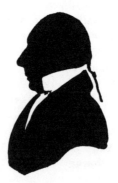
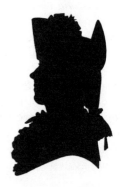

Dr John Calef   Dr Frederick L. Bohme   Dr Alexander Gordon

Dr John Calef (1726–1812) served at the Siege of Louisbourg in 1745. He commanded the Fort at Annapolis Royal during 1778–79 and died at St Andrews, New Brunswick, in 1812. Silhouette by an unknown artist. Dr Frederick Ludovic Bohme (ca.1751–1831) came to the Clements area in 1783 after serving with the Waldeck Regiment in the American war. He practised in Clements Township until he died in 1831. Silhouette by an unknown artist. Dr Alexander Gordon (ca.1753–1803) arrived in Halifax in 1783 with the 42nd Regiment. He later served in Sydney and Charlottetown before returning to Halifax in 1800. He died at sea. Silhouette by unknown artist.

CHAPTER THREE

Poor Relief Takes Precedence over Health Care, 1763–1775

The Treaty of Paris, which Great Britain and France signed on 10 February 1763, ended the Seven Years' War and diminished the importance of Halifax as a military and naval base for the next twelve years. The departure from Halifax of military and naval forces began immediately after the capture of Louisbourg in June 1758, and gradually, the number of soldiers and seamen in the town dwindled from approximately 22,000 in May 1758[1] to about 2,200 by August 1762.[2] Two consequences of the transition from military and naval base to civilian town were a dramatic lessening in the demand for goods and services in Halifax and the emergence of unemployment. A third consequence was the appearance of destitute and helpless people, mostly women, whom Chief Justice Jonathan Belcher described[3] in 1761 as "the great Concourse of dissolute abandoned Women, followers of the Camp, Army, and Navy." It is probably not well known that the regiments sent to Halifax during the middle years of the eighteenth century were accompanied by a surprisingly large number of women and children. For instance, Col Peregrine Lascelle's 47th Regiment is said[4] to have included, in addition to 290 soldiers, 130 women and fifty children. Almost twenty years later, in January 1769, Rev. John Breynton pointed out[5] that 750 soldiers of the 14th and 29th regiments were stationed in the town along with a total of 475 "women and children of the Army." A most revealing letter[6] on this subject was written by Governor William Campbell to Lt Col James Bruce, officer commanding the forces in Nova Scotia. He complained to Bruce that a number of idle, helpless, and indigent women had been left in Halifax by departing regiments and that these women now represented a heavy burden on the inhabitants of the town, who had to pay for their support and maintenance. Governor Campbell requested that Bruce order all regiments to take their women with them at the time of departure.

Although settlers during the first three years of Halifax's history were victualled, that is, provided with food and services, for approximately one year after their arrival,[7] almost from the beginning there were persons referred to as idle, helpless, and poor. Given that 420 servants[8] arrived in Chebucto with the Cornwallis settlers in late June 1749, it is clear that the problem of the poor was imminent. One of the first mentions of assistance to the poor in Halifax appears in the minutes of Council, 24 February 1749/50, where it is reported[9] that Isaac Smith was fined five pounds and that the money was to be "for the use of the poor." In October 1750 (o.s.), two months after the arrival of Lascelles's Regiment, Council decreed[10] "that every person who shall have a licence given to him to keep a public house shall ... pay each six pounds per annum to the use of the poor of the settlement." Two days later, Council decided[11] that "the penalty on all persons convicted before the Governor and Council of retailing spirituous Liquour without Licence ... [is to] pay ten pounds [for each offence] ... one-half to the Poor of the settlement."

By December 1752, three regiments of soldiers were stationed in Halifax while less than half of the civilian population was still victualled at government expense. The growing numbers of "camp followers" and poor prompted the Reverend John Breynton to preach a charity sermon at St Paul's "for the benefit of the Poor and distressed in this place. Tis hop'd all charitable dispos'd persons will favour and contribute towards a design so laudable."[12] That the problem must have been serious is evident from a memorial presented to Council[13] by the justices of the peace of Halifax, in which the idea of establishing a workhouse was raised for the first time:

As there are many idle and disorderly persons within the Town of Halifax, who have no visible means of support themselves and are daily, through idleness and a Vagabond way of Life committing Thefts and Petty Larceny, whereby to subsist themselves, and as there are also many disorderly servants who by means of the abovesaid people are enticed to defraud and pilfer from their master, and absent themselves without leave from their service and there is no other Punishment provided without sending them to Prison, where they remain useless and Idle, and are a charge to the Government, and uncapable of paying any charges of Prosecution, or where they are servants are a charge to their Masters who suffer also by the loss of their time, The Justices whould [sic] humbly represent to your Excellency and this Honourable Council, that they apprehend if a Bridewell or Workhouse

were erected, to which such offenders might be committed and there employed in hard labour, and also be subject to such Punishment as your Excellency and Honours shall think reasonable ... Such people do ... pay for
their subsistance ... by picking of oakum, and making Netts for the Fishery.

It was resolved that the Justices should be directed to look out for a
proper place for the same [a workhouse] to be erected upon, and to form a
Plan for the Building for that purpose and to make an Estimate of the Expense of Building and inclosing the same, and they make a Report thereon
as soon as possible, and of such rules and regulations for the Government of
the same as they think necessary.

The *Halifax Gazette* of 23 December 1752 communicated this plan to
the citizens of Halifax. "We are credibly informed that a House of
Correction is thought of being built forthwith for the suppressing of
Petty Larcenies, and other Evils that daily happen through the Idleness of several persons of both sexes, who refuse to labour at their
proper callings for reasonable Prices."

Nothing appears to have been done immediately in response to
the memorial, since on 26 March 1753, Council decided[14] "that until
the House of Correction shall be erected to receive such corporal
punishment as aforesaid [disorderly people] be committed to His
Majesty's Gaol in Halifax." The estimate[15] for supporting the "civil
establishment" of Nova Scotia, sent to the Lords of Trade in October
1753, indicated that a workhouse was one of the buildings to be constructed in Halifax during 1754. It was to be a log structure, forty
feet by thirty feet, located in an acre of ground surrounded by a
high picket fence. There was also to be a building for the keeper as
well as a kitchen and a brewhouse. In the description of the
masonry, it was stated that the "stone work for the under-pinning
and Black Hole and digging the Foundation [would cost] £22 and
18 shillings." The total cost of the workhouse was estimated at £295,
thirteen shillings, four pence.

The Lords of Trade disallowed[16] the costs for the workhouse as
set forth in the estimate, so Council decided to appropriate an existing building as a temporary house of correction. On 27 June 1754,
Council passed[17] an Act for Establishing a House of Correction or
Workhouse in Halifax. It recommended that the stone house located on Hospital Street should be used and that Richard Wenman
should be appointed as keeper. One month after the grant for building the workhouse had been disallowed, Col Charles Lawrence reiterated to the Lords of Trade the necessity of having such a facility.[18]
He reminded them that Halifax, as a new settlement, seemed to act
as a magnet to a great number of dissolute people.

It appears that Richard Wenman kept the workhouse in the stone house on Hospital Street during the latter part of the 1750s, receiving twenty pounds in September 1756 for his services.[19] The building was found, however, to be too small for the number of inmates. In June 1758, Lawrence laid before Council a proposal[20] for building a larger workhouse, a description of which had been submitted by Josiah Marshall:

Dimensions and manner of Building a Workhouse, vizt, 50 feet long, 20 feet wide, and 8 feet high in the clear, to be made of hewed timber, laid close, with a Roof double boarded and shingled, the walls inside to be lined round with Plank, the Floors each of them to be laid with plank, supposed to have 4 windows on each side containing nine lights of glass to each window and 3 iron grates, two partitions of plank with a stair case in the Entry and a Whipping Post, to have one outside Door with a good lock and Iron Barr, to have two Doors within with a good lock to each, to have a stack of chimneys at each end, the above building to be set on a good dry wall which shall be sunk at least 2½ feet in the ground to prevent its being hurt by the frost.

Marshall indicated that he could build the proposed workhouse for two hundred pounds. Council adopted his proposal and ordered Charles Morris to administer the contract. The expense would be defrayed out of duties that had been collected on spirituous liquors,[21] which amounted, in October 1758, to £2,204. Three years earlier, the Lords of Trade had allowed[22] an amount of £295 for the building of a workhouse, but this was not mentioned in Council's deliberations in June 1758. It is likely that Josiah Marshall's proposal was not carried out, since in October 1758, the newly established Nova Scotia House of Assembly[23] was ordered to prepare a bill for the establishment of a workhouse.[24] In the same month, a committee of the legislature was struck to search for a piece of land to be used as the site for the workhouse.[25] On 13 December, the House passed an Act for Erecting a House of Correction or Workhouse within the Town of Halifax. It received Governor Lawrence's assent[26] the next day. The workhouse specified by the Assembly differed from the one agreed to by Council six months earlier in that it was to be larger and constructed of masonry rather than wood.

Application had been made[27] by the House to His Excellency the governor in October 1758 "for a quantity of four acres of that land lying between the Governor's farm and Fort Cornwallis." This was probably the lot of land "were [sic] the Jews burying ground was,"[28] which had found favour with the committee in charge of finding a site for the workhouse, and "which piece of land His Excellency said might be laid out when they pleased." This lot is shown (Figure 15)

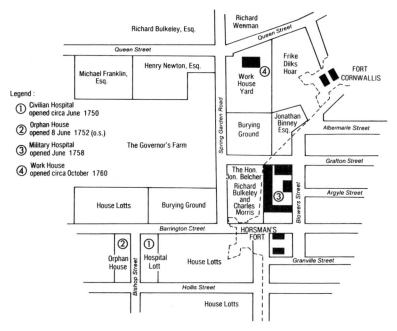

Figure 15
Location of the civilian hospital, military hospital, orphan house, and workhouse,
circa 1762. Drawn from a plan of the town of Halifax, *circa* 1762, which was
traced in December 1931 from the original in the Crown Lands Office.

as part of a plan of Halifax said to have been drawn in the year
1762.[29] Richard Short's drawing of a portion of the town (Figure 16)
shows the workhouse as the building in the right foreground with
two tall chimneys surrounded by the remnants of a fence.

On 25 November 1758, the Assembly asked the governor to appoint a committee of both Houses to manage the building of the
workhouse. His Excellency agreed. An initial appropriation of five
hundred pounds from the fund amassed from duties on spirituous
liquors was granted[30] by the governor on 19 December 1759.

Council introduced two additional bills with important implica-
tions for the workhouse, and for the poor. The first, which received
Governor Lawrence's assent[31] in August 1759, Bill for Regulating
and Maintaining an House of Correction and for Binding out Poor
Children. It read in part:

That the Overseers of the Poor of the town of Halifax be, and accordingly
they hereby are authorized and impowered, when and so soon as the said

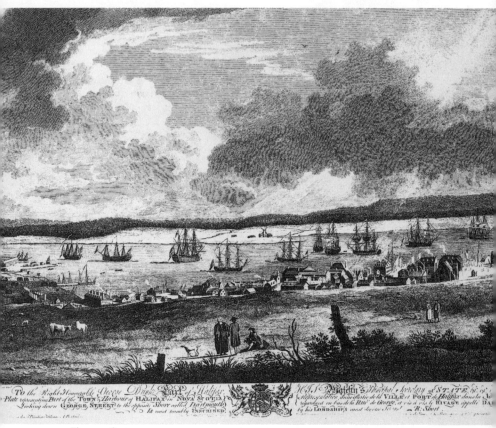

To the Right Honourable George Dunck Earl of Halifax

Plate representing Part of the Town & Harbour of HALIFAX in NOVA SCOTIA
Looking down GEORGE STREET to the opposite Shore called Dartmouth
Is most humbly INSCRIBED

H.I.S Majesty's Principal Secretary of STATE &c &c
respectfully shewe d'une partie de la VILLE et PORT de Halifax dans la
regardant en bas de la Rue de George, et vis à vis le RIVAGE appellé Da
by his LORDSHIP'S most devote S—t—t   R. Short

Figure 16
Richard Short's drawing entitled "A Plan representing Part of the Town of
Halifax in Nova Scotia looking down Prince Street to the opposite Shore." (Art
Gallery of Nova Scotia)

House of Correction shall be built and finished, to agree with some discret and fit persons to be the master and keeper, and needful assistants for the care of the same. And to provide, as there shall be occasion, suitable materials, tools, and implements, necessary and convenient for keeping to work such persons as may be committed to the said House, and generally, to inspect and direct the affairs of the said House ...

That it shall and may be lawful for the Justices of the Peace in their General Sessions, or for any one Justice of the Peace out of Court, to send and commit to the said House of Correction, to be kept, governed, and punished according to the rules and orders thereof, all disorderly and idle persons and such who shall be found begging, or practising any unlawful games, or pretending to fortune telling, common drunkards, persons of lewd behaviour, vagabonds, runaways, stubborn servants and children, and persons who notoriously mispend their time to the neglect and prejudice of their own or their family's support ...

That no person committed to the said House of Correction shall be chargeable to the government, for any allowance, either at going in or coming out or during the time of their abode there, but shall be maintained out of their earnings, and the remainder thereof shall be accounted for by the master or keeper ...

That if any person or persons committed to the said House of Correction be idiots, or lunatic, or sick or weak, and unable to work, they shall be taken care of and relieved by the master or keeper of the said House, who shall keep an exact account of what charges ...

That the pay of the said master or keeper of the said House of Correction and the charge for any materials, tools, or implements purchased ... shall be defrayed out of the surplus of the earnings of the labour done in the said House.

That the said overseers of the poor shall take order from time to time, by and with the consent of two or more Justices of the Peace for the County of Halifax for setting to work the children of all such, whose parents shall not, by said overseers, or the greater part of them, be thought able to keep or maintain them, or any poor orphans, or by indenture to bind any such children or orphans as aforesaid to be apprentices, where they shall see convenient, till such man child shall come to the age of twenty one years, and such woman child to the age of eighteen years.

The office of overseer of the poor for Halifax had been created[32] on 22 March 1759, pursuant to an Act for Preventing Trespasses, and in April, four persons had been chosen by a committee of Council to act as overseers.[33] Mention of idiots and lunatics was the second time the government had shown some compassion towards the mentally ill. On 28 April 1752 (o.s.), one Ensign John Fleming of Warburton's

Forty-fifty Regiment "had been found to be a Lunatic" by a special inquest of jurors.[34] He and his brother were given free passage to England so that "said John Fleming [could] be secured in a Hospital of Bedlam[35] or some other Hospital in England approved for the cure of Lunaticks." In the Lords of Trade Instructions[36] to the first three governors of Nova Scotia, no direction had been given concerning the care of the poor, or persons considered to be idiots and lunatics.

The second act, also passed on 13 August 1759, was an Act for Relief of the Poor in the Town of Halifax. It gave the overseers one hundred pounds to be used for poor relief. The overseers, apparently feeling that they had not been given the necessary authority to carry out the functions outlined in the two bills, sent a memorial[37] to the House in January 1760, stating:

That they had no authority of themselves to send any poor to the Workhouse, either to be relieved or set to work, nor to release them from thence, that there is no provision made for relieving the Poor, other than being sent to the Workhouse, or by Voluntary subscription, which being unequal, is attended with very great inconveniences, and is disagreable to the publick, who say that every one ought to pay their equal proportion towards relieving the said Poor. That there are many Industrious Families with children who only want Temporary Relief and are not proper objects for a Workhouse and that the vessels who come from different parts of the continent frequently bring into this Port, lame, aged, and distressed people, who become a great burthen to the place.

The concern expressed in the last sentence had been for some time a worry of Council and the House of Assembly. It induced them to pass an Act to Prevent the Importing [of] Disabled, Infirm, and other Useless Persons into this Province, to which the governor assented[38] on 18 March 1760. Another outcome of the memorial was an Act in Addition to an Act Intitled an Act for the Relief of the Poor in the Town of Halifax, passed[39] by the House on 17 March 1760 and given the governor's assent on 31 March. This was the first instance of a poor tax being levied on the citizens of Halifax.

The workhouse was probably in the final stages of completion in April 1760, for Council minutes[40] record a resolution "that the sum of fifty pounds be paid out of the Public Treasury to the Overseers of the Poor in order to purchase materials and Implements for setting to work the persons in the Workhouse." The total expense, including fencing the workhouse grounds, was £726.[41]

In the Act for Regulating and Maintaining an House of Correction or Workhouse and for Binding out Poor Children, reference was made to "setting to work the children of all such whose parents shall not, by the said overseers, or the greater part of them, be thought able to keep or maintain them, or any poor orphans; or by indenture to bind any such children or orphans as aforesaid to be apprentices ... that the children maintained and supported in the Orphan House at the expense of the Crown, shall remain and be under the direction of the Governor as heretofore, and bound out in such manner as he shall order and direct." This meant that in late 1760, there were in Halifax two institutions for the care of orphans and abandoned children. As described in chapter 2, the Lords of Trade wrote[42] to Jonathan Belcher in March 1761, complaining that some of the inmates of the orphan house on Bishop Street (see Figure 15) were not actually orphans but children of poor people, and that this increased the expense to the public of supporting the house. Belcher responded that he would limit the number of children in the orphan house to twenty-five.[43] Existence of the workhouse meant, therefore, that additional orphans or poor children in the town had a second institution into which they could be admitted for care and apprenticeship.[44]

HALIFAX WAS NOT THE ONLY TOWN IN NOVA SCOTIA that had experienced difficulty in supporting its poor. On 17 July 1761, Council sent down a resolution for the relief of the poor in the townships of Liverpool, Annapolis, Granville, Horton, Falmouth, and Newport.[45] On 20 July 1761, the House ordered that money be borrowed to support the poor in the new settlements. Problems of supporting the poor in these settlements and in Halifax were compounded by information[46] that His Majesty had disallowed the Act to Prevent the Importing [of] Disabled, Infirm, and the other Useless Persons into this Province. Jonathan Belcher had been informed,[47] but without explanation, of the disallowance of the act. In a letter to George III, dated 15 April 1761, the Lords of Trade explained, "As the words, descriptive of the persons, whose coming into the Province it is the object of this Act to prevent, appears to us too loose and general, and as the Provisions of the Act make the Master of every vessel liable to suffer unreasonable hardships at the discretion of the Overseers of the Poor, who are even in cases where the disability or Infirmity of any persons on board may have happened by common casulty [sic] in the course of the voyage. We think it our duty humbly to lay the said Act before your Majesty for your Royal Disallowance."

By the 17 April 1762, some inhabitants of the new townships of Onslow, Truro, and Yarmouth were said[48] to be in "distressing and indigent circumstances" and in "want of supplies and provisions."

Mr Hinshelwood, by order of the lieutenant governor and in consequence of the state of the new settlements, laid before the House the
state of the old duty fund, by which it appeared that a balance of
£350 remained. The governor agreed that this amount be applied to
help such persons in the new settlements "as stand most in need of
supplies." On 17 August 1762, the House voted that fifty pounds be
borrowed from the public money of the province to supply "the
present distressed condition of the Poor in the Township of Halifax
... till a Law can be passed for making an assessment upon the inhabitants of Halifax." Surprisingly, Council did not agree and also
turned down[49] the Act for the Relief of the Poor of the Town of
Halifax, passed by the House on 25 August 1762. Lieutenant Governor Belcher, in his address[50] to the House of Assembly in April
1763, dealt with the dilemma of providing for the poor thus: "You
must have been so sensible of the casual nature of Duties upon spirituous Liquors that you cannot be surprised or disappointed at the
insufficiences of that Fund, either for Redemption to this Loan, or
in the least to answer the annual just demands from the Public ... By
the absolute dependence on these Duties we rely upon the consumption of a noxious manufacture, which it is the very object of the Laws
to restrain, nor would it be an unpolitical wish, that we could wholly
prohibit." The House was undeterred. On the same day as Belcher's
address, it resumed consideration of the poor-relief bill rejected by
Council in the previous session. This time, the Council and governor
agreed[51] to the bill. Two additional bills[52] dealing with the poor
were adopted in 1763. These were an Act to enable the Several
Townships within this Province, to Maintain their Poor, and an Act
to enable the Inhabitants of Townships to assess themselves for the
relief of the Poor, both of which received assent on 26 November
1763. The latter act transferred the burden of supporting the poor
from the provincial government to the township officers.

Jonathan Harris[53] was appointed keeper of the workhouse by the
overseers of the poor in October or November 1760. After less than
a year's experience, he wrote to the Assembly in June 1762, "setting
forth the great difficulties he labours under for want of a supply
from the Government to keep at work such as are able and to purchase provisions for the support of the poor and indigent." The
Assembly sent a message to Council desiring that it join in an
application to the lieutenant governor for the payment of £205 due
to Jonathan Harris, which he received in full in August 1762. Earlier, in February and July, Lieutenant Governor Belcher had directed[54] Benjamin Green, the provincial treasurer, to provide the
overseers of the poor with funds amounting to a hundred pounds
for artificers and materials employed at the workhouse "necessary

for keeping to work such persons as have been committed to the said House." Jonathan Harris sent a second memorial[55] to the House in October 1763, expressing his continued dissatisfaction with the lack of funding. He recalled that for three years he had attempted to support a number of helpless men, women, and orphan children, and asked for relief. As a result of this memorial, the original act regulating and maintaining the workhouse was amended[56] in November, to read:

That from and after the publication hereof, the ordering and governing [of] the said House of Correction or Workhouse shall be in the Justices of the Peace in their Quarter Sessions (except three rooms which shall be reserved for the reception of the poor, under the direction of the Overseers of the Poor) ...

One of which Justices in rotation shall visit the same at least once every week, to see that such persons as shall be committed thereto, are kept diligently at work; and to rectify any abuses that may be found in the management thereof.

That it shall be in the power of The Overseers of the Poor of the Town of Halifax only to send such sick and weak persons to the Workhouse, there to be relieved by their direction, and the expense thereof to be defrayed out of such taxes or poor's rate, as shall be granted and collected for the Town of Halifax.

The act was also amended to provide support for the poor residing elsewhere in the province.

The reservation of three rooms "for the reception of the poor" was an outcome of deliberations by a joint committee of the Council and House, which reported[57] in November 1763 that "the persons entitled to receive alms, should be separated from those committed to the House of Correction for being disorderly." This was the first instance in which the poor in Nova Scotia were identified by government as a distinct group and given specific living accommodation separate from that of criminals.

Since the civilian hospital had not been funded[58] by the Lords of Trade since 1758, and since the allowance for a surgeon, midwife, and medicine had also been removed from the estimate of the "civil establishment" in March 1761,[59] the workhouse, after 1760, was the only institution for the reception of the sick poor. When, in November 1763, the poor were separated from people held in the workhouse for petty crimes, the three rooms set aside for the poor represented the only civilian hospital facility in Halifax.

There were, however, two other hospitals in Halifax in 1763: the naval hospital and the military hospital. Charles White was surgeon at the naval hospital from 1761 until 1771,[60] when he was succeeded by George Greaves.[61] On 7 October 1772, Admiral John Montague wrote[62] from Boston "that the person to act as surgeon to the Hospital at Halifax is the Dispenser of Medicine and by no means qualified as a surgeon." Montague mentioned the "necessity of a good surgeon being at Halifax where the ships are to careen and refit." George Greaves was still surgeon at the naval hospital in July 1774, with only two patients.[63] The military hospital (Figure 15) came into being in June 1758, after Warburton's 45th Regiment had vacated its barracks to join the British forces that carried out the attack on Louisbourg.[64] As John Knox wrote, "The barracks evacuated by the 45th Regiment [are] being prepared as a hospital for the reception of the sick that are unable to proceed on the expedition, [and] every corps is forthwith to send their sick to that Hospital where the Deputy Director will receive them." The names of the directors and surgeons of the military hospital from 1763–74 have not been identified. It would be expected, however, that the surgeons of the various regiments[65] stationed in Halifax during that period would have treated their patients in that hospital.

Neither the naval nor the military hospital appears to have been available to the civilian population; consequently, hospital facilities for civilians, other than the poor, were non-existent in Nova Scotia during the 1760s. The lack of adequate medical care was highlighted in a letter written by the Reverend John B. Moreau[66] to the Society for the Propagation of the Gospel in 1762: "The Phisicians [sic] here tell me that I can't live another winter, if I stay in this Province. I hope the venerable Society will give me leave of absence for a year to go to Bath." In May 1766, Governor Montague Wilmot wrote[67] to the Lords of Trade asking to return to Europe because of his ill health. He indicated that he had gout and explained that "the physicians assure me that I cannot survive another winter in this country and I am to expect relief only from Bath waters." Governor Wilmot was buried in Halifax twenty-one days later.[68] In September 1766, Lieutenant Governor Michael Francklin recommended[69] to the Lords of Trade that Dr John Phillipps, who had been a surgeon at Lunenburg since 1757, should be allowed to go to England "because of his present ill state of health ... to seek advice of the most able and skilful phisicians [sic]."

In June 1764, the newly appointed Governor Wilmot wrote[70] to the Lords of Trade about the desperate state of the provincial treasury:

The [General Assembly] appropriated the Duties on Spirituous Liquors for several years, [paid] bounties and premiums on catching and curing fish and on the clearing and fencing of land, [and] with [the] sum of money in the Treasury ... they erected a jail, and a workhouse of masonry. This Workhouse in which there is also a Poor House is now maintained at no less than £500 per year from these funds besides the assessment of £100 per year from the inhabitants of this Town and is the receptacle for all the old, the infirm, the decripid [sic], and the indigent who have come in this Province at different periodes [sic] within these fifteen years, together with the dissolute and abandoned which are too frequently imported. From these Funds are paid the officers of the General Assembly and the Expenses attending the Sessions ... to which is to be added several considerable sums given from thence to the support of indigent persons in the New Settlements ... The Annual Revenue of the Duties having considerably decreased ... The General Assembly had recourse to borrowing on interest by which there is a Debt of more than Twelve thousand pounds accumulated at this time.

For the first time, the term "poor house" appears in the records of Nova Scotia.

Sometime during Governor Wilmot's administration[71] (5 October 1763 to 23 May 1766), Dr Thomas Reeve was appointed[72] "to take under his care, the sick in the Workhouse of the Town of Halifax." Dr Reeve wrote in a memorial to the House in June 1766 that he was "praying that some allowance may be made him for his care, trouble, and great [personal] expense for medicines." On 30 June, he was paid sixty pounds for his services[73] and a similar amount the next year.[74] On 1 July 1768, Dr Reeve was paid[75] for attendance "to [the] sick in the Poor House." Although the House of Assembly had informed[76] Reeve in 1770 that "there will be no future allowance for such purposes," his allowance was continued until October 1774, when he received a final payment of sixty-four pounds for his services.[77]

One might have expected that Dr Alexander Abercrombie, who had been surgeon to the civilian hospital from 1750 to 1760 and was much respected by government officials,[78] would have been appointed, rather than Thomas Reeve, as surgeon and apothecary to the poor. Since 1 May 1755,[79] Dr Abercrombie had been providing attendance and medicines to the children in the orphan house, but he had received nothing for these services until 8 July 1768, when he was paid a hundred pounds. He continued to be paid twenty pounds per year as surgeon to the orphan house, until his death on 31 March 1773.[80] Dr Abercrombie was held in high regard. His obituary read:

On Wednesday last died here, in the 51st year of his age, Alexander Abercrombie, MD, in his Profession, as an eminent, skillful, benevolent and successful Physician, a blessing to the Province, a Friend ever stedfast [*sic*] and amiable, and one who in every quality of mind, and for Prudence in Conduct, could be more easily admired thro' his life by all, than sufficiently extolled, honored, and lamented by any, under the irreparable Public Loss by his Death. His obsequies were respectfully performed last Saturday, and attended by a numerous Train of sincere mourners of every rank and order of the Town.

Dr Abercrombie was succeeded by Dr John Philipps, who, in April 1773, was appointed[81] "to take care of the sick children in the Orphan House." Abercrombie had provided medicines, advice, and attendance to the Indians in the vicinity of Halifax and, in September 1763, had submitted[82] a bill covering the period from 1 October 1760 to 22 September 1763. He was paid fifty pounds. For medical assistance to Indians[83] for the period from 27 September 1763 to 22 May 1766, he received an additional seventy-two pounds. On 26 September 1766, Dr Abercrombie was officially "appointed to the care of such of the Indians as apply to the Government in case of sickness of hurts and wounds." On that same date he was appointed[84] surgeon to the orphan house.

On 14 June 1765, a joint committee of Council and House ordered[85] "that the Workhouse be shut up by which a saving will be made of at least £165 per annum." On 2 July, Council endorsed this decision by declaring[86] "that the Keeper of the Workhouse have notice that the Government will not grant any supplies or maintain it and that he shall shut up the same, and apply to the Justices for further orders." This was in reaction to a revelation in the House, on 7 June, that the provincial debt had risen to £16,000. The severe deficit provoked Benjamin Green, administrator of the government, to write[87] to the Lords of Trade in August 1766:

I humbly hope your Lordships will pardon the mention of one thing more, which is done at the desire of the principal inhabitants of this place, who esteem themselves greatly interested in obtaining your Lordships favourable Regards for their Relief which is, That the Repeal of the Act of the Legislature here for preventing the scum of all the colonies from being admitted into this Province without Restriction has caused such an Inundation of persons, who are not only useless but very Burthensome to the Community, being not only those of the most dissolute manners, and void of all sentiments of honest Industry, but also infirm, decrepit, and insane, as well as extremely indigent persons, who are unable to contribute anything towards their own maintenance, that the Industrious Inhabitants, especially in the Town of Halifax, esteem themselves subject to a grievous Tax thereby, and are disabled from affording the Relief they are willing to do to their own honest poor, the Expence of whose support, especially in the Winter Season, is very considerable, and, if I have not been misinformed, the passages of persons from Jails, Hospitals, and the Workhouses, in the neighbouring Colonies, have been paid for, and other Encouragement given them to embark for this place, since it has been known that we were obliged to receive them.

Further evidence that members of the House despaired of the increasing debt appeared in October 1766, when they rejected[88] claims by the overseers of the poor totalling £445 for provisions for the workhouse, and by Jonathan Harris on account of the poor house; however, Council declared in November that it could not agree with the House on the matter and the claims had to be honoured. The House reconsidered and agreed to pay £248 for the workhouse and £197 for support of the poor house.

By January 1767, the provincial debt had grown to £23,500. On the third day of that month, a memorial[89] from the overseers of the poor pointed out that several of the poor maintained in Halifax belonged to different parts of the province and that three hundred pounds would be needed to support them during the winter, an amount too great to assess the inhabitants of Halifax. The overseers asked for relief, and Council resolved that "the Overseers of the Poor should proceed to assess the inhabitants of the Town of Halifax in proportion to their abilities and that whatever sum shall be deficient to make up what is necessary for the support of the Poor after making the assessment, such sum shall be paid out of the Treasury." A further memorial[90] from the overseers was read in the House in July, "setting forth that by the great increase of the Poor in the Province, the sum granted by the Town of Halifax last January for the support of the Poor [during] the current year, is greatly insufficient to answer that purpose and praying relief." This great increase was probably what prompted the magistrates to ask[91] Council that "the Hospital may be granted for the use of an Alms House and for some other public uses." As a result, Lieutenant Governor Michael Francklin proclaimed,[92] on 19 November 1767, that "the House built and formerly used for an Hospital may be occupied for ... the use of an Alms House [and] hereby empowering Hibbert Newton, Esq., Mr Francis White, Mr Edward Nichols, and Mr Phillip Brehm, Overseers of the Poor of the Town of Halifax to occupy and use the said House for the aforesaid purpose during pleasure." The increase in the numbers of poor in Halifax induced the Council and House to reintroduce the Act to Prevent the Importation of Impotent, Lame, and Inferior Persons in this Province," which had been disallowed by King George III in 1761. It received second reading on 19 June 1768.[93] Lieutenant Governor Francklin, writing to Lord Hillsborough, explained[94] that the act was necessary since the frequent importations of poor people and camp followers led to heavy taxes for the people of Halifax and placed a heavy burden on provincial funds. Governor Campbell forwarded[95] the bill to Lord Hillsborough in January 1769. At the Court of St James in May 1769, the king disallowed it for the second time.[96] This contentious act is set forth in Appendix 4.

On 10 March 1768, Jonathan Harris, keeper of the workhouse, was buried from St Paul's. Sometime prior to November 1768, he was succeeded[97] by Thomas Fitzpatrick, who had been keeper of the gaol[98] in 1763. Fitzpatrick continued as keeper for about two years until, in October 1770, John Woodin was listed[99] as keeper. The situation must have been desperate. In 1769, Richard Tritten, one of the overseers of the poor in that year, stated in a memorial[100] to the House that thirteen pounds had been advanced for rugs, blankets, shirts, etc., for the use of the poor house, "at which time there was no bedding in the Poor House for the people to sleep on."

The second attempt to establish the Act to Prevent the Importing of Impotent, Lame, and Infirm Persons into the Province failed and on 2 April 1770, Council was so informed.[101] The reason,[102] essentially the same as in 1761, was that it "would subject the Masters of Vessels to penalties and inconvenience which in reason they ought not to be exposed to." This was bad news for Governor Campbell and Lieutenant Governor Francklin, for the provincial debt had increased[103] from £16,000 in June 1765 to £23,500 by June 1770.

During the two-year period 1770—71, Governor Campbell authorized Benjamin Green, the provincial treasurer, to pay out more than a thousand pounds in support of the poor house.[104] To make matters worse in terms of the provincial debt, a number of Halifax residents refused[105] to pay the poor tax in 1771, which led to at least one resident being brought before the Supreme Court.[106] A large outlay of money from government coffers to maintain the poor continued through 1772, 1773, 1774, and into 1775. During this period the provincial debt remained at over twenty thousand pounds, and John Woodin, keeper of the workhouse, constantly petitioned the House for an allowance to support the poor. On one occasion, he submitted a memorial[107] listing the poor-house inmates during the period from April to September 1773. The three women and nine men described as having "no legal settlement in Halifax" presumably were in addition to the poor of Halifax, who would be classified as legal settlers. Unfortunately, Woodin did not indicate the total number of persons in the poor house in 1773. The memorial which was signed by the overseers of the poor, did indicate that a nurse named Hall and a cook (unnamed) were working there in October 1773.

Some relief for the poor came from money collected at a benefit performance[108] of a comedy entitled *The Suspicious Husband*, presented "by the Gentlemen of the Army and Navy." The proceeds were distributed "to the indigent Families and other old and poor people." Also, in November 1773, the overseers of the poor called[109] a meeting of the freeholders to discuss poor relief. The following advertisement, which appeared in the *Nova Scotia Gazette and Weekly Chronicle* of 8 February 1774, may have resulted from that meeting.

"Employment for the Poor;

Halifax Work-house, 7 Feb., 1774
This is to give Notice that any number of Persons whether men, women, boys, or girls, that are willing to pick Oakum, or spin, shall have Employment, good Usage, good Victuals and Drink, and a good warm Stove Room to Work and Lodge in if required, without Confinement by applying to the Master of said House.

John Wooden"

In 1774, an Act for Punishing Rogues, Vagabonds, and other Idle and Disorderly Persons was passed.[110] It dealt with people who refused to work, with beggers, and with lunatics. It recommended that those found to be furiously mad should be kept safely locked up in a secure place. The act concluded hopefully, "That nothing herein contained shall ... restrain any friend or relative of such lunatics from taking them under their own care."

Once the grant for the hospital and money for surgeons and midwife had been discontinued, the only remaining charitable institution in Nova Scotia was the orphan house. On 20 March 1764, the Lords of Trade turned their attention to that establishment. To Governor Wilmot, they wrote:[111]

With respect to the allowance for an Orphan House, we have no conception how it is possible that the cloathing[*sic*] and maintaining 25 charity children should, exclusive of the profits of their labor, amount to £354 per annum. Such a charge appears to us to bear no proportion under any difference in circumstances to what would be judged a reasonable allowance in this Country, and therefore it will be your duty to make the most careful and diligent enquiry into the state of this Establishment and to make all possible savings upon it either by checking any abuse which may attend the conduct of it upon the present plan, or by putting the charity under more frugal and reasonable regulations.

Response[112] to this request for enquiry was given by the Reverend John Breynton:

The strictist enquiry has been made into the State of the Orphan House and the Expense attending it. The Charge indeed seems great but if all circumstances are considered the allowance will not appear unreasonable or extravagant.

The Articles of Provisions, cloathing and servants wages have been during the last seven years full as dear again as in England but as the Colony will soon be able to furnish many of the necessarys of life at a much cheaper rate, a considerable saving may be expected next year.

In Regard to the Labour of the Orphans, no Profit can arise from thence. Were they to continue in the Orphan House as they do in the Charity Schools in England to the age of 12 or 14 years and where manufactures are carried on to advantage some Emolument might be expected but as Hands are so much wanted here for agriculture, fishing and servant children (if not disqualified by Diseases) are commonly bound out at seven or eight years old, an age incapable of attempting to spin work either wool, flax, or Hemp without greater waste than the Profit of their Labour will amount to.

By this Apprenticing the Orphan so young there necessarily follows a quick succession in the Orphan House of Helpless children and often, infants which require Wet nurses at 10 shillings per week besides other Expenses.

This explanation seemed to satisfy the Lords of Trade. For the next ten years, they continued to allow in the annual estimates an expense of £384 for the orphan house. It is clear, however, from the following account by Governor Francis Legge, that the money was not used efficiently. He described[113] the orphan house as:

a very necessary and beneficial charity. At my first arrival I paid a visit to the House and found it in a very ruinous condition, and the children by that means suffering greatly with the cold, enquiring into the reason, the keeper informed me that he had expended at different times very considerable sums which the Government had not refunded him.

I therefore thought this matter an object worthy [of] my attention and care which induced me to make a diligent enquiry into the expense of maintaining twenty-five children intended to be supported. I appointed a committee of Council to examine into the affair who reported that some saving might be made out of the Parliamentary allowance sufficient to repair the buildings and keep them in repair and recommended to me the appointing persons [of] reputation, to make a thorough enquiry which accordingly I have done, and invested them with powers to agree with any person upon examination considered what would be necessary and proper for diet and clothing.

They have in consequence of my orders made a contract with the keeper for two hundred and fifty pounds for the same number of infants ... What now remains is a decayed inhospitable building just falling into ruins.

Governor Legge had appointed,[114] in April 1774, a committee consisting of Mr Morris, Mr Bulkeley, Mr Butler, and Mr Burrow, to report on the orphan house. They submitted their report on 12 May. Four days later, Doctor Philipps, Mr John Fenton, and William Smith were appointed governors of the orphan house to "consider the cheapest manner for which the several necessary articles of provisions, cloathing, etc., may be provided and to establish a regular course of Diet to be provided weekly." On 18 November 1774, Legge wrote[115] to Lord Dartmouth that "the Orphan House is refitted, and rendered comfortable for the children, who are now protected from the inclemency of the weather."

As noted earlier, the Lords of Trade disallowed the allowance for a midwife in the estimate of the civil establishment of Halifax for 1761, but it was 1764 before this item was removed from the estimate submitted by the governor.[116] Midwives were included in the estimates for Lunenburg for every year until 1767; in that year two midwives[117] were paid five pounds each for their services. Curiously, Mrs Ann Catherwood, who had been midwife at Halifax during the period 1750–59, received what the estimates referred to as a pension of twenty-five pounds in the years 1767, 1768, and 1769, at a time when payment was disallowed for the services of a midwife in Halifax.

Removal of the position of midwife from the 1764 estimate meant that the residents of Halifax, including the poor, had to rely upon their own resources for attendance provided during childbirth. The chronic circumstances are reflected in a petition[118] that Eleanor Fallon, midwife, presented in November 1769 to the House of Assembly. She stated that she was frequently called upon to attend the poor women in the town at the time of a delivery. She requested some compensation for her services. The House considered the state of the province's funds and decided to deny the petition. Eleanor

Fallon died in late 1771 or early 1772, since her estate was administered[119] in Halifax on 9 March 1772. On 1 November 1774, Elizabeth Fleming advertised in the *Nova Scotia Gazette* that she had "perfectly learn'd the art of a midwife and [was] particularly approved of and strongly recommended by Doctor Hill,[120] and others to come to this place." It is not known whether residents of Halifax responded. During the first twenty-five years of settlement by the English in Nova Scotia, only three surgeons indicated that they practised midwifery. Henry Meriton advertised[121] in 1753 that he was a man-midwife, and John Grant stated[122] on 13 January 1755 that "he has practised midwifery in Halifax which was not common to other surgeons in Halifax." John Phillipps, surgeon in Lunenburg during 1757–66, indicated in a memorial[123] to Council that he was acting as man-midwife in that town.

It is not surprising that there were both midwives and men-midwives in Halifax in the 1750s. The monopoly that midwives held over the birthing process in Great Britain began to be eroded in the seventeenth century.[124] The emergence of the man-midwife, or *accoucheur*, can be dated from the publication of the first original English work on midwifery by Dr William Harvey, which appeared in 1651. Through his book, Harvey, who had earlier become famous for his treatise on the circulation of the blood, placed midwifery on a scientific basis for the first time. Shortly after Harvey's book appeared, the Chamberlen family of physicians in England secretly invented the obstetric forceps, and very soon it became well known that the Chamberlens' mortality rate for deliveries was much lower than the usual rate among midwives.[125] Women continued to dominate midwifery, however, until about 1733, when the secret of the forceps became generally known and the instrument began to be used by *accoucheurs*. Among midwives, however, custom and the absence of formal training ensured that they did not adopt forceps to aid in deliveries, and this eventually diminished their control over the childbirth process. Dr William Smellie was undoubtedly the most well known man-midwife in eighteenth-century England. In 1735, he began to use forceps in deliveries and, during the 1740s, is said to have delivered over a thousand babies.[126] He also began to give lectures on reproductive anatomy and midwifery in the 1740s, and Henry Meriton, mentioned above, who came to Halifax with Cornwallis in 1749, was one of his pupils. In 1752, Dr Smellie published his well-known book, *Treatise on the Theory and Practice of Midwifery*. By the middle of the eighteenth century, "the man-midwife had advanced from merely being an attendant on the emergencies of childbirth to gaining a hold on the greater part of the best-paid midwifery."

The Act Regulating and Maintaining the House of Correction, passed in 1759, required that persons regarded as lunatics or idiots were to be taken care of by the master or keeper of the workhouse. In 1766, Benjamin Green, writing[127] to the Lords of Trade concerning the disallowed Act to Prevent the Importing of Disabled, Infirm, and other Useless Persons into the Province, included the insane as among "the scum of all the Colonies being admitted into this Province without Restrictions."

In July 1772, the Lords of Trade communicated[128] to Governor Campbell that "the King having been pleased with the advice of His Privy Council to signify to us His Majesty's Pleasure that we should in all future draughts of Commission for Governors in the Plantations insert a clause giving them, as Chancellors, the necessary powers to issue commissions for the care and custody of Ideots [sic] and Lunaticks." The instructions[129] to Governor Francis Legge, dated 10 June 1773, contained accordingly a clause "to provide for the Custody of Lunatics and their Estates without taking the profits thereof to our own use."

DURING THE FIRST NINE YEARS AFTER THE FOUNDING OF HALIFAX, Nova Scotia was governed by governor and Council. After 1758, the elected House of Assembly joined the governor and the appointed Council in enacting the province's laws. Only one surgeon, Dr Robert Grant, was appointed to the Council during the period 1749–74. He had come to Halifax in 1749 as a surgeon's mate on the *Charlton* and, in June 1756, was sworn[130] in as a member of Council. He continued to attend Council meetings[131] until June 1758, after which he moved his business of victualling HM Ships of War to Louisbourg and later to Quebec. On 16 August 1759, Grant was replaced[132] on Council because of inattendance. Robert Grant was one of a group of councillors who wrote to the Lords of Trade, on 12 March 1757, complaining of Governor Lawrence's delay in calling an Assembly.[133] This was the only incident of note involving Grant as a member of Council.

Four physicians and surgeons were elected to the House of Assembly from 1758–74: John Steele and Samuel Willoughby, who were elected in 1761 and sat in the Third Assembly (1761–65); John Day, who held a seat in both the Fourth (1765–70) and Fifth (1770–85) assemblies; and John Philipps, who represented Halifax County in the Fifth Assembly. Neither John Steele, who died during his first year in the Legislature, nor John Philipps had remarkable careers in the Legislature. Samuel Willoughby, who represented Cornwallis Township in both the Third and Fifth assemblies, seems to have been an eccentric personality. He refused to take his seat in the Third Assembly and was expelled[134] on 21 June 1762. In the Fifth Assembly, he was suspended[135] between October and December 1774, pending a trial for usury, and on 28 June 1776, his seat was declared vacant.

Of the four who were members of the House of Assembly prior to 1775, John Day was the only one to take an active part in its deliberations. He was a leading figure in the House during 1765–68 and even more so from October 1774 to July 1775. He took his seat as the member for Newport Township when the Fourth Assembly convened on 28 May 1765 and was appointed,[136] three days later, member of a committee to examine the provincial treasurer's accounts. The regard which the members of the Assembly had for John Day is indicated by his appointment on June 3 (six days after first taking his seat) to the committee responsible for preparing the address to the governor. The address recommended that the offices of Impost and Excise lay before the House an explicit and particular account of their receipts and payments for the past year, the money in their hands, and the notes due to the Town of Halifax. Their object was to determine the actual state of the expenditures, revenues, and debt of the province, preliminary to devising a plan for reducing the provincial debt of £16,000.

Dr Day was member also of the joint committee of the House and Council, established on 11 June 1765, to discuss the public accounts. One Committee suggestion was that £165 per year could be saved by closing the workhouse. As noted above, however, this did not happen. Dr Day was one of four members of the House who argued, in an address to Benjamin Green, commander in chief of the province from May to August 1766, "that the poor inhabitants of the new settlements cannot pay Taxes, and that the building and maintaining of a Light-House, a Work-House, Market-House, and Gaol, and for opening roads, cannot be defrayed out of public funds and ask that an application be made to the King for relief."[137] The committee accused Green, who was also provincial treasurer, of making unauthorized expenditures and suggested measures for controlling estimates and expenditures. One suggestion was to place the collectors of duties on commission rather than on salary.

On 24 July 1767, John Day presented to the House a bill entitled An Act to Explain, Amend, and Reduce into One Act, the Several Laws Now in Force Relating to the Duties of Excise on Rum and Other Distilled Spirituous Liquors Sold in this Province. He also brought before the House a bill to amend an act passed in 1762, entitled An Act for Regulating and Maintaining an House of Correction or Workhouse within the Town and for Binding Out Poor Children. Although this bill was received and read in the House on 2 November 1768, for some unknown reason it was not mentioned again during the Fourth Assembly. In fact, John Day was not mentioned as being in the Assembly after 21 November 1768, and he probably removed his family to Philadelphia early in 1769.[138] He was a druggist[139] in Philadelphia during 1770–71, and on 22 September 1772, the *Nova Scotia Gazette* records that he and his family arrived back in Halifax on the schooner *Dolphin*.

During the Fifth Assembly, John Day was elected as a member for the Town of Halifax in a by-election held in August 1774. On 6 August, he inserted one of the first election advertisements, if not the first, in a Nova Scotia newspaper.[140] It read: "As it is probable that a Writ may shortly be issued to choose a Representative for the Town of Halifax in the room of Col Charles Proctor, deceased, permit me to offer myself a Candidate on this Occasion. Should I be the object of your choice, give me leave to assure you that I will exert the utmost of my abilities faithfully to serve the public." On 30 August 1774, the same newspaper indicated that John Day had been elected "by a great majority." The by-election appears to have passed relatively unnoticed by the Halifax community. A person calling himself "A Friend of Truth" wrote in the *Gazette* on 6 September, "You say that Col John Day was elected a Member for this Town by a great majority. The Public would be glad to know who opposed him."

Dr Day took his seat on 6 October 1774. Two days later he was appointed to a committee to prepare a Bill to Regulate the Proceedings of the Courts of Judicature, and to a second committee to consider the establishment of a loan office and a paper medium of exchange. Between 8 October 1774 and 15 July 1775, John Day served on ten committees, brought in four bills, and was the acknowledged leader of the House. He led the fight against Council over the "farming" of duties, stating that, "if the Duties at all the Outposts of this Province were farmed, it would more than double the present Revenue received from those places." One of the bills he introduced resulted in an Act relating to Wills, Legacies, and Executors, and for the Settlement and Distribution of the Estates and Intestates. Also, in June 1775, he reported for the committee to draw up an address to Governor Legge condemning a plan to reduce to nine the quorum of the House and increase to ten the representation for Halifax town and county.[141] He wrote that the plan was "replete with mischief, [and] subversive of real representation." Governor Legge did not think very highly of John Day and complained to Lord Dartmouth that "Day, a member, who had resided for some time in Philadelphia, and imbibed republican principles, is one of the agent victuallers of the army and assisted by Tonge, the Naval Officer, framed a petition to the King for lessening the power of the Governor, Council, and officers of Government, to throw the whole weight of power into the hands of The Assembly." Day's strong leadership in efforts to prevent the Halifax oligarchy from gaining complete control of the House brings to mind Joseph Howe's role, some fifty years later, in the movement to introduce representative government. John Day died on 29 November 1775,[142] having "lost his life on board a vessel bound from Nova Scotia to Boston with supplies for the Garrison in that place during the American War."[143] Day's estate papers[144] show that he was worth a substantial amount, £1,704, at the time of his death and that he had a personal library of two hundred and twenty volumes. Among these were at least six books that would be classified as medical, including *A Discourse upon the Institution of Medical Schools in America*, written by John Morgan and published in 1765 by Bradford in Philadelphia.

IT WAS NOTED IN CHAPTER 2 that, in December 1758, John Day had advertised[145] that he had drugs and medicines for sale at his store on Hollis Street. Prior to 1768, Day's was one of only two Halifax newspaper advertisements for drugs and medicines. In 1768, Ward's Medicines were listed[146] for sale and 1769 saw[147] the first advertisement having to do with the care of teeth: "Monsieur Jarbove's most excellent Anodyne Water for Teeth." In 1773, Keyser's Pills were advertised[148] in the *Royal Gazette*, which also, as of November 1774, regularly carried Dr John Philipps's advertisement[149] for drugs and medicines. The only other advertised item claiming medicinal value was Velmo's Vegetable Syrup.[150]

Smallpox does not appear to have been prevalent in Nova Scotia from 1763–74; only one incident of a smallpox scare has been noted. In June 1763, a brig bound for London from St Christopher's put into Halifax for a refit after it had sprung a leak.[151] The master of the brig had died of smallpox at sea, and the ship had been ordered to anchor on the Dartmouth side, where it was washed down with vinegar. There was no appearance of the smallpox after the brig had been refitted in the Halifax careening yard. That Nova Scotia had been spared from smallpox epidemics during this period can be surmised from *An Essay on the Present State of the Province of Nova Scotia with some Structures on the Measures Pursued by the Government from its first Settlement by the English in the year 1749*. This anonymous twenty-four-page pamphlet,[152] signed on the last page by "A Member of the Assembly," is thought to have been printed in 1774.

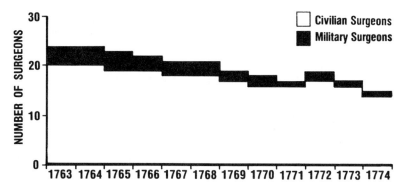

Figure 17
Civilian, naval, and military surgeons in Nova Scotia, 1763–74.

Total number of surgeons in Nova Scotia during period: 31
Number of surgeons who departed Nova Scotia during period: 10
Number of surgeons who died in Nova Scotia during period: 6

It has been suggested[153] that John Day was the author, for it contains statements very similar to those made in Day's committee reports to the House, and the terminology suggests that it was written by someone with medical training.

It is clear that the great financial burden of the workhouse and the increasing number of poor people in Nova Scotia between 1763 and 1774 were important components of the crippling provincial debt. Money that had previously been used to fund the civilian hospital and to pay for its surgeon, medicines, and the salary of a provincial midwife was diverted to provide a refuge for the numerous camp followers, infirm, decrepit, insane, and the indigent. Consequently, the number of physicians and surgeons able to make a living at their profession in Nova Scotia during this period dwindled from twenty-four to fifteen. Figure 17 shows the decline, compared to the previous decade, of medical personnel in the province, as well as the small proportion of military surgeons relative to civilian surgeons. The largest group of settlers to come into Nova Scotia at the time was immigrants from Yorkshire.[154] Only one Yorkshire immigrant by the name of Stapleton was listed[155] as being in the medical profession, and it does not appear that he remained in the province.

There has been frequent mention in this chapter of idiots, lunatics, and mad persons and how they were treated, or mistreated. Arnold Chaplin has written[156] that there was "no department of medicine during the reign of George III at a lower ebb than in that of the care and treatment of the insane." As in Nova Scotia, mad people in European countries were dealt with by being securely locked up and subjected to various repressive measures such as beatings, starvation, and incarceration in dungeons or blackholes to control them. Throughout the eighteenth century, there was no serious effort to provide the mentally ill with medical treatment. Furthermore, it was not the medical profession but a number of concerned legislators who recognized that something must be done to alleviate the deplorable living conditions and brutal treatment experienced by the mentally ill. The first movement in this regard began after 1763, the year in which a report was presented in the British House of Commons on the condition of the madhouses in London. As Porter has pointed out, lunatics in the eighteenth century were mainly confined in private madhouses, and the "trade in lunacy" proved to be quite lucrative.[157] The owners of these madhouses frequently charged high fees, and had absolute control over the discipline and welfare of the inmates. It was not until 1774 that a bill was introduced and passed by the British Parliament, requiring that madhouses be inspected annually by visitors appointed by the College of Physicians. Unfortunately, conditions in madhouses did not improve, and it was not until the second decade of the nineteenth century that the teachings of Dr Philippe Pinel,[158] a French physician, began to effect a positive change in the attitudes of the public and the medical profession towards the mentally ill. It is possible, also, that the well-known attacks of insanity experienced by George III, in the latter years of his reign, invoked a degree of public empathy towards those afflicted with mental illness.

THE YEARS 1763–75 can be summed up as a period during which the health-care system declined while the provincial debt increased dramatically. The Lords of Trade gradually reduced their annual provincial grant to the point where monies for a provincial midwife, medicines, and surgeons was eliminated. Since the civilian hospital had been closed in 1759, the citizens of Halifax were left without any medical services whatsoever. The increase in the provincial debt can in large measure be attributed to the policies of the Lords of Trade, particularly their refusal to halt the influx of camp followers, indigent, and destitute people into Halifax from various places around the world. As a result, Halifax became a magnet for numerous poor people, and its workhouse and poor house became filled with transient poor. The expenditures required to support these people caused the provincial debt to rise to £23,500 by 1770 and remain at that level until the outbreak of the American Revolution.

The air is salutary for men and Beast, no Province in America is equal to it, intermitent Disorders, and glandular obstructions are here unknown, and I believe there are as few Premature Deaths in Proportion to the Numbers who pay the Debt of Nature, as in any Part of the World. It must however be allowed that sedentaries with relaxed Fibres and chronick affections, find this climate much too severe for them, but well-fed and labourious Husbandmen, preserve Health and Vigour to an extreme old age.

Figure 18
Description of Nova Scotia as a healthy place to live by an anonymous author.

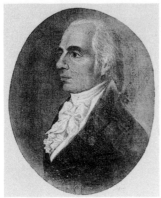

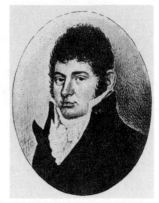

Dr Joseph Norman Bond (1758–1830) arrived in Shelburne in 1783 and later practised in Yarmouth from 1787 until his death. Portrait by unknown artist. (Yarmouth County Historical Society Museum)

Dr John Halliburton (ca.1737–1808) came to Halifax in 1782 to be surgeon at the naval hospital. He was appointed a member of Council in 1787, and practised in Halifax until his death. Portrait by unknown artist.

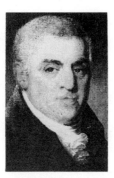

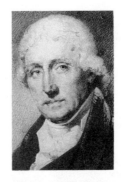

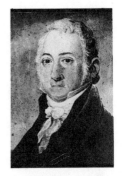

Dr William J. Almon   Dr James Boggs   Dr Joseph Prescott

Dr William James Almon (1755–1817) served with the Royal Artillery during the American War. He came to Halifax in 1783 and practised there until shortly before his death, which occurred in Bath, England, in 1817. Oil on canvas by Robert Field. (Laleah Almon, Toronto). Dr James Boggs (1740–1830) came to Port Mouton in 1783 and after spending a few years in Guysborough, settled in Halifax where he practised until his death. Artist unknown. (Dr George Bate, Saint John, and Olga Grant, Rothesay). Dr Joseph Prescott (1762–1852) was born in Nova Scotia and served in the American War as an assistant surgeon at the hospital in New York. After the war he practised in Windsor, Shelburne, Lunenburg, and Halifax, where he died. Oil on tin-plate attributed to John Weaver. (Nova Scotia Museum)

CHAPTER FOUR

A New Order
of Medical Men:
The Loyalists,
1775–1784

The skirmish at Lexington and the battle, on 19 April 1775, at Concord, Massachusetts between British troops and the minutemen[1] of
the Massachusetts Militia heralded the beginning of dramatic change
in all aspects of life in Nova Scotia, including health care. During the
next decade the population of Nova Scotia tripled, and a total of 170
physicians, surgeons, and apothecaries (55 civilian and 115 army
and navy) came into the province. By 1800, only an eighth of these
medical practitioners, twenty-one in number, were still residing in
Nova Scotia. These surgeons formed the nucleus of the province's
medical profession during the last fifteen years of the eighteenth
century. Their progeny, especially the offspring of Dr William J.
Almon and Dr Joseph N. Bond, provided a substantial part of the
leadership that regularized the practice of medicine in Nova Scotia
in the nineteenth century. Thanks to the American Revolution, the
level of health care in Nova Scotia improved significantly, for many
of these Loyalist medical personnel were highly qualified.

The American Revolution dominated every aspect of life in Nova
Scotia from 1775 to 1783. The transfer to Halifax of the headquarters of the British army in April 1776 and the influx of civilians from
Boston marked the beginning of eight years of constant movement
through Halifax of British and Hessian regiments and Royal Navy
squadrons. Ironically, the major smallpox epidemic of 1775–76 was
a major factor in the cancellation by the Americans of an invasion of
Halifax. There were numerous difficulties associated with the establishment of the various military, naval, and prison hospitals in Halifax during the war, which had also wrought havoc with the lives of
the thirty-thousand Loyalists, including fifty-five surgeons, who arrived in Nova Scotia in 1783.

The battles at Lexington and Concord were the outcome of a series of acts adopted by the British Parliament to control its colonies in North America during the previous century. The Navigation acts of 1660–63, the Sugar and Molasses acts of 1733, the Stamp Act of 1765 (repealed in 1766), and the Townshend Act of 1767 applied economic restrictions that stifled manufacturing in the colonies and placed taxes on official documents and certain commodities, all without according the colonists direct representation in the British Parliament. As a result, the colonies were alienated.

The tax on tea, in particular, created much hostility and led to the famous Boston Tea Party: on 16 December 1773, 340 chests of tea, carried by three British ships in Boston Harbour, were thrown overboard by a mob. This caused the British to close the port of Boston to trade, and gave rise, in September 1774, to the First Continental Congress in Philadelphia.

Immediately after Lexington and Concord, the repulsed British troops retreated to Boston, where they were surrounded by a force of sixteen thousand minutemen. The British force was sufficient, however, to defend Boston for the next eleven months. During this period, on 10 May 1775, the Second Continental Congress declared war on Great Britain.

During the summer of 1775, Halifax contained about 1,800 civilian inhabitants.[2] Four companies of the 65th Regiment had left Halifax for Boston on 27 April 1775, leaving three companies in garrison at Halifax, totalling only seventy-seven officers and men.[3]

On 31 July 1775, Governor Francis Legge wrote,[4] "The buildings of the Navy Yard have been set on fire, but timely discovered and extinguished ... It is certain without doubt a malicious design to destroy the yard. There remain here only thirty-six effective men ... I would propose that a Regiment of one thousand men be raised for the defence of this Province to be composed of Germans, Neutrals, and Irish, without regard to their religion. The concerns raised by Governor Legge indicated Halifax's vulnerability to attack by the rebel forces. In addition to Halifax, both Windsor and Annapolis indicated, during July 1775, that they were under threat of attack.[5] Both towns asked for a supply of arms and ammunition, as well as troops, "to apprehend any pirates from Macchias [sic] who may attack." General Thomas Gage, stationed in Boston, cognizant that Nova Scotia was unprotected from attack, ordered[6] the formation of two new regiments in early June 1775. These were the Royal Highland Emigrant (Eighty-fourth) Regiment, and the Royal Fencible Americans. The former was to consist of two battalions, one of which, under the command of Lt Col John Small, was to be raised in Nova Scotia and Newfoundland.[7] The regiment of Royal Fencible Americans was to be raised in Nova Scotia and commanded by Lt Col Joseph Gorham.[8]

The summer of 1775 was filled with apprehension and anxiety for Governor Legge and Nova Scotians in general, due both to a prevailing expectation of attack by the army of General George Washington, and to a second fearful scourge: the smallpox. It is unclear when the smallpox first appeared in Halifax during 1775, or how it was brought into the town. The first burial from St Paul's Church in which the cause of death was given as smallpox was recorded on 23 July 1775. Most of those who died of smallpox and were buried from St Paul's probably were recorded as such by the Reverend Mr Breynton, for he wrote,[9] "The Labours of my function were likewise greatly augmented by the breaking out of the Small Pox amongst us last Summer. When that Distemper (so peculiarily [sic] fatal to Americans) began to spread, I applied every effort to promote Inoculation, preached a sermon upon the occasion and raised a subscription towards Inoculating the Poor. I flatter myself I have been Instrumental in saving many lives in this Province."

Figure 19 shows the number of deaths[10] that occurred in Nova Scotia during each month for the two-year period 1775–76. Whereas prior to August 1775 the average number of deaths per month was nine, the average number from August 1775 to March 1776 was forty. Figure 19 indicates also that during the five-month period from August to December 1775, there was a total of 237 deaths in Nova Scotia, 144 of which (sixty percent) were attributed to smallpox.

On 4 July 1775, a notice appeared in the *Nova Scotia Gazette and Weekly Chronicle* proposing a method of inoculation. The anonymous author suggested that the heads of poor families who could not afford the services of a practitioner should inoculate their own family members by using the procedure described. The method began with a lengthy period of abstinence from meats, spices, wine, and all seasoned food prior to the inoculation, a "Vomit of Tarr" three days before, and calomel in a pill on the day of the inoculation. The actual inoculation consisted of creating small punctures in the skin with a "lancet dipped in variolus matter." For a number of days after, the writer advised that the inoculated person be purged with jalap, and should drink barley water sweetened with brown sugar.

Concern about the spread of smallpox prompted the House of Assembly to order preparation of a bill to prevent the spreading of contagious distempers. The bill[11] underwent a number of revisions before it received Governor Legge's assent on 17 November 1775.

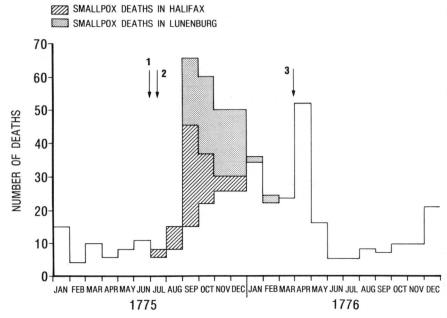

Figure 19
Total number of deaths in Nova Scotia during the period 1775–76.

1 Mention of smallpox in Halifax, 4 July 1775.
2 Bill to prevent spreading of contagious distempers passed 12 July 1775.
3 Arrival of General Howe with 12,060 civilians and military personnel from Boston
   on 2 April 1776.

Whereas an earlier act had dealt mainly with diseases brought to
Nova Scotia by ships and applied, therefore, to ports such as Halifax, Lunenburg, and Yarmouth, this act applied only to towns and
villages located outside of the town of Halifax. It directed that those
infected or recently inoculated be quarantined: "Provided that any
person or persons desirous of being Inoculated (for the Small pox)
themselves or of having their families Inoculated, may Proceed
therein, provided that the house or place wherein they dwell or reside, during the time of their being infected with Small pox shall be
at least one hundred and sixty rods distance from any other house
or dwelling ... A flag [should be] hung out at their said House, to the
End that all persons may take notice thereof and avoid, if they see
cause, going near such houses or places." Within Halifax, Dr George
Greaves was advertising[12] by August 1775 that he operated an inoculation hospital in a house in the North Suburbs. This was the first

private hospital operated in the province. Greaves's advertisement read:

The happy Effects of inoculating for the Small Pox is too well known to need any arguments to persuade a reasonable Person to prefer Inoculation, to taking this Disorder in the natural way. The Subscriber G. Greaves has made himself fully acquainted with every Improvement lately adopted by the most eminent Practitioners of this Age in said Disorder, therefore all such as choose to put themselves under the care of said Subscriber are desired to apply as soon as possible – The Charge to each Patient is Ten Shillings, being for inoculating, medicines and Attendance, through the whole course of the Disease.

Geo. Greaves

N.B. G. Greaves has a very commodious House well situated in the North Suburbs which he has furnished with Cradles and Beds, for taking in private Patients for Inoculation and a Nurse to attend at the Rate of Six Dollars each Patient received into said House, Diet to be provided at the Patients own Expense, or otherways pay One Shilling per Diem if victualled by the above Subscriber.

On 8 August, Dr John Philipps and Dr William Faries, surgeons at the naval hospital, inoculated two hundred persons against smallpox. The notice[13] describing this event indicated that the patients ranged in age from one fo fifty years, and that not one patient died as a result of the procedure. It is possible that either Philipps or Faries was author of an article, published 29 August 1775 in the *Nova Scotia Gazette and the Weekly Chronicle,* entitled "Advice and Instructions concerning inoculation addressed to the industrious poor of Halifax." The article appeared under the pseudonym G. Tiplady of the "Halifax Yard," who wrote, "I am satisfied that the smallpox is the true and genuine smallpox."

The smallpox which broke out in Halifax in late June or early July 1775 spread rapidly to other parts of Nova Scotia, including Lunenburg. Rev. Peter de la Roche, rector of St John's Anglican Church, Lunenburg, described[14] the smallpox epidemic:

The Settlement was visited in the fall of last year with a dreadful plague; I mean the Small pox, which had never been here since the settlement began ... As soon as it was spread enough to be certain that inoculation could not be charged with the further propagation of it, I gave the example and inoculated my eldest child ... But this method was not relished by the generality ... I dare say, above a thousand more have had it in the natural way, and dreadfully too; tho' but few have died (not above eighty), owing to the poor and frugal diet of the settlers their lives long and to the robust labouring people, as also to the favourable season of the year, for it happened between the heats of the summer and the beginning of winter.

The smallpox spread also to Windsor and environs, as indicated in a memorial[15] from Michael Head, surgeon of that town. Head listed the names of fifty-eight persons whom he had inoculated, and asked to be paid for his services.

On 29 August 1775, Richard Bulkeley, the provincial secretary, wrote[16] to Isaac Deschamps in Windsor, providing the following direction to prevent the spreading of the smallpox: "It should be earnestly recommended to the Magistrates and Principal Inhabitants to use their influence in prevailing on the people to enter mutually into such regulations as may prevent the small pox from being generally contiguous at this time."

As mentioned earlier, Nova Scotians not only were besieged by a smallpox epidemic but were under threat of invasion by the rebels. On 11 August 1775, General George Washington wrote[17] to the Committee of the General Court of the Massachusetts Bay indicating that he was low in ammunition and would not attempt an attack on Nova Scotia under such conditions. Colonel Thompson had proposed that one thousand men, four armed vessels, and eight transports were needed to destroy Nova Scotia: "We are lately informed that there is not to exceed two hundred British Troops in Halifax."[17] Thompson's figure of two hundred was very close to the actual figure indicated in Governor Legge's Letter[18] to the Earl of Dartmouth, written 17 October 1775: "It was given out by the rebels, that they intended a descent on this Province ... that their design was to destroy the Navy Yard here and cut off all supply of wood, hay, and provisions from the troops at Boston." Legge mentioned the two recently created regiments and the authorization of a third, which was to be called the Loyal Nova Scotia Volunteers.[19] He put his present strength at only 126 men fit for duty. Since His Majesty's Forces at Halifax were reported,[20] four days later, to number 390 soldiers, over 200 must have been sick, probably with the smallpox. The militia, which was not much trusted by Governor Legge,[21] was also rendered ineffective by the smallpox.[22]

Halifax, then, was woefully underdefended during the summer and fall of 1775. However, it was at least in part the presence of smallpox that saved the town and, indeed, the province from capture and occupation by the rebels. As a resident of New Jerusalem, Maine, described it in December 1775, "Thirteen thousand men had been embodied by the Congress to subdue Nova Scotia, and particularily Halifax, and that they were prevented from pursuing their design while the men of War lay in the Bay of Fundy, and that they believed Halifax would have been taken long since had it not been for the smallpox being there which at present deterred the Liberty Army."[23] Governor Legge confirmed this statement in a letter to the Earl of Dartmouth,[24] though according to Legge, the number of men in the attacking force was much smaller:

By persons from New England I am also informed that Congress had allotted out five thousand men for the attack on this Province, that the smallpox at Halifax and the Frigates in the Bay of Fundy had hitherto prevented them, but it was their determined intent to have this Province in their possession, or to destroy it, that it should be of no use either to the Army or Navy. A State of the King's Forces within this Province by which you will percieve that the whole number amounts to nine hundred and eighty, but by reason of sickness, new recruits and others absent, there remains no more than four hundred and forty six men fit for duty.

Because of the importance of Halifax as a naval and army base and a source of supplies for the British troops in Boston, and once Montreal had been taken[25] by the rebels on 13 November, martial law was proclaimed[26] in Nova Scotia on 30 November 1775. General Howe wrote[27] to Governor Legge on 18 December that Brigadier General Eyre Massey and the 27th Regiment had been dispatched from Ireland to defend Halifax.

The outbreak of hostilities and the subsequent raising of three provincial regiments led to an increase in the number of medical personnel in Nova Scotia from sixteen to twenty-one in 1775. William Fletcher, surgeon to the 65th Regiment of Foot from June 1770 until January 1777, was in Halifax with his regiment during that year.[28] William Faries, the assistant surgeon at the naval hospital in August 1775, had been in Halifax as early as 1772 with the 65th Regiment.[29] It is not known when Dr Faries left the 65th Regiment and became associated with the naval hospital. William Pringle, who later married a daughter of Richard Wenman, was appointed[30] surgeon's mate in the Loyal Nova Scotia Volunteers on 25 December 1775 and continued[31] in that regiment until at least January 1781. A fourth army surgeon in Halifax in 1775 was Patrick Dundon.[32] It is unclear what regiment he was with at that time, but on 23 May 1776, he was appointed[33] surgeon to the 52nd Foot, which was then stationed in Halifax after having been evacuated from Boston on 2 April 1776.

Among the first group[34] of Loyalists to arrive in Halifax in May 1775 was Dr John Prince. He and his family embarked[35] from Salem, Massachusetts, on 22 April and arrived in Halifax on 8 May

1775. Shortly after, he took the oath of allegiance, as was required of all civilians entering the province.[36] In August, Dr Prince was described as a merchant and trader at Halifax.[37] It is unlikely that he ever practised as a physician in the town, although he had practised in Salem for the previous fourteen years. Rev. Jacob Bailey recorded[38] in his journal in 1779 that Dr Prince "had acquired in the space of five years [in Halifax] a large fortune by merchandise."

Dr John Philipps was probably the most prominent surgeon in Halifax in 1775. He was surgeon and a trustee of the orphan house,[39] surgeon to the naval hospital,[40] and, as of 25 December 1775, surgeon by appointment to the Loyal Nova Scotia Volunteers.[41] In addition to the two hundred civilians that he and Dr William Faries inoculated on 1 July 1775, he inoculated nineteen children on the same day in the orphan house.[42] Dr Philipps had been in Halifax since 1758. Although not the most senior surgeon there in 1775, he was probably the most influential and well known.[43]

The year 1776 began in Halifax with a continuation of the same fears that had plagued residents in the autumn of 1775: invasion by the rebels, and the smallpox. Commodore Mariot Arbuthnot wrote[44] to Howe in January "that the Garrison [in Halifax] is not more than 500 ... but is very sickly." Later in the month, General George Washington advised[45] the Congress that "whatever may be the determination of Congress upon the subject [attack on Nova Scotia], you will please to communicate it to me immediately, for the season most favourable for the enterprise is advancing fast, and we may expect, in the Spring, that there will be more troops there, and the measure be more difficult to execute." Washington must have been further encouraged to attack after receiving an unsigned petition,[46] dated 8 February 1776, from Cumberland, Nova Scotia. The petition conveyed the sympathy of the people in northern Nova Scotia for the proposed attack on the province and the petitioners promised to fight alongside the attacking force.

During the early months of 1776, Governor Legge encountered opposition among the inhabitants of Truro, Onslow, Cumberland, Amherst, and Sackville to two acts passed in late 1775.[47] The Militia Bill[48] and the bill to raise a tax to help pay for the militia[49] were opposed universally by inhabitants in the townships. They were unwilling to leave their families unprotected and felt that they were not financially able to pay the tax. The petition of the inhabitants of Cumberland explained: "Those of us who belong to New England, being invited into the Province by Governor Lawrence's Proclamation it must be the greatest piece of cruelty and imposition for them to be subjected to march into different parts in arms against their friends and relatives."

The residents of Halifax were also fed up with Governor Legge's policies. Nineteen leading citizens, including John Prince, merchant, petitioned[50] the king, George III, on 2 January 1776, to the effect that they, as Loyalists, had quit their possessions in the colonies now in revolt and had sought refuge in Nova Scotia, where they were being treated by Governor Legge in an abusive and discouraging way.

General Sir William Howe was aware of the internal strife in the province. This, combined with the fact that he was surrounded by the rebel army and unable to obtain an adequate supply of provisions for his men in Boston, caused him to evacuate Boston and to move his headquarters to Halifax. He outlined his plans to the Earl of Dartmouth:[51]

Halifax, tho' stripped of provisions during the winter, and affording few conveniences to so numerous a Body, is the only Place where the Army can remain until supplies arrive from Europe. My first attention will be paid to the Defences of the Town, and His Majesty's Dockyard, and to enable Governor Legge to overcome the spirit of Disaffection which has lately appeared in the northern parts of Nova Scotia, after which I conclude that three Battalions, with Goreham's and Maclean's Corps will be a sufficient force for its Protection.

A document[52] recording the "State of the Regiments, Officers included, at Boston" on the day of the evacuation indicated that General Howe had under his command a total of nineteen Regiments of Foot, the 17th Light Dragoons, the Royal Artillery, and two battalions of marines, totalling 8,906 army personnel. These troops, as well as 1,124 civilians in the town of Boston and environs[53] and approximately 2,030 women and children of the army,[54] 12,060 people in all, were evacuated from Boston in seventy-eight ships and several smaller vessels on 17 March 1776.[55] Two of the ships, the *Richmond* and the *Two Brothers*, carried the hospital.[56] This armada was escorted on its passage from Boston to Halifax by a Royal Navy squadron under the command of Rear Admiral Molyneux Shuldham, whose squadron consisted of fourteen ships.[57]

The medical personnel evacuated with the civilians from Boston were William Brattle, physician; Peter Oliver, physician; William Coffin, apothecary; Sylvester Gardiner, physician; John Jeffries, physician; Nathaniel Perkins, physician; William Lee Perkins, physician; and Bartholomew Sullivan, doctor. Of these eight civilian doctors, only two, Brattle[58] and Jeffries,[59] remained in Halifax for longer than a few months. The other six were in Halifax during the summer of 1776, but left[60] the province in the late summer and fall for England and New York. Howe wrote[61] to Germain, in April 1776, that many of the principal former residents of Boston who were now under the protection of the army in Halifax had no means of subsistance and were eager to find passage to Europe, Rev. Mather Byles, one of the Boston evacuees, described his predicament[62] on May 1776:

I had not the least suspicion that the Army would ever have evacuated Boston. That astonishing event has now taken place and the Retreat has been so sudden and precipitate, that it has totally ruined multitudes who thought themselves perfectly secure in the British Protection. Of that number I am one, not being allowed to bring away furniture, or anything that I possessed, but a couple of beds, with such articles as might be contained in a few trunks and boxes. I now see myself an exile for some time from my native country, pent up in one wretched chamber in a strange place, together with my five motherless children, deprived of every other earthly enjoyment, and entirely at a loss as to my future Residence and Subsistence.

It is estimated that, in addition to the twenty-one medical personnel in Nova Scotia prior to the arrival of General Howe's armada, and the eight civilian doctors listed above, there were approximately sixty surgeons and surgeons's mates with the nineteen regiments which arrived in Halifax on 30 and 31 March 1776.[63] There would also have been fourteen naval surgeons in Admiral Shuldham's squadron, one per ship. The total number of medical personnel in Nova Scotia in April 1776 was, therefore, in the order of one hundred.

Sometime prior to 24 May 1776, Dr John Jeffries was appointed surgeon to a hospital, located on George's Island, that had been established shortly after the arrival of the troops from Boston. This hospital was in addition to the general military hospital located on Blowers Street (Figure 15) and was established to quarantine soldiers with the smallpox.[64] Jeffries was assisted by two surgeon's mates, a Mr Goldthwaite[65] and a Mr Morehead.[66] The hospital was probably discontinued some time after Howe's army left Halifax for New York on 10 June.

James Dickson had come to Halifax with Rear Admiral Shuldham's squadron on 2 April 1776 and, twelve days later, was referred to as surgeon and agent on board the *Richmond* hospital ship.[67] Later in the month, he was described as surgeon of the *Chatham*, Admiral Shuldham's flagship, and appointed[68] to replace Mr Charles White as surgeon and agent for the care of the sick and hurt belonging to His Majesty's Ships in Halifax harbour. On 28 May and again on 7 June, James Dickson signed a report indicating he was treating patients on the *Two Brothers* hospital ship.[69] According to Commodore Arbuthnot,[70] Dickson left with Admiral Shuldham for New York on 10 June 1776. Arbuthnot described the wretched condition of the hospital facilities for navy personnel in Halifax:

The Hospital my Lord is another Distress that I am deficient in Language to express my feelings about. Provisions are at this place, and the Circumstances of the Place such, that no part of the Orders of the Commissrs of Sick and Hurt have been able to have been complied with: thay have conceived that the inhabitants of the Place would have received them and that the Surgeon would have lodged and boarded them for fifteen pence a day: no person is to be found that will receive those people, neither can a proper place be procured to make an Hospital of, without hiring an old house, and put in repair at the Kings Expence perhaps about 150 Pounds, not that at present do I know of such a one: but if some Care is not taken before the Winter, very disagreeable will be the Lot of those poor People who may be put sick on shore: The Commissrs of the Sick presuming that Boston would be the place where the greatest part of those Men would remain sent the Surgeon to that place & thought little of this the Contrary is the fact for when the Fleet sailed from hence last, Mr Dickson of the Hospital Ship, put all his miserable Objects on shore to us to be taken care of and if a place could have been found, we should not have had fewer that [*sic*] One hundred since here I have been; this I have represented to Admiral Shuldham & now beg your Lordships Excuse for this long detail.

General Sir William Howe and Admiral Molyneux Shuldham left Halifax for New York, with 140 vessels and 8,000 troops, on 10 June 1776.[71] General Washington was advised[72] of Howe's departure from Halifax and that nearly twelve hundred sick personnel had been left behind in Halifax. Shortly after Howe's departure, Commodore William Hotham arrived in Halifax with thirteen transports carrying a regiment of Hessians and two companies of the Guards.[73] The Hessians were part of the first division of Hessian troops, consisting of 7,800 men, under the command of Lieutenant General De Heister. Sir George Collier and five men-of-war escorted the force to America, having left Shiphead on 20 May. This armada consisted of ninety-two sail, eighty-six of which were transports.[74] Their destination was New York, but because of foul weather, ships were dispersed and Hotham's thirteen transports put into Halifax. The Hessian troops and the Guards arrived in New York from Halifax on 15 August 1776. With the addition of the Hessians, the Guards, and the 42nd and 71st Highland regiments, which had arrived in Halifax on 8 June, General Howe's army consisted of 23,000 effective men.[75]

At the Council meeting of 3 June 1776, Lieutenant Governor Arbuthnot told the councillors[76] that "a considerable number of women and children amounting to 2,030 persons are to be left in Halifax on the embarkation of the Army." By 27 June, General Massey informed[77] Germain that "the wives and children of soldiers are [to be] sent with the invalids to England." He mentioned that this would greatly relieve the distresses of the vast number of women and children left behind by the army. This was not carried out, however, since on 6 October, Massey wrote[78] that "all of the women and children of the Army are still in Halifax and almost naked." Presumably, a number of these women and children would be taken into the poor house kept by John Woodin[79] and given medical attention by Dr Thomas Reeve.[80]

In addition to the hospital operated by Dr John Jeffries on George's Island and the two hospital ships mentioned earlier, there were at least four other hospitals in Nova Scotia in 1776, two in Halifax, one in Windsor, and one in Liverpool. Major Gilfred Studholme, major of brigade, wrote to Major General Massey from Windsor on 6 November 1776, describing Fort Edward as containing a barracks that could lodge six officers and 150 men. The fort contained also a hospital that could hold twenty-six patients.[81] George Frederick Boyd, who had been appointed surgeon to the Second Battalion, Royal Highland Emigrants on 8 May, was probably surgeon at the Fort Edward Hospital.[82]

In January 1776, an inoculation hospital had been established in Liverpool, where smallpox had broken out. A number of Liverpool residents were inoculated, but it appears that the procedure itself caused the disease in some of these people. As a result, "the people meet concerning the smallpox and generally sign an agreement not to be inoculated."[83] The smallpox was also a cause of conflict in Horton. In June 1776, Andrew Davidson and John Bishop were found guilty[84] of "Introducing the smallpox to this Town contrary to a law of this Province." Both Bishop and Davidson "acknowledged they did inoculate their family, but pleaded they did not understand the law."

The general hospital (Figure 15) must have been very busy during and after General Howe's two-month stay in Halifax. If, as General Washington had been informed, Howe did leave twelve hundred sick soldiers at Halifax upon his departure on 10 June 1776, they would have been under treatment in the general hospital. Dr John Jeffries was surgeon there[85] by 16 December 1776 and remained in that important position, as well as becoming purveyor to the hospital, until early 1779.

It was mentioned earlier that on 12 December 1775, Dr John Philipps had been appointed[86] surgeon of the naval hospital. Its exact location at that date is not known; however, sometime in late 1776 or early 1777, the hospital was moved to George's Island. It is quite possible that the quarantine hospital on George's Island, operated, by Dr John Jeffries in May 1776, became the site of the naval hospital referred to here. The first mention of the naval hospital being located on George's Island is found in the journal of Sir George Collier.[87]

It was in about 2 Months after that He [General Massey] took the strange Resolution of turning all the sick seamen from off George's Island (abreast of the Town) where the Naval Hospital was under Pretence of fortifying it; had I been as mad as himself I could by Force have prevented this inhuman Measure from being executed, but a Civil War of this kind woud [sic] have been as blameable as new; the poor sick Seamen were accordingly turnd off the Island and carried ashore below the Town in a heavy Rain – some of these unhappy Men were at the point of Death, others with Fevers and various other Disorders; there are amongst them some whose Wounds were still open and dangerous; Wounds they had received in the Service of their Country, fighting like brave men; their Treatment however from this frantic madman was the same with the rest, all were indiscriminately forcd into the Boats, and landed in heavy Rain in wh[ich] they remained 24 Hours before any Shelter coud [sic] be found by the Surgeons for them ... I ordered a Man of War to get ready to sail for New York, in order to lay the affair before Lord Howe and the General, and request that either this absurd Bedlamite or myself might be recalld.

The account of this incident by the surgeon in charge of the naval hospital, James Dickson, appeared in the *Nova Scotia Gazette and Weekly Chronicle* of 6 October 1778. Dickson had apparently returned to Halifax from New York sometime prior to 15 May 1777, possibly with Sir George Collier in September 1776, and had taken over from John Philipps as surgeon in charge of the naval hospital, He wrote:

Naval Hospital on George's Island
May 16th, 1777.

Sir,

Yesterday about 12 o'Clock after I had visited the Hospital and gone on board the *Rainbow* with eight recover'd Men, that I had discharged from the Hospital, Major Lyons, Town Major, Lieut Needham, and Mr Hill, Surgeon to the Marines, went to the King's Naval Hospital on George's Island with two Boats, and in consequence of Orders from General Massey, ordered every Man, (be their State of Health ever so infirm and weak), that could possibly walk, into their Boats, and landed them during a heavy Shower of Rain at the ... gun Battery, and there left them to [fend] for themselves ...

I am very apprehensive from the Condition I know the Healths many of them are in, that this cruel Treatment must be fatal to them, as it was not in my Power to provide any Place to receive them, and the constant Rain all day yesterday and all last Night, must make their remaining ever since in the streets very dangerous.

I had a Message deliver'd to me by the Steward of the Hospital, that if the Storehouses were not clear'd in three or four Days, that the Medicines, Instruments, Bedding, and other Stores shoud be turn'd out into the Streets by the General's Orders, and that Sir George might gather them up.

I must beg you will please to direct what is to be done with these sick People who are wandering now about the Streets, as I have endeavor'd tho' without succeeding to find a place, to shelter them from the Inclemency of the Weather.

I am, Sir,
Your most Humble Servant,
James Dickson.

On his Majesty's Service,
    To Sir George Collier.

As a result of the confrontation between Sir George Collier and Major General Massey, the naval hospital was returned to George's Island; on 29 May 1777, James Dickson was described as the hospital's surgeon, at that location.[88] Later, in October and December 1777, John Scott was referred to as a surgeon at the naval hospital.[89]

The incident of the forced removal of patients from the naval hospital on George's Island followed an earlier bizarre but little-known fracas between Collier and Massey, which occurred in Halifax in early November 1776. One of Collier's ships had been sent with provisions for some of Massey's soldiers stationed at Fort Cumberland. Because of inclement weather, the ship did not complete its mission. General Massey was enraged. As Collier wrote:[90]

He swore. He cursed and behaved like a frantick Mad Man, blaming the Capt. of the Man of War for not arriving at the Port He was bound to, tho' Massey knew no more of sea Matters than a Savage of the Woods. He behaved too with personal rudeness to the Capt. when He went to wait upon Him, which the other came to complain of to me, I mentioned it afterwards in a gentle manner to Massey reminding Him that Sea officers were only accountable to me for their Conduct.

I took care however his neglect shoud [*sic*] be remedied and his Garrison supplyd and we rubbd on a little longer with the appearance of being upon tolerable terms, however He took occasion to be offended at something or other (I really have forgot what it was) but He sent his Aide de Camp Capt. Wade to desire me to meet Him the next Morning with Pistols behind the Citadel Hill – I must with shame acknowledge his Folly made me so angry that I consented to meet Him, and went at the app[ointe]d time accompanied by Capt. [Andrew] Barkley – the Genl and Capt. Wade joined us as we were going to the Ground the 2 Seconds lamented that so slight a misunderstanding shoud [*sic*] have brot [*sic*] us into the Field, and wishd Matters might proceed no further – I own I saw the Impropriety of it, and the fatal consequences which must follow from the 2 Chief Officers of Navy and Army going out to fight at a time, when we were surrounded by Enemies of our Country – I made this Observation to Genl Massey and told Him I flattered myself from wh[at] He saw That He would not ascribe the motive of what I was going to say since I was ready to give him satisfaction if He desired it, but that I thought certain Ruin must attend whoever survived, as his Maj[est]y would certainly never pass over so great an Injury offered to his Service and must naturally conclude both Parties undeserving to command who coud [*sic*] behave so very improperly. I added that I was not in the least conscious of having given Him offence, or at least not intended, and advised Him to reflect for a few minutes before He took his Resolution in saying which I left Him by himself and walked 20 yards backward and forward with the 2 seconds. When I rejoined Him he appeared irresolute and undetermined. I repeated what I had said and He replyd that he woud [*sic*] not make any Ansr [*sic*] till the Lt Governor had given his Opinion upon it –

We all four accordingly walked to the Lt Govrs and I let Massey tell [th]e Story his own way, the Govr blamd him and was rejoicd to have the Termination left to his decision, He instantly obligd us to shake Hands, and promise to remain Friends for the future; this Reconciliation on my part was truly sincere, on Masseys I fear it never was as the sequel shewd.

The "sequel" was the removal of patients from the naval hospital on George's Island. Collier's statement about being "surrounded by Enemies" was indeed true, for General Howe sent him to Halifax to provide extra protection to "our very important settlement." Lieutenant Governor Mariot Arbuthnot had received word on 13 August 1776 that the rebels of New England were proposing to invade Nova Scotia.[91] Lord George Germain, in a letter[92] from Whitehall dated 11 December 1777, referred to the rivalry between Collier and Massey and indicated concern over its possible effect on the success of a rebel invasion. It appears, however, that the duel between Collier and Massey was not made known to the secretary of state for the colonial department, since no mention of it appears in the state papers.

Compared to 1775 and 1776, very little happened in Nova Scotia in 1777, either from a military or a medical standpoint. No new regiment or naval squadron arrived in Halifax, nor does it appear that any new doctors arrived in the province.

Dr Thomas Reeve, the last remaining of the thirty-six medical personnel who arrived with Edward Cornwallis in 1749, died in late July 1777.[93] He had been a surgeon in Halifax during the first twenty-eight years of its existence and, during the 1750s, had also been an apothecary and surgeon's mate at the civilian hospital.[94] Sometime during Governor Wilmot's administration, Dr Reeve was appointed[95] "to take under his care, the sick in the Workhouse of the Town of Halifax." He continued to act in that capacity until shortly before his death, submitting a bill on 21 June 1777 for attending sick poor persons.[96]

A doctor by the name of Parker Clark, who had been resident in the province since at least 1770,[97] had been among the followers of Jonathan Eddy who, in November 1776, in company with rebels from Machias, had attacked and almost captured Fort Cumberland.[98] They were prevented by the timely arrival, on 26 November, of marines from Halifax and of soldiers belonging to the Royal Highland Emigrants from Windsor.[99] Dr Clark was among those arrested two days later. He was brought to Halifax, along with Richard John Uniacke, stood trial on 18 April 1777, and was found guilty of treason.[100] His sentence of execution was "respited," or temporarily delayed. Dr Clark must have escaped, or been pardoned, since in 1785 he was granted[101] land at Eddington, Maine. He died at Ipswich, Massachusetts, on 19 September 1798, aged 80.[102]

One of the prisoners taken by Jonathan Eddy's rebel forces before they were dispersed by the troops from Halifax and Windsor was Dr Walter Cullen. He was a surgeon's mate of the Royal Fencible Americans, having been commissioned in that regiment on 2 May 1776.[103] By late December 1776, Dr Cullen was reportedly[104] held prisoner in New England. He remained there until shortly after 12 January 1778, when he was part of a prisoner exchange.[105] Replacing Dr Cullen at Fort Cumberland was James Silver, a surgeon of Marines,[106] who is recorded as having treated one Mr Samuel Wethered, who had been hit by a cannon ball from the garrison of Fort Cumberland during the rebel attack in November 1776. For services rendered, Silver was paid fifty pounds from Wethered's estate.[107]

The decisive battle at Saratoga on 17 October 1777 caused Lieutenant Governor Arbuthnot to write[108] to Lord George Germain about his concern for the defence of Nova Scotia. He pointed out that he presently had a force of only a thousand men (six hundred Marines and four hundred Highlanders) to defend Halifax and guard the four hundred rebel prisoners held in the town. He requested that arrangements be made to remove the rebel prisoners. The officer commanding the army in Halifax in November 1777, Major General Eyre Massey, wrote[109] a pessimistic letter to his superior, General Howe, in which he commented on Burgoyne's misfortune and predicted an imminent invasion of Halifax by the rebel army.

There was a significant epidemic of smallpox in Nova Scotia during 1777, particularly among the army and the rebel prisoners. Captain Alexander McDonald of the Second Battalion of the Royal Highland Emigrants wrote[110] on 6 May: "You will be very likely surprised at the Expence of the hospital but I can declare to you upon honor that I have paid every farthing of it & can produce vouchers for the same we had above an hundred men sick all winter & almost lost as many." A second mention of sickness in that year appears in General Massey's letter to Lord Germain, dated 22 July 1777: "I have now 400 rebel prisoners and more daily brought in by men-of-war, above 180 of them sick, I may say dying. The care of the prisoners with the detachment now in service makes me very weak, but such troops as I have fear no enemy as I am well supported by good officers."

E.D. Poole, in *Annals of Yarmouth and Barrington, Nova Scotia, in the Revolutionary War*,[111] printed orders, dated 25 March 1777, sent by John Hall Sr of Granville to his son John Hall Jr, who was commanding a small schooner bound for Halifax with cider and potatoes. The postscript of his father's letter read, "You are to give the American prisoners at Hallefax [sic] 20 or 30 Bushel of potatoes at your arrival thare as I hear they are Kept Vary, Vary Short." John Hall Jr had Zachariah Foot carry the potatoes on board the guardships that housed the prisoners in Halifax harbour, and Foot wrote, on 10 May, that he did so because "Mr Hall's son had not [yet had] the small pox." This statement suggests that John Hall Jr and Zachariah Foot had been informed that the smallpox existed among the prisoners on the guardships, and Foot went on board because of some degree of immunity which he had developed due to a previous encounter with the disease.

In August and September 1777, Dr John Jeffries recorded in his diary,[112] "I inoculated 127 Rebel Prisoners of all ages ... all of them recovered of the small pox." Jeffries had two methods of inoculation: he "used a lancet moistened with the pus, and made two or three scratches with the infected lancet," or he "used a bit of thread laid on an incision." The thread was contaminated with pus taken from a patient diagnosed as having the smallpox.

Between July and September 1777, a Boston newspaper, the *New England Chronicle*, reported the deaths of sixty persons from the frigates *Hancock* and *Boston* who were prisoners of war at Halifax. In the paper's view, these people had died of "starvation."

A further mention of sickness in 1777 appears in Simeon Perkins's diary,[113] in which he records on 26 August that a resident of Liverpool had recently returned from Halifax and described the prisoners there as being sick with smallpox and yellow fever. This is the first mention of yellow fever in Nova Scotia. Yellow fever is caused by a virus transmitted by mosquito bite and is characterized by haemorrhage, jaundice, and vomiting.

In another regard, Captain Alexander McDonald mentioned in a letter of 11 June 1777 that his wife would soon be in need of a midwife. He asked Donald McLean to send [to Halifax] "one of the best midwives in New York."[114] This suggested that Halifax was then without a midwife, or that Halifax midwives were unacceptable to McDonald and his wife. A midwife by the name of Ann, wife of William Scott, had been buried from St Paul's on 17 April 1776. She was fifty-six years of age and had resided in Halifax since at least December 1763.[115] There would have been numerous midwives throughout Nova Scotia at the time, but only two have come to light. One was a Mrs Harris of Horton, who is recorded as providing midwifery services in the Falmouth area in January and February of 1776.[116] The other was Mrs Elizabeth Doane of Barrington, described[117] as having "filled an important niche in the scattered fishing settlement. There was no physician, and being skilled in the use of roots and herbs, and in nursing, she was soon acting as nurse, doctor, and midwife."

As early as February 1778, Lord George Germain had indicated[118] to Lieutenant Governor Arbuthnot that "a reinforcement consisting of 2,500 men is proposed to be sent out in the spring to Nova Scotia." The first regiment designated was the 70th Regiment of Foot, which, on 10 February 1778, consisted of 677 men (including officers), sixty women, and twelve servants.[119] The other two regiments were designated on 21 March 1778, when General Sir Henry Clinton, Howe's successor as commander-in-chief, was sent secret instructions[120] from Whitehall stating that the newly raised regiments, consisting of 2,700 men commanded by Colonels McLean and Campbell, were preparing to sail from Glasgow for Halifax. The three regiments were to be accompanied by a number of medical personnel, including a new staff for the general military hospital. On 16 April 1778, fifty tons of hospitals stores, a surgeon, an apothecary, and four hospital mates were ordered [121] for the hospital at Halifax and directed to be transported to Nova Scotia on the *Dunmore*. [122] Prior to their arrival, Dr John Jeffries and two mates provided the medical services at the general hospital. [123] Dr Jeffries, according to General Massey, [124] "has taken unusu'l pains in the Execution of his Duty here, had all the soldiers' wives and children of the Army under his care, and by my orders inoculated above 500 children, since which he had all the Rebel prisoners under his care with yellow fever and horrid Disorders, I think he merits the attention of your Excellency as he was promis'd to be provided for by General Howe."

The three regiments – the 70th Foot, the 74th (known as the Argyle Highlanders), and the 82nd (the Duke of Hamilton Regiment) – arrived in Halifax on 12 August, [125] along with the new staff of the general hospital, all in good health. The hospital staff consisted of John Marshall, surgeon; Peter Bernard, apothecary; James Kay(e), hospital mate; John Crawford, hospital mate; William Digby Lawlor, hospital mate; and James Bowman, hospital mate. [126] John Jeffries, initially part of the hospital's new establishment, held the position of purveyor. The purveyor was, essentially, the hospital's administrator, and Jeffries was paid twenty shillings per diem, as compared to ten shillings per diem paid to the surgeon, John Marshall. Sir Henry Clinton disapproved [127] of Dr Jeffries's appointment "on account of a Garrison Establishment being sent out from England which was thought sufficient for that place," and directed Brig. Gen. Francis McLean to eliminate the position of purveyor.

On 5 November 1778, Lord Barrington conveyed to Lord Germain [128] the concerns of Dr John Marshall, surgeon at Halifax, over the conditions of the rebel gaol and hospital. [129] Marshall had earlier written to Dr Robert Adair, inspector of regimental infirmaries for the British army, that "herrings salted up in casks [would] best convey some idea of the situation of the prisoners. Deaths are extremely frequent." [130] Germain directed Lieutenant Governor Richard Hughes and Brigadier General McLean [131] to alleviate the suffering of the prisoners and to prevent the fever and disorder from spreading to British soldiers:

I have received a letter from Lord Barrington inclosing an extract of a letter from Mr Marshall, surgeon to the Garrison at Halifax, relative to the mode in which the Rebel Jail and Hospital are conducted there, which seems not only to be prejudical to the Health of the prisoners, but also to that of His Majesty's Troops to whom they are contiguous. I am to acquaint you as is his Majesty's Pleasure that Lord Barrington should give directions by the first conveyance to the proper officers upon the Staff to take care that the Rebel Prisoners may no longer be liable to Diseases which a want of space and air and cleanliness must necessarily occasion, and I have received His Majesty's command to instruct you to concur and co-operate as far as lies in your power to keep the healthy persons separate from the sick, and to give every degree of attention to remove the grievance complained of.

And with respect to the Regulations which would probably prevent His Majesty's Troops from suffering the evil which they were exposed to from the proximity of the Rebels, the General Hospital Orders are given to the proper Department at Halifax, to substitute Regimental Hospitals in room of a general one.

The decision to decentralize the hospital facilities in Halifax had been transmitted[132] on 5 November 1778 by Lord Barrington to Brigadier General McLean: the "General Hospital at Halifax is contrary to His Majesty's Intentions." And Dr Robert Adair had directed[133] John Marshall that "no general hospital is to be formed."

A second large contingent of soldiers arrived in Halifax between 15–18 November: Lieutenant Colonel de Seitz's Regiment of Hessians and the King's Orange Rangers.[134] The Hessian Regiment remained in Halifax during the next year, but one detachment of the King's Orange Rangers was dispatched to protect the town of Liverpool.[135] There had been in Halifax a small detachment of Brunswick Troops, prior to the arrival of the Hessians, and it was ordered to spend the winter at Lunenburg under the command of Lieutenant Colonel Von Specht. Included in the Brunswick detachment were four surgeons, but I have been unable to identify them.[136] At its meeting of 18 November 1778, Council dealt with the problem of where to house the Hessian regiment and resolved[137] that they be quartered in barns, outhouses, and public houses in the North Suburbs of Halifax.

Very little is known about the activities of the civilian surgeons residing in Halifax and elsewhere in Nova Scotia during 1778. John Philipps continued to provide medical attention to the children of the orphan house and to sundry indigent sick and diseased persons in the gaol.[138] Dr Edward Wyer,[139] who probably arrived in Halifax in 1777, succeeded Dr Thomas Reeve in July 1777 as surgeon to the poor house. Wyer submitted an account of £90 in June 1778 for his attendance and medicines for the poor, sick, and hurt persons of the province who had no legal settlement.[140]

A third doctor who had practised as a physician and surgeon in Halifax,[141] but who had spent most of his twenty-six years in Nova Scotia as a member of the Anglican clergy, was the Reverend Thomas Wood, who died on 14 December 1778. The inscription of his headstone in the Old Parish Burying Ground at Annapolis Royal indicates that, between 1752–78, he was a major figure in the religious, cultural, and literary life of Nova Scotia:

Rev. Thomas Wood,
Born in New Jersey,
Physician and Surgeon
Ordained 1749. From 1752 a Missionary of the S.P.G. in Nova Scotia. Ministered in English, French, German, and Micmac. First visited this Town 1753.
Assigned to the Townships of Annapolis and Granville.
Lived there laying the Foundation of the present Parishes from 1764 to his death Dec 14, 1778 aged [illegible].
Divine blessing crowned his apostolic zeal, posterity reveres his memory.

Although yellow fever, not the smallpox, was stated as the sickness among rebel prisoners in the general military hospital in September 1778, the smallpox was rampant throughout parts of Nova Scotia during that year. At least two people in Cornwallis Township, King's County, requested that they be exempted from jury duty because of their fear of contracting the disease. Robert Kinsman wrote[142] that he had never had the smallpox, and, since it was so common throughout Horton and Cornwallis, he asked to be excused from this duty because he feared he would contract the disease from persons in the courtroom.

In May 1779, the naval hospital on George's Island, which two years earlier had been temporarily abandoned by Major General Eyre Massey's orders, was transferred to a building located on the Halifax waterfront. Brig. Gen. Francis McLean wrote[143] that, "as the position of George's Island constitutes the Principal Defences of this Harbour, Forces very Desirous of Garrisoning and putting it into the necessary state of Defence which I could not do while it remained occupied as a Naval Hospital accordingly represented the necessity of removing the sick to the Officer Commanding the Navy here, who readily consented to it and gave the necessary directions immediately."

The building that housed the naval hospital on the Halifax waterfront was described[144] by Lieutenant Governor Sir Andrew Snape Hamond in August 1781: "I was particularly struck with the miser-

able accommodation which this place affords to such sick and wounded
seamen as are so unfortunate to be sent here for cure. There are at
present 107 patients in what is called the Hospital, a great part of
which number inhabit a decayed storehouse built upon piles in the
water which has scarce a roof and a floor to it ... It is located between
the dockyard and the Town surounded [sic] by rum shops."

The decision to construct defensive works on George's Island was
prompted by news that Nova Scotia was under threat of attack by the
rebels.[145] Brig. Gen. Francis McLean of the 82nd Regiment, officer
commanding the British army at Halifax, was ordered to lead a
force to Penobscot to oppose there an attack by the rebel army. Mc-
Lean left Halifax on 12 June 1779 with 640 soldiers, 440 of whom
were of the 74th, and 200 from the 82nd Regiment.[146] With the departure of McLean, Halifax was defended by approximately 1,500
soldiers,[147] consisting of the 70th Regiment, a Hessian regiment,
and a detachment of Brunswick Troops that had returned to Halifax from Lunenburg[148] in April 1779.

THREE DIFFERENT PATENT MEDICINES[149] were advertised for sale in
Halifax during 1779: Keyser's Pills, Maredants Drops, and Sal
Salutis. Keyser's Pills had first been advertised in the *Nova Scotia
Gazette and Weekly Chronicle* in September 1773. In February 1779, an
advertisement from the store of George Townsend and Company,
also in the *Gazette*, described the well-known efficacy of the pills in
curing venereal disease in a "secret manner." In May 1779, the
printer of the *Gazette*, Anthony Henry, advertised that he had for
sale a few bottles of Maredants Drops, which, as the paper reported
later, were invented by Mr Norton, surgeon, of London.

The third patent medicine was advertised by Thomas Brown in
the *Gazette* in August 1779. Brown's advertisement not only outlined
the attributes of Sal Salutis but gave an opinion of existing, but unidentified, competitive medicines. Brown stated that he had

lately received from England for Sale, the Genuine and much approved SAL
SALUTIS; or SALT OF HEALTH. A Medicine which upon an accurate knowledge of its composition and experience of its salutary effects, can be safely
pronounced to be competent to the cure of most disorders incident to human
life.

It has been objected to many Medicines given to the Public, that though they
have, in some cases, performed surprising Cures, their effects have been, at
other times, violent and dangerous; insomuch that numbers are deterred

from taking them, on account of the risque, and others never take them but in desperate cases, when their constitutions are so far gone as to induce them to run the hazard of every thing that has the appearance of success. This danger does by no means apply to the SAL SALUTIS, or SALT of HEALTH, as it operates in no sudden, extraordinary manner; but rather as an alternative, by its attendant and saline powers; and makes the stomach so much a Physician of what it will bear, that the quantity can be increased or diminished, without the least risque or danger.

In short, without entering into a Physical Analysis of all the properties of this Salt, let it suffice to say, that as the preservation and restoration of health form the greatest blessing of Life, and that both form a chymical process of this Salt, as well as the most repeated and confirmed experience of its effects, it is recommended as one of those beneficent dispensations of Providence, which, in its various bounties, it has been graciously pleased to bestow upon mankind.

DISORDERS for which this Salt is particularly a Medicine.

For the JAUNDICE, and all BILIOUS CASES,
LEPROSY, SCURVY, KING'S EVIL, &c.,
MALIGNANT SCURVY,
HECTIC FEVERS, CONSUMPTIVE WEAKNESSES,
   and universally decayed HABITS OF CONSTITUTION.
FRESH COLDS, RHEUMATISM, &c.,
FEMALE WEAKNESSES, &c.,
DRY GRIPS and CONSTIPATIONS of the BOWELS,
STRANGURY HEAT, and DIFFICULTY of MAKING URINE,
OUTWARD ULCERS, and ULCERATED LEGS,
SEA SCURVY, YELLOW FEVER, Yaws, and other Disorders, incident to MARINERS, as well as all those who reside in WARM CLIMATES.
If it was necessary, abundance of Cures by this Salt, might here [be] added to prove the superior virtue and usefulness of this innocent and bountious [sic] gift of nature.

The first advertisement of drugs and medicines in the province from outside of Halifax was placed in the *Gazette* by Michael Head, surgeon, of Windsor, also in August 1779.

An extensive regimen was carried out by Dr Jesse Rice[150] in his treatment, in April 1779, of Simeon Perkins's daughter: "Doctor [Jesse] Rice, of Yarmouth comes to my House, & prescribes for my Daughter Nabby, having an eruption on the skin, occasioned by two great Quantity of salts in the Blood. He has ordered Flower of Sulphur, & Magnesia Alba, equal parts, to be given every night, a tea spoon full, if that is Ineffectual, then to give her Creamor Tartar, & Othips Mineral, one third more Creamor Tartar than of the Othips Mineral, – half a Tea Spoon full."

Another type of advertisement related to health care, which appeared for the first time in a Nova Scotia newspaper in 1779, sought a "wet nurse." Because of poor diet as well as illness, mothers frequently were unable to nurse their newborn. Beginning in 1779 and continuing as late as 1821, the *Gazette* and other Halifax newspapers[151] carried advertisements requesting the services of wet nurses and advertisements from anonymous young women offering their services as such. The first advertisement for a wet nurse appeared in the *Gazette* in June 1779. It sought a woman with "a good breast of milk" to come and live with a family in Halifax. Numerous advertisements were submitted by young women who probably had great difficulty finding employment of any type. For example: "A Young Woman with a good Breast of Milk, would be glad to take a child to suckle, or go out into a family. Enquire of the Printer."[152]

Dr Edward Wyer performed the first lithotomy recorded in Halifax, on 16 July 1780. His successful removal of a stone from the bladder of the son of Capt. Richard Tritton was described, two days later, in the *Nova Scotia Gazette and Weekly Chronicle*. This operation had become very common by 1745, the year that the Company of Surgeons of London was formed. Zachery Cope, the historian of its successor, the Royal College of Surgeons of England, writes,[153] "Stone in the bladder was common and the operation for its extraction by perineal incision (lithotomy) was frequently performed. Since it had to be done on the conscious patient, whose movements were controlled by strong attendants, speed of performance was desirable. Cheselden often performed the operation in two minutes, and in favourable circumstances sometimes extracted the stone from the bladder in less than a minute."

The first indication that the thermometer was being used to diagnose patients in Halifax appeared in the *Nova Scotia Gazette and Weekly Chronicle* of 4 January 1780.[154] Gabriel Fahrenheit (1686–1736) is said to have invented the mercury-in-glass thermometer in 1714. However, use of the thermometer in clinical applications did not begin until 1758, when Anton de Haen (1704–96) of Vienna first employed[155] it as a diagnostic aid.

Patent medicine were advertised[156] in America as early as 1708 and, during the 1750s and 1760s, became very popular in the thirteen colonies. Newspaper advertisements for such medicines were very common. An English list of patent medicines published in 1748 numbered two hundred and two proprietary medicines, many of which found their way to the American colonies. "Americans dosed themselves with galenicals and chymicals, and swallowed complicated concoctions containing disgusting ingredients in their efforts to drive away the ills that attacked them. These ills were many. Respiratory ailments, dysenteries, and malaria were the chronic diseases taking the greater toll year in and year out than did the more feared smallpox and yellow fever, which occasionally struck with epidemic force."[157] After the two Continental Congresses, held in September 1774 and May 1775, all exports from Great Britain to the American colonies, except Nova Scotia, were halted, including patent medicines. Although medicines such as Keyser's Pills and Sal Salutis had been advertised in Nova Scotia prior to 1780, it was not until that year that the *Nova Scotia Gazette and Weekly Chronicle* began regularly to include in its pages long lists of patent-medicine advertisements. The issues of 4 January and 2 May 1780 advertised various nostrums.[158]: essence of peppermint, Maredants Drops, Dr Bateman's Pectoral Drops, Jesuit's Drops, Dr Hooper's Female Pills, Dr Anderson's Scots Pills, Lockyer's Pills, Stoughton's Elixir, Daffy's Elixir, Dr Bostock's Elixir, Dr Radcliffe's Strengthening Elixir, Dr Frauncess's Strengthening Elixir, Godfrey's General Cordial, Fryar's Balsam, Bateman's Golden and Plain Scurvy Grass, and Ladies Court Plaisters. Of these, Dr Anderson's Scots Pills and Daffy's Elixir had been in existence since the middle of the seventeenth century, while Dr Bateman's Pectoral Drops were patented in 1726 and Dr Hooper's Female Pills in 1748. The secret composition of these medicines was guarded by their proprietors, but in some cases, they did state that their medicines contained "twenty-two ingredients," or "twenty-six botanicals, some from the Orient and some from the English countryside." Some patent medicines were marketed under a number of different names for the same concoction.[159] Daffy's Elixir, for example, was listed in the *Pharmacopoeia Londonensis* in 1721 under the title "Elixir Salutis" and, later, in the *Pharmacopoeia Edinburghensis* as "Compound Senna Tincture."

Other interesting advertisements appeared in the *Gazette* during 1780. Someone using the pseudonym "Doctor Rare" advertised[160] a cure for the gout:

The following receipt for the gout is exactly transcribed from a very ancient Dutch Author, which I wish to be published in your paper, for the benefit of such as are subject to the honourable Malady.

for the GOUT

Take an ould Fat Goose, prepare her as if you would roast her. Then take a kitten or young cat, flea it, cast away the head and entrails thereof, and contund [?] the flesh thereof in a Mortar, add as then thereto fat bakone One ounce, three quarters of an Ounce of Wax, as much Rosine, and whyte Frankinsence; beat all these together, and replenish therewith the Goose; broach her, and sow [sic] her fast to the spit least any thing fall thereout; roast her, and receive the droppings thereof in a dripping pan; when as now the Goose is dressed and roasted that she droppeth no more, throw her as then away, least any body eat thereof. And this Salve or Unctione cureth the Gout.   Doctor Rare.

The first advertisement by a person offering veterinary services to the public of Halifax appeared in October 1780:[161]

This is to inform the Public, a person in town will undertake to cure (no Purchase no Pay) any of the following Diseases in Horses, viz: Canker in the Mouth, Blindness by having the Poll Evil, Fistula upon the Weathers, Slip Shoulder'd, Stiffle, Mangy Face, Ring Bone, Splinter Bone, Spavin, Blood Spavin, Canker in the Feet, Strain in the Lines, Strangles, Cropping, Docking, Nicking, Grease Malanders, Quitets, Founder'd, or any other disease incident to Horses. Those Gentlemen who may be inclin'd to favor him with their Commands are requested to apply at Mr Dougherty's, Blacksmith and Farrier, opposite the House of Malachy Salter, Esq., at the Entrance of Irish Town.

Even though Dr James Lind had, as early as 1753, alerted[162] the Admiralty about the importance of citrus fruits and their juices in preventing scurvy, the disease was still causing death and suffering among thousands of naval personnel as late as 1780. The first advertisement indicating the availability of lemon juice for sale in Halifax appeared in May of that year in the *Gazette*. The juice sold for four shillings a bottle.

WITH RESPECT TO THE POOR HOUSE AT HALIFAX, a very detailed set of records exists for the period 31 May 1779 to 30 September 1780.[163] Nathaniel Russell had succeeded John Woodin as keeper and master of the poor house in September 1778, and from 9 September 1778 to 31 May 1779, he was paid £315 for maintaining several poor, sick, lame, blind, and lunatic persons who had no legal settlement in the province.[164] During the succeeding fifteen months from June 1779 to September 1780, a total of seventy people (fifty-three men and eighteen women) were cared for in the poor house, ten of whom died there.

The monthly returns indicate that the number of poor-house inmates varied from a high[165] of thirty-seven in September 1780 to a low of thirteen in October 1779. The cost of maintaining them varied from £24 9s. to a high a £36 3s. per month. This money was spent for "fire, candles, poultices, gruels, wines, etc." In addition to the maintenance cost of £480, Dr Edward Wyer was paid £81 for his attendance and medicines for poor persons,[166] and Robert Collins, mason, was paid £71 for repairs he had made to various public buildings, including the poor house, during 1779.[167]

Although a Hessian regiment had arrived[168] in Halifax in November 1778 and would have had a regimental hospital established soon afterwards, notice of the Hessian hospital did not appear until 30 January 1781. According to the *Nova Scotia Gazette and Weekly Chronicle* of that date, it was located "in the street leading to the new Great Barrack." The new Great Barrack, probably the South Barracks, was under construction[169] as early as 1778 at the south end of Albemarle Street. It was probably under the supervision of either Dr J.C. Helmerich[170] or Dr J.F.T. Gschwind,[171] both of whom are known to have been in Halifax in 1781.

The only new hospital established in Halifax during 1779 and 1780 was one for the reception of rebels and other prisoners. John Marshall, surgeon, mentioned[172] in May 1780 that he had not been paid for attendance and medicines "for the reception of Rebel and other prisoners" for the last six months. It is likely that, after Lord George Germain ordered[173] Brigadier General McLean in November 1778 to substitute regimental hospitals for the general military hospital, a separate hospital for rebel prisoners was established in an attempt to reduce the spread of disease. Where this hospital was located is not known, though on 17 January 1782, reference was made to a prison hospital "opposite to and at a small distance from the Naval Hospital with a narrow and much frequented street or road between them."[174]

Sir Andrew Snape Hamond, who was sworn in as lieutenant governor of Nova Scotia on 31 July 1781, inspected the naval hospital in August and described it as "a decayed storehouse built upon piles in the water [and] which has scarce a roof or floor to it."[175] He recommended to the commissioners of the Sick and Hurt Board that a new hospital be built to accommodate 150 to 200 patients and that £2,500 be allocated for its construction and furniture. Seven days later, before he had received authorization to build a new naval hospital, Sir Andrew directed[176] George Thomas, naval storekeeper at Halifax, to pay William Gorham and his wife Mary £128 for the land on which to build it. Hamond reiterated the need for a new hospital in a letter[177] to Rear Admiral Samuel Graves:

I beg leave to acquaint you that the condition the seamen are in here for want of proper accommodation, when sent on shore sick or wounded for cure, is so very wretched, that, in my opinion, it is absolutely necessary something should instantly be done for their relief. An old rotten store built up on the waters edge and with scarce floor or roof to it is the present Hospital, nor can any better Quarters be hired, so crowded is the Town at this time with inhabitants. I have written to the Admiralty representing the necessity that an Hospital should be built and if you are pleased to give your sanction to that measure I will set about erecting a building immediately. I purpose that it be of wood.

On 20 December 1781, Hamond wrote to Rear Admiral Robert Digby:[178]

The present hospital has been patched up for the winter and put in as good condition as possible. The accommodation for the men however is still miserable, yet for this wretched place Government pays an annual rent of £150 stirling. The situation I propose for the new Hospital is a Field of about 3 acres leading down to the waters side immediately above the dockyard ... The plan of this intended Building I have the Honour to enclose, and I am informed by the Master Shipwright and other intelligent people that the expence will not exceed £3,000. As it is absolutely necessary for the workman to have the winter before them, in which season only they can provide the materials, I have for a month past advertized to have proposals given in for erecting the work, but as yet no tender has been made me, nor has anything else been done than merely the purchasing and planning out the ground.

Sir Andrew's advertisement appeared in the *Gazette* on 11 December 1781: "Whereas a Naval Hospital is intended to be built early in the Spring in the Field above Mr [John] Butler's Stil-house; notice is hereby given, that Sir Andrew Hamond will be ready to receive Proposals at his Office in the Dock-Yard, from any Persons willing to contract for erecting the Building, (a Plan of which may be seen at the Storekeeper's Office) or he will engage with any Person who will undertake to furnish a certain Number of House Carpenters to be employed under the direction of the Builder." Sir Andrew had received authorization[179] to build the new naval hospital from Rear Admiral Digby sometime prior to 1 January 1782. By 7 January, he had awarded the tender for building the hospital.[180]

James Dickson was the principal surgeon at the naval hospital as well as surgeon to the sick prisoners of war.[181] His assistant, Dr William Faries, who had been in Halifax since 1772, died in February 1781.[182] John Handasyde[183] replaced Dr Faries on 4 August 1781.[184] He and James Dickson cared for patients in both the naval and the prison hospitals, which were adjacent to each other. Prisoners who were not considered to be in need of medical attention were kept on a prison ship, the *Stanislaus*,[185] which had been anchored in Halifax harbour since 10 August. The *Stanislaus* was inspected by John Loader, the master shipwright, for its suitability for use as a prison ship,[186] and Loader was instructed by Sir Andrew to renovate it for prisoners.[187] On 29 August, prisoners were transferred to the *Stanislaus* from various temporary facilities in Halifax.[188] Sir Andrew had also planned to hire a ship to serve as a prison hospital and wrote[189] to the board of the Hospital for Sick and Hurt Seamen that as a temporary measure, he had fitted up an old storehouse "on the Banks of the River" to house sick prisoners. This old storehouse was quite likely the prison hospital mentioned earlier, on the water's edge near the naval hospital. In October, Sir Andrew reported that there were seventeen French and twenty-four rebels sick at the prison hospital, while there were five hundred and ten Americans and ninety-five French prisoners on the *Stanislaus* prison ship.[190]

THE SMALLPOX WAS REPORTED IN LIVERPOOL in the summer and in Halifax by the fall of 1781. Simeon Perkins, the diarist of Liverpool, recorded the presence of the disease in July and later referred to a child being moved to the "smallpox house" in Liverpool on 5 September 1781.[191] This house, back in the woods from Birch Point, belonged to Thomas Brown. Doctor Morehead had recommended to the overseers of the poor for Liverpool that John Doggett, who had the smallpox, be moved to that house on 29 July. Doggett died there eight days later, on 6 August.

Another Thomas Brown, who resided in Halifax, wrote[192] in September in answer to an enquiry from the Reverend Jacob Bailey of Cornwallis: "You ask how it happens that the Small Pox is so prevalent in Halifax – I answer that it chiefly operates on Infants whom our Gentlemen of the faculty did not choose to try their skill upon till the summer was nearly past – indeed several adults, new comers, have been inoculated.

In April 1781 John Marshall, surgeon of the general military hospital of the garrison, had represented[193] to Brigadier General Camp-

bell, who had replaced Francis McLean,[194] "the danger the troops
incur of becoming infected with the smallpox and other diseases by
having sick naval Prisoners of war sent to the said Hospital for cure:
And whereas in order to obviate the inconveniences which it is apprehended might thereby arise, and because His Majesty's Naval
Hospital is more contiguous to the Prison Ship and much more conveniently situated for the reception of such Prisoners than the said
General Hospital, I have thought proper to place their care under
your direction."

There is no evidence to indicate how serious the smallpox outbreak was in either Halifax or Liverpool. It may have been, however,
that Richard Wenman, who by then had managed the orphan house
in Halifax for almost thirty years and was buried from St Paul's on
30 September, died of the dreaded disease. He was succeeded by
Samuel Albro,[195] who was described by Mr Jonathan Binney, one of
the persons appointed to assess applicants for the position of keeper
of the orphan house, as "the first person fit for that trust." Another
person[196] who died late in August 1781 in Halifax, possibly of the
smallpox, was Dr George Francheville, who had been a resident of
Halifax since 1751. He had been a surgeon of Ordnance, served at
Fort Cumberland during the siege of Beauséjour, and, before offering his services as a civilian surgeon in Halifax, had been a surgeon
of the Royal Artillery.

A Dr John Harris had arrived in Nova Scotia from Philadelphia in
June 1767 and resided at Pictou until 1777, when he removed to
Truro.[197] He became an object of suspicion to the authorities in November 1781, thanks to his brother Matthew Harris of the township
of Pictou, whom the provincial secretary had been instructed[198] to
arrest and bring to Halifax on grounds of treasonable activities. Former lieutenant governor Michael Francklin, who had issued the instruction, added that "the Doctor of Cobequid" had also given
indications that he favoured the rebel cause. There is no evidence
that Dr Harris, who had been elected the member of the House of
Assembly for Truro Township in a by-election in June 1781, was
ever charged with treason.

James Dickson, who had been the principal surgeon of the naval
hospital since 1777, died on 13 January 1782.[199] John Handasyde,
his assistant since August 1781, was appointed[200] surgeon to His
Majesty's Naval Yard at Halifax on 1 January 1782. On 14 January,
Hamond informed[201] Rear Admiral Digby that he had appointed
Handasyde principal surgeon and agent of the naval hospital, "until
your pleasure is known." Rear Admiral Digby, however, had in mind

someone else, and on 9 March 1782, appointed Mr John Halliburton instead.[202]

Halliburton had joined the Royal Navy[203] as a surgeon's mate in
May 1758 and quite likely visited[204] Halifax briefly while he was surgeon to a navy ship in 1763. He is known to have practised in Newport, Rhode Island, where he was in charge of a naval hospital from
January 1773[205] until at least November 1778.[206] Dr Halliburton
escaped to New York on 2 February 1782, after having supplied
Sir Henry Clinton with information about the rebel and French
Forces occupying Rhode Island. In recognition of his intelligence-
gathering services, carried out under great danger to himself and
his family, Halliburton was later given the option of being in charge
of the hospital in New York or in Halifax.[207] On 12 April 1782, he
accepted the position as principal surgeon and agent of the naval
hospital at Halifax and continued to serve in that capacity for the
next 25 years.[208]

On 1 January 1782, John Loader, the master shipwright who had
inspected the *Stanislaus* for its suitability for use as a prison ship, was
appointed[209] to superintend the building of the new naval hospital,
and Mr William Lee, the building contractor, began to gather materials for construction.[210] Later in January, the artificers and labourers belonging to the Naval Yard, some of whom were probably helping to build the hospital, entered into an agreement to have four
pence per month deducted from their pay so that, should they require it, Mr Handasyde could provide them with medical attendance.[211] This is one of the earliest examples of a medical insurance
agreement in Canada.

On 24 April 1782, the Admiralty finally sent Sir Andrew authorization to build the naval hospital, and the navy board sent along a
plan for construction.[212] By 16 May, Hamond wrote that "the Hospital building is now in such a forward position that the frame will be
erected next month."[213] Alexander Thomson, Esq., the purveyor of
the hospital, was directed in August to buy bathing tubs for the hospital:[214] "The surgeon of His Majesty's Naval Hospital at this Port
[is] representing that men are frequently landed from Ships of War
in a very unclean condition and their skins foul and dirty."

On 23 September, bedding and chests of medicines were sent to
the new naval hospital[215] and, on 13 November, it was announced[216]
that the hospital "will be ready to receive patients by Christmas." The
hospital establishment included: one head surgeon (John Halliburton); one purveyor (Alexander Thomson); one dispenser and assistant surgeon (John Handasyde) at a hundred pounds a year; one

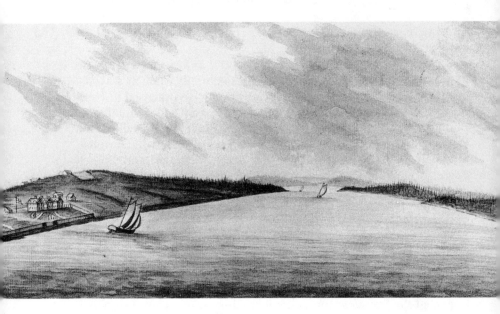

Figure 20
"The Hospital and Entrance of Bedford Basin," by James S. Meres. A pen-and-ink drawing measuring 161 cm by 363 cm, done from the *Pegasus* in October 1786. The original is in the Log Book of the *Pegasus*. (National Archives of Canada, C-2555)

additional surgeon's mate (Richard Wood) at five shillings per day for every additional fifty patients; one matron and head nurse (Jane Kennedy) at twenty shillings per week; one nurse for every ten to twenty men, at five shillings per week; one cook; one porter; and two labourers.[217] A pen-and-ink drawing of the new naval hospital (Figure 20) was done in October 1786 by J.S. Meres, who was on the *Pegasus*.[218] The drawing shows a fine structure that was later described[219] as "the glory of architecture in Halifax." The plan of the Naval Yard (Figure 21), drawn by Charles Blaskowitz in 1784, locates the new hospital north of the Yard near the narrows leading into Bedford Basin.

The old naval hospital was advertised for sale in the *Nova Scotia Gazette and Weekly Chronicle* on 26 November 1782: "To be sold, a large house with lot 50 feet in front and 250 feet deep, picketed in. Situated in the North Suburbs of Halifax leading to the Careening Yard now let to Dr Haliburton for the use of the Government as a Hospital at a rent of £50 per annum, being a compleat [*sic*] Estate and capable of great improvement. For further particulars apply to William Slater, merchant in Halifax."

Another hospital, referred to as the Red Hospital, was advertised for sale a month later in a December issue of the *Gazette*; it was described as a large house leading to the Careening Yard. The Red Hospital was located very close to the water's edge, as described in a petition[220] from Samuel Sparrow, in which he asked for a water lot "opposite to the Red Hospital." This hospital could have been used as the prison hospital, or it could have been used as one of the many regimental hospitals that had existed in Halifax since the outbreak of the American Revolution in 1775. In any event, the Red Hospital dated from at least 1766, for in July of that year, Francis Elliot was granted a license to occupy the beach between the Red Hospital and Mr William Fury's lot to the north of Barnard Wharf.[221] Also, the *Gazette* of 24 July 1769 advertised "a house for sale situated on the beach near the red hospital."

THE *STANISLAUS* PRISON SHIP caused much concern among Halifax's civilian, military, and naval population during January 1782. On 12 January, Lewis Davis, surgeon of the King's Rangers, wrote[222] to Doctor John Marshall:

Permit me to acquaint you that lately I have had a great number of sick that exceeding the number of sixty which I entirely impute to the contagious putridity which reigns on board the Stanislaus Prison Ship. Every week one or

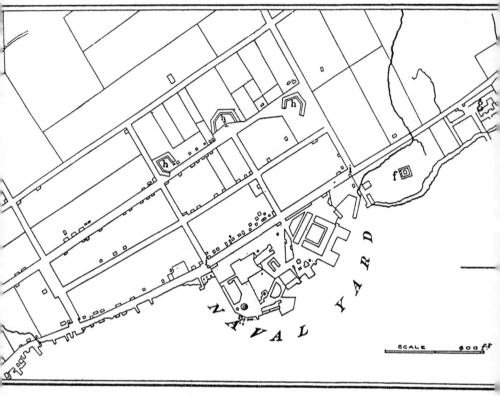

Figure 21
Plan of the Naval Yard, Halifax, drawn from the original prepared by Captain
Charles Blaskowitz in 1784. The original is held by the Public Archives of Nova
Scotia. The plan presented here appears on the inside front cover of the
Collections of the Nova Scotia Historical Society, vol. 13. The Naval Hospital (letter g)
appears in the upper right corner of the plan.

two of those men (or little party) we have on Board as guards are brought to my Hospital senseless.

Permit me to request your being so obliging as to represent this matter to Brigadier General Campbell and to point out to him the necessity there is of withdrawing the aforesaid Guard from that Ship, as it is my sincere opinion that the Garrison otherwise might be greatly injured by it.

The next day, Davis was examined before a board of surgeons appointed by garrison orders to enquire into the matter and report.[223] Davis called the disease on the *Stanislaus* "Jail Fever." He explained that the guard party consisted of seventeen men and that they stayed on the prison ship for a week. As many as thirty of his men were sick at one time. Several died. Davis described the symptoms of the disease: "A shivering headache, delirium, tremor of the hands and tongue. Sudden prostration of strength, a white or parched tongue, blackness of the roots of the Teeth. A Remarkable offensive breath and livid lips. The skin was a dirty yellow hue before death." The report of the hospital staff and regimental surgeons[224] concluded that jail fever had found its way into some of the regimental hospitals. It recommended that the guard should be withdrawn from the *Stanislaus*, the prisoners sent away, and the ship laid up or destroyed. The report described the *Stanislaus* as being "improperly ventilated and filled with stums [?] from foul and diseased bodies." The guard was withdrawn and, when weather permitted, the prison ship was put under the scrutiny of a guard vessel[225] that was anchored nearby, "agreeable to what I understand is the practice at New York."

Doctor John Philipps was directed by Council in January 1782 to attend the King's Troops, who were thought to have a malignant putrid fever. He declared it to be an inflammation pleurisy of which, at that point, only one person had died.[226] The *Gazette* noted on 22 January, and again on 29 January, that the rumour that a malignant putrid fever was gaining ground in the town was without foundation. It is unclear whether the fever was epidemic among the civilian population.

On 13 May, Hamond wrote to Brigadier General Campbell[227] that "directions have been given for moving the Prison Ship and Guard Vessel to a situation between the Eastern Battery and St George's Island for the convenience of the two Corps you have appointed alternately to take in charge the security of the Prisoners." In an attempt to convince the officers and surgeons of the army in Halifax that the *Stanislaus* was, in fact, free of epidemic diseases, Sir Andrew directed the surgeon of the naval hospital and the surgeons on three ships in the harbour to inspect it on 19 July 1782.[228] They reported favourably that the prisoners were being treated well and that no epidemic disease was found.

On 23 September 1782, Sir Andrew Snape Hamond wrote in a letter[229] to Major General Paterson, commander of His Majesty's Forces in Nova Scotia, that he felt a guard should be mounted immediately on the prison ship to prevent further escape of naval prisoners. The letter implied that Dr Marshall felt otherwise, presumably because of the danger of contracting infectious disease. Hamond requested that Paterson "order a guard to do duty on board the Prison Ship." The *Stanislaus* continued as a prison ship in Halifax harbour until at least 13 December 1782,[230] though in October, 232 of its prisoners were dispatched to Boston on the *Albany*[231]

It appears that fever did indeed exist among the troops in Halifax. In the fall of 1782, Dr William Paine was sent from New York to Halifax by Sir Guy Carleton,[232] "in consequence of a malignant Fever then raging amongst the Troops at Halifax." He commenced duty as physician to His Majesty's hospitals in North America in October, stationed at the general hospital at Halifax.

Dr Paine was born in Worcester, Massachusetts, on 5 June 1750 (o.s.), graduated in arts from Harvard in 1768, was awarded an MD by Marischal College, Aberdeen, in 1774, and qualified[233] as a licentiate of the Royal College of Physicians (LRCP) of London in 1781. At the time of his arrival in Nova Scotia, Dr Paine was the most highly qualified medical doctor to have practised in the province, for he was the first to have both the MD and the LRCP qualifications. He remained in Halifax until June 1784, when he removed his family to Passamaquoddy.[234] Although he had been banished from Massachusetts, he was accepted back into his home town in 1789, where he lived and practised until his death in 1833.

THE AMERICAN WAR OF INDEPENDENCE in effect came to a close with the defeat of General Earl Cornwallis[235] at Yorktown, Virginia, on 19 October 1781. The combined strength of American and French troops on land and the French fleet at sea were too much for the besieged British forces.[236] Many months passed before a treaty of peace could be concluded between the United States and Great Britain and it was not until a year after the Battle of Yorktown that the first Loyalist refugees began to leave the United States for the British colonies to the north.

Although the majority of Loyalists arrived in Nova Scotia in 1783, two separate groups came in late 1782: three hundred refugees arrived at Annapolis Royal from New York in October,[237] and in December, a further five hundred and one arrived in Halifax from Charlestown, North Carolina.[238] It was recorded in the Council minutes of 16 December[239] that a considerable number of refugees from the colonies in rebellion had arrived from Rhode Island and South Carolina, with many more to follow.

As noted earlier, approximately thirty thousand persons arrived in Nova Scotia from New York and other parts of the American colonies, during the period May to December 1783. By October 1783, a total of 20,880 civilians and 8,400 disbanded soldiers had been transported, primarily from New York, to five settlements[240] in Nova Scotia: Saint John (14, 162); Port Roseway (8,896); Digby (2,530); Halifax (928); and Cumberland (493). These figures show that approximately half the Loyalist refugees and disabled soldiers settled in Saint John and vicinity. This significant population led, in July 1784, to the creation of the province of New Brunswick.[241]

Listed in Appendix 5 are the names of fifty-two Loyalist surgeons who came to Nova Scotia in 1783. Seven of them – Joseph Falt, George Holland, John Hoose, Andrew Seidler, John C. Sieger, Johannes Skener, and John F.T. Stickells – had been in the German service and therefore had not resided previously in the American colonies. The remaining forty-five, possibly excepting Dr Joseph N. Bond, were practising or serving in the American colonies before the outbreak of hostilities in April 1775.

On 15 July 1783, Royal Assent had been given to an act of the British Parliament[242] setting up a Loyalist Claims Commission. Claims were to be submitted in London by 25 March 1784, but it was not until 2 March 1784 that the *Nova Scotia Gazette and Weekly Chronicle* printed the act and brought it to the notice of Nova Scotian Loyalists. Specifically, it was an "Act for appointing Commissioners to inquire into the Losses and Services of all such persons who have suffered in their Rights, Properties, and Professions, during the late unhappy dissentions in America, in consequences of their Loyalty to His Majesty, and attachment to the British Government." Over two thousand claims were received under this first act, and 1,700 under the second act, which was passed in 1785. Among the 3,700 claimants were eighty-one doctors, a surgeon's mate, a dentist, two medical students, and a midwife.[243] As noted in Appendix 5, only seventeen of the fifty medical personnel who arrived in Nova Scotia in 1783 made claims that have survived. It is likely that most of the others did not own property or have a practise in the thirteen colonies prior to, or during, the war. Of the Loyalist physicians and surgeons who came into Nova Scotia between 1775 and 1782, nine submitted claims. A summary of the claims for loss of property, loss of income per year, sum allowed by the commissioners, and pensions awarded to these twenty-six physicians and surgeons appears in Appendix 6. A comparison of the averages for the four categories with those of all other claimants indicates that Loyalist physicians and surgeons had not been better off financially than farmers or tradesmen.

The claims for loss of income and of real and personal property submitted by some of these surgeons provide a vivid illustration of the terrible disruptions of war. A.C. Leiby writes[244] about Dr James Van Buren, who settled, after the war, in Granville Township:

Dr James Van Buren of Hackensack had once been an ostensible neutral. Evidently a lukewarm adherent of the conferentie [?] church, he had once seemed moderately favourable to the American cause, and when the beaten American troops retreated from Fort Lee he was asked by Washington himself to treat the sick and wounded, which he did with every evidence of zeal. When the British seized Hackensack, he set up a hospital for the 26th Regiment stationed there, an act which in itself was laudable enough. Where the British were concerned, however, he did not stop at medical care, he went along as a guide for British General Grant on some of his expeditions from Hackensack and, as has been said, was imprisoned by the Americans for doing so. He was, however, soon released, and returned to Hackensack, apparently confident that he held the friendship of Whig and Tory alike. For the next two years he studiously avoided quarrels with his patriot neighbors, insisting that he had helped General Grant only as necessity required. This pretence ended once and for all in October 1778. When Cornwallis and Grey returned to New York, James Van Buren went with them.

Isaac Goodman, who eventually settled in Conway Township, near Digby, wrote[245] in his claim, that he "went to America in 1774. He went to Rhode Island to settle as a surgeon. The Americans wanted him to go into their Army and because he refused it they put him into prison. When Sir Henry Clinton came there he was made a surgeon to an Hessian Regiment. He was wounded in an Engagement on Green's farm but he is not lame." Peter Huggeford, who later practised in Saint John and Digby for a few years before returning to New York, received similar treatment[246] from the rebels. "He was taken violently from his family in 1776 by the rebels and kept in prison for seven months before he escaped. The rebels sent his wife and eight children from their home and his real estate and personal estate was confiscated."

The arrival of so many disbanded soldiers in Nova Scotia during the later part of 1783 led to severe difficulties for the overseers of the poor, particularly in Halifax. They submitted to the governor and to Brigadier General Campbell a memorial[247] "for assistance in looking after the many disbanded soldiers who nightly are packed up on the streets in a perishing state and sent to the Poor House afflicted with various disorders. Governor Parr was informed that in addition to the disbanded soldiers,[248] "a number of orphan children, mostly of soldiers, having remained in the Poor House in the city [New York], who would probably be left destitute on the removal of the King's Troops from hence, I have directed them to be sent to Halifax, and to be bound as apprentices to the Rev. Mr Breynton ... They amount to 13 boys and 1 girl." At a meeting of the House of Assembly in October 1783, a member reported[249] further that

there are some infirm and helpless soldiers (or men that have been soldiers) left in an Hospital lately belonging to the Military and that they are in a perishing condition. It was resolved to wait on the Governor and represent to him the state of the suffering sick and discharged soldiers who are in the different Regimental Hospitals ... Article II [in the Report of the Committee appointed by the House of Assembly for the Examination of the State of the Public Accounts] was read and it was resolved that the money expended for the support of the Poor for the last 15 months past is an enormous sum, and that it be recommended to the House to appoint a Committee to draw up a plan for the better regulation of the Poor House in the future."

The *Gazette* of 14 October 1783 confirmed the dilemma of the poor, stating that they "suffered very much [during] the last year."

As mentioned earlier, Dr William Paine was, in 1783, director of all hospitals for the British army in Halifax. In February 1783, Paine received directions[250] from Dr J.M. Nooth, the superintendent general of hospitals for the forces in North America and the West Indies. It read:

An order was sometime since sent to Halifax to discontinue the General Hospital there, as it was supposed that the sick of the Garrison could be properly accommodated in the Regimental Hospitals. It was at the same time ordered by the War Office that Mr Marshall, surgeon, and Mr Bernard, Apothecary, should remain at Halifax to give their advice whenever it might be wanted in the Garrison, and that the Hospital stores should be kept there, under the care of the apothecary to be in readiness to furnish a General Hospital whenever the Exigencies of the service might require it.

For some years therefore no General Hospital has been kept open at Halifax and till the late arrival of the Recruits [1,964 German officers and men who arrived[251] in Halifax on 13 July 1782], it was by no means thought necessary ... You as senior officer, will have the control and Direction in all Hospital matters ... No General Hospital therefore is to be established at Halifax, unless the service shall render it indespensibly [*sic*] necessary.

You are therefore to take care that proper houses be procured for the sick and wounded and that these Hospitals be furnished by a person appointed as acting Purveyor for that purpose.

Two days after Dr Nooth sent this letter, Sir Guy Carleton wrote[252] to Major General Paterson: "The appointment of a Purveyor of the Hospital at Halifax has been already disapproved of by Sir Henry Clinton, and cannot be allowed. As Mr Marshall is not satisfied with his situation, you will let him return to Europe by the first opportunity. Mr [James] Kay, and Mr [Walter] Cullen, who are Regimental Surgeons, are also paid as Hospital Mates. If so, you will discontinue them and reduce them to their Regimental Pay and duty. If the two mates sent from the Hospital here [New York] are not sufficient, you shall have more."

On 17 June 1783, the War Office informed Carleton[253] that the medical establishment for Nova Scotia and Newfoundland would be limited, after 24 June, to one surgeon at ten shillings per day, and three hospital mates at seven shillings and six pence per day. It was directed that Mr Marshall be offered the appointment as surgeon. On 27 August, Carleton wrote[254] that Dr John Marshall had gone home and that Donald McIntyre,[255] one of the assistant surgeons, had been appointed surgeon of the hospital at the request of Major General Campbell. Carleton also recommended that the medical establishment be augmented because of the multitude of refugees who had arrived in Nova Scotia.

Four months after these reductions at the army hospitals had taken place, the Admiralty directed[256] that the naval hospital at Halifax be reduced to a peacetime establishment on 31 December 1783. Dr John Halliburton continued as surgeon and agent of the naval hospital.

The Careening Yard, or dockyard, had its own surgeon in 1783 in the person of George Rutherford. He had been surgeon to the prison hospital in New York and took up his appointment as surgeon to the dockyard[257] sometime before October 1783. His request to return to England was granted in November 1783 and his successor at the dockyard was Dr Duncan Clark, formerly of the 82nd Regiment, who remained in the post until as late as October 1785.[258]

THE FIRST RECORDED MEASLES EPIDEMIC in Nova Scotia broke out in Halifax, Liverpool and probably elsewhere during the summer and fall of 1783. On 17 June 1783, the *Gazette* carried a detailed front-page description of measles, its cause, symptoms, regimen, and treatment. The anonymous author of this article recommended that decoctions of liquorice, with marshmallow roots, sarsaparilla, and infusions of linseed, be taken as a drink, in addition to bleeding and vomiting, to treat the disease. Further advice included the administration of syrup of poppies to children who develop a troublesome cough while afflicted with measles, and a daily ride on horseback for adults who continued to have a cough after the measles subsided. On 25 July 1783, Simeon Perkins recorded in his diary[259] that measles had broken out in Liverpool; in October, two of Hallet Collins's children died of the disease.

Another item of medical interest that appreared, in 1783, for the first time in the records of Nova Scotia was a "Receipt for the bite of a Mad Dog." It followed a newspaper account of the distressing death of a three-year-old boy in New Haven, Connecticut, who had been bitten by a mad dog.[260] The prescription read:

Take of the leaves of rue picked from the stalks and bruised six ounces; garlick picked clean and bruised six ounces: venice treacle, or mithridate, and scrapings of pewter, of each four ounces. Boil all over a slow fire, in two quarts of strong ale, until one pint is consumed. Strain it, and keep it in a bottle close stopped and give of it nine spoonfuls warm to the person seven mornings successively – Six spoonfuls will cure a dog, and nine days after the bite apply some of the ingredients to the wound – Ten or twelve spoonfuls may be given to a horse or bullock, and from three to five to a sheep or hog.

Between 19 April 1775 and 31 December 1783, a total of 170 physicians and surgeons arrived in Nova Scotia. Fifty-five were civilian doctors, while 115 were surgeons to regiments, naval or military hospitals, or to ships of the Royal Navy. In addition to the fifty-two physicians and surgeons who came in 1783 (Appendix 5), five civilian surgeons arrived during the period 1775–82 (see Table 4) were still residing in the province at the end of 1783, as were twelve other surgeons who accompanied various regiments to Halifax during the American Revolution (Table 5).

All in all, sixty-six physicians and surgeons had come to Nova Scotia during the revolution and were still in the province at the end of

Table 4
Civilian Surgeons Who Came to Nova Scotia in 1775–82

Year of Arrival	Physician/Surgeon	Previous Home	Settled in
1775	John Prince	Massachusetts	Halifax
1776	Edward Wyer	England	Halifax
1779	Jesse Rice	Massachusetts	Yarmouth
1782	William Baxter	Connecticut	Cornwallis

Sources: For Prince, see Minutes of Council, 4 August 1775 (PANS RG1, 189:303); for Wyer, see Valuation of Real Estate Within the County of Halifax, 1775–76 (PANS RG1, vol. 411); for Rice, see Memorial of Sundry Settlers in the Township of Yarmouth, 30 June 1783 (PANS RG1, vol. 223, Document 5); for Baxter, see King's County Deeds (PANS RG47, 1:400).

Table 5
Regimental Surgeons Who Came to Halifax during the American Revolution

Year of Arrival	Physician/Surgeon	Regiment/Ship	Settled in
1776	George F. Boyd	Eighty-fourth	Windsor
1776	Walter Cullen	Fencibles	Halifax
1778	Duncan Clark[261]	Eighty-second	Halifax
1778	John Fraser[262]	Orange Rangers	Windsor
1778	James Kay	Seventieth	Windsor
1779	John Bolman	Hessian	Lunenburg
1781	Lewis Davis	King's Rangers	Halifax
1781	John F.T. Gschwind	Hessian	Halifax
1782	Frederick L. Bohme	Waldeck	Clements
1782	John Halliburton	Naval Hospital	Halifax
1782	William Paine	Army Hospital	Halifax
1782	Stephen Thomas[263]	Orange Rangers	Liverpool

Sources: For Boyd, see Drew, Roll of Commissioned Officers; for Cullen, see Massey to Germain, 20 December 1776 (PANS CO217, vol. 53, Document 13); for Bolman, see Petition of John Bolman for compensation for medical services given at Lunenburg, 1779–80 (PANS RG1, 531:25); for Kay, see Establishment for the General Hospital at Halifax, 24 November 1778 (PANS RG1, vol. 368, Document 58); for Davis, see St Paul's Anglican Church Marriages, Davis to Margaret Hurd, 31 October 1781 (PANS MG4); for Gschwind, see Halifax Supreme Court Records (PANS RG39, series C, Box 25); for Bohme, see Muster Roll of Discharged Officers and Discharged Soldiers and Loyalists at Bear River, 26 June 1784 (PANS RG1, vol. 376); for Haliburton, see Petition of John Halliburton, 9 June 1807 (PANS Adm. 1/497); for Paine, see Second Report, 803, Archives of the Province of Ontario.

1783. By 1800, only nineteen (twenty-nine percent) were still in Nova Scotia, six having died, and the remaining forty-one (sixty-two percent) having left.

The general and staff officers at Halifax who had been appointed by His Excellency Sir Guy Carleton were listed on 1 January, 1784.[264]

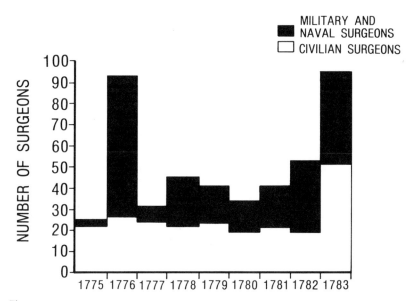

MILITARY AND
NAVAL SURGEONS
CIVILIAN SURGEONS

Figure 22
Civilian, naval, and military surgeons in Nova Scotia, 1775–83.

Total number of surgeons in Nova Scotia during period: 191
Number of surgeons who departed Nova Scotia during period: 62
Number of surgeons who died in Nova Scotia during period: 13

They included the surgeon Donald McIntyre and surgeon's mates Peter Browne, James Boggs, John Gemmel,[265] John Gould, Christopher Carter,[266] and Jonathan Ogden from hospitals in Halifax, and the surgeon Abraham Van Hulst[267] from a hospital in Annapolis Royal.

The total population of Nova Scotia on 1 January 1784 was calculated[268] to be 41,700, including 14,000 "old inhabitants which were completed at the beginning of 1783," and 27,700 Loyalists. Some of the Loyalists recently arrived in Halifax from New York were described[269] as "destitute of almost everything." However, as noted at the outset of this chapter, Nova Scotia benefited greatly from the influx, at the end of the American Revolution, of a large number of well-trained Loyalist physicians and surgeons. Figure 22 shows that the number of physicians and surgeons in Nova Scotia increased from twenty-five in 1775 to ninety-five in 1783. Only nineteen of the twenty-five present in 1775 were practising among the civilian population, compared to seventy-six of the ninety-five in 1783. The population figures for Nova Scotia in 1775 and 1783 indicate that the ratio of the number of persons in the province to the number of practising doctors decreased from 737:1 in 1775 to 605:1 in 1783. Whereas only four of the nineteen doctors practising in 1775 (twenty-one percent) are known to have attended a medical school, or to have sat an examination and qualified as a surgeons,[270] twenty-three of the seventy-six practising in 1783 (30.3 percent) are known to have had formal university training,[271] attended a hospital medical school,[272] or been examined by a recognized college of physicians or surgeons.[273] In addition, since at least twenty-eight of the remaining fifty-three physicians and surgeons practising in Nova Scotia in 1783 had been born in the thirteen colonies and had received their medical and surgical training through apprenticeship, it is likely that the majority were well prepared for their profession. The acceptance of the credentials of Loyalist doctors such as William J. Almon, James Boggs, and John Boyd is evidence that at least some of the graduates of the apprenticeship program in the American colonies in the eighteenth century were deemed to have training equivalent to men who had studied in Great Britain.[274] The training of doctors will be discussed further in the next chapter.

Thus, it can be said that in 1783, for the first time in the history of Nova Scotia, there was a sufficient number of well-trained doctors in the colony. At the same time, however, there was no civilian hospital by the end of the war, and many of the inhabitants of Nova Scotia, old and new, could not afford to pay for medical attendance. An adequate level of health care had yet to be achieved.

CHAPTER FIVE

Health Care and Poor Relief at the End of the Century, 1784–1799

Thus far this book has shown how the existence and condition of health-care facilities for the civilian population of Nova Scotia, particularly in Halifax, were determined during the last half of the eighteenth century primarily by four entities: government, the military and navy, the poor, and the civilian practitioners. The presence of and interaction between these four factors led to the establishment of twenty-five different hospitals in the Halifax area during this fifty-year period. As shown in Appendix 8, twelve of them were military hospitals, five were naval, two were for prisoners of war, and six were established for civilians. Over half of these hospitals were temporary and were closed within two years of opening, while the average lifespan of the twenty-five hospitals was just over eight years. Only three of the hospitals still existed at the end of the century: the hospital for the Maroons at Dartmouth; the hospital in the poor house; and the naval hospital. The longest-surviving civilian hospital consisted of two rooms in the poor house and was established in 1764, whereas the hospital associated with the orphan house, a children's hospital, existed from 1752 until 1784.

As indicated in chapter 1, the initial plan by the Lords of Trade was to provide adequate health-care facilities in Halifax including a general civilian hospital, surgeons, a midwife, and medicines. Within a year of the opening of the general hospital, however, the Lords of Trade were questioning the need for its continued existence. During the latter part of the 1750s, Governor Lawrence in particular pleaded constantly with the British government, to continue the hospital's funding. As described earlier, with the arrival in Halifax of numerous regiments during the latter half of the 1750s and the establishment of the general military hospital in 1758, government officials in London eliminated the grant for the civilian hospital, claiming that both civilians and the military could be treated in the military hospital. Furthermore, by the end of the 1750s, the line items in the annual grant for the pay of surgeons and a midwife and for the provision of medicines had also been eliminated. This transfer by the British government of the support of health-care facilities for the civilians in Nova Scotia to the local government bodies took place at the onset of a fifteen-year period (1760–75) during which the province, and especially Halifax, was in a state of socio-economic decline, its population decreasing to a low of 1,800 in the summer of 1775.[1]

The decrease in the annual grant from Whitehall to Nova Scotia, the departure of the military and navy, and the dramatic increase in the number of poor and indigent people, many of them left by departing regiments, were the main reasons why Halifax's economy deteriorated in this period. The local government found that it could not fund health-care facilities at all and concentrated on establishing a Bridewell and a poor house to care for the numerous poor and the ever-increasing criminal element in Nova Scotia. Not only had the military and navy left many of these poor and indigent people in Halifax but, with their departure, they had also deprived Halifax and Nova Scotia of significant income, primarily from the sale of food, rum, and supplies. The provincial debt rose steadily during the period, reaching a figure in excess of twenty thousand pounds in the early 1770s.

This pattern was to repeat itself during the period 1775 to 1796, in that during the American Revolution, a large number of military and naval personnel once again arrived and were stationed in Halifax, and once more the economy of Halifax and Nova Scotia flourished and the provincial debt decreased. Immediately after the end of the war, however, the problem represented by the large number of transient poor, abandoned camp followers, and disbanded soldiers again became very serious, and the Bridewell and poor house became severely overcrowded and very expensive to maintain. As before, the provincial debt became almost unmanageable and was only brought under control by the introduction of a provincial capitation tax in 1791. The revenue from this poll tax, which continued to be collected annually until 1796, was not sufficient, however, to allow the Council to establish and maintain an adequate civilian hospital, and it was not until 1859 that such a facility was available to the citizens of Halifax.

This concluding chapter carries these and other issues, such as the diseases and epidemics with which the medical community had to deal, through the years 1784 to 1799, the end of the period under study. With regard to the medical profession itself, there was an abortive attempt, in the last decade of the eighteenth century, to pass a bill to regulate the practice of medicine in Nova Scotia. Similar legislation was in effect, at the time, both in the United States and in Lower Canada, yet it wasn't until the nineteenth century that regulation became a fact in Nova Scotia. I shall examine the reasons for this, not the least because they shed light on the calibre of medical practitioners in the province. To round out the picture, I shall touch briefly on some of their extra-medical activities, notably the participation of various medical men in provincial politics.

Finally, I shall end on a demographic note by presenting a unique set of statistics on the mortality of all Nova Scotians between 1749 and 1799, including average age at time of death, infant and child mortality, death rate, and causes of death.

ALTHOUGH SCOTTISH EMIGRATION to the Island of Cape Breton did not begin until the early years of the nineteenth century, many settlers from both the Lowlands and the Highlands of Scotland arrived at the ports of Pictou and Halifax during the last quarter of the eighteenth century.[2] In general, the passengers on these emigrant ships were extremely poor and in a sick and destitute condition, and support of the poor became, once again, a major expense on the public purse. Lieutenant Governor Parr described one large group of Scots who arrived at Pictou in September 1791: "Lately 650 persons have arrived at Pictou in the North East Part of this Province, from Glasgow. In general they are in a wretched condition ... I have been obliged on my own credit to furnish them with provisions to save their lives, and to prevent their emigration to South Carolina, whither they have been strongly solicited."[3]

Seven years earlier, in September 1784, Parr had complained to Lord Sydney about the wretched condition of the passengers who had arrived in Halifax on the *Sally*.[4] He wrote: "I beg leave to represent to your Lordships that the ship *Sally* Transport arrived in this Harbour about three weeks ago with a number of persons on board, many of them in a sick and weak condition, and without cloathing [*sic*], thirty-nine of them had died on their passage, and twelve died in a few days after their arrival. They numbered at the time of embarkation to about 300 and had been sent by your Lordships directions. In what quality am I to receive them?" Later in the same month, Dr Donald McIntyre, surgeon to the garrison, informed Parr that the passengers on the *Sally* were very sick and destitute. He asked Parr to have them accommodated in the poor house,[5] but Parr responded that the poor house was full and could not accommodate any more people. On 9 October 1784, Parr requested that Secretary of State Evan Nepean use his office to prevent the lord mayor of London from sending more poor, indigent people to Halifax, stating that "they are unwelcome guests to infant settlements."[6] One of the passengers on the *Sally*, C.N.G. Jades, complained to Nepean that he had contracted yellow fever from the convicts travelling on the *Sally*. It does not appear, however, that this fever spread to the citizens of Halifax.[7]

Members of the House of Assembly attempted to support the poor by initiating various bills, all of which the Council refused to uphold. For instance, a Bill for the Maintenance and Support of Transient Poor, Maimed and Disabled Seamen and Soldiers, and other distressed People, which Mr Uniacke laid before the House on 17 November 1784, was passed and sent to Council on 20 November.[8] On 8 December, Council informed the House that the Bill was not acceptable and ordered that it "lie on the Table."[9] In the next session, on 16 December 1785, the House revised the same Transient Poor Bill, which, on 21 December, Council rejected for a second time.[10] The House set up a committee of five members on 22 December 1785 to confer with the Council about the necessity of such a bill. There is no indication in the minutes of the House for the session that any subsequent deliberations took place. In the 1786 session, a Bill for the Maintainance of the Transient Poor was presented by the solicitor general and, on 28 June 1786, read for the second time.[11] The bill was not mentioned further in the minutes of the 1786 session.

On 16 June 1786 the committee that the House had appointed to take into consideration the present state of the poor house at Halifax submitted its report.[12] It included three recommendations that, had they been implemented, would have altered radically the procedure for dealing with criminals, the poor, and the sick in Halifax. The committee found "the [poor] House in exceeding good order and managed with cleanliness, prudence, and economy, except on the part of the Doctor [Dr W.J. Almon] whose charges are very extravagant." The report continued:

The Expenses of supporting that House for the year 1785 has been upwards of £1,200 exclusive of the Doctor's charge which amounts to £260, during which period 175 persons of both sexes have been relieved of which number 43 remained in the house at the end of the year on the Province account [transient poor] and 8 on the Town account together with four orphans. The expenses of the House for this year will be equal to the last.

Almost the whole of those relieved in the Poor House are not objects of charity but persons whose abandoned and profligate way of life has compelled [them] to seek relief in that way.

The first recommendation made by the committee was that the trustees be empowered to sell the former orphan house at public auction and use the proceeds to build a small stone building that would contain cells for capital criminals. This building would serve as a provincial gaol. The second recommendation dealt with the establishment of a small public hospital, but it unfortunately continued the practice of including the hospital, for the general public, as part of the poor house. The proposed hospital was to be a new building on the poor-house grounds and consist of four rooms. It was to be under the direction of the overseers of the poor.

The third recommendation was the most radical: "That there shall be no established Poor House but that paupers and orphans shall as usual be under the care of the Overseers of the Poor who shall put them out to board with such families and in such way as thay [sic] shall think best for the benefit of the Publick." Unfortunately, none of these recommendations was implemented, with the result that the transient poor, in particular, became a crippling burden on the Council and House.

For the fourth year in a row, on 12 November 1787, a bill entitled an Act for the Relief and Settlement of the Poor was presented and read for the first time; second reading took place on 15 November. As in the previous session, it was not mentioned again in the minutes of the session.[13] Some of the consequences of the lack of legislation dealing with the poor and the existence of such a large number of poor persons in Halifax are described by a correspondent who attended the Supreme Court session of July 1787:

That the lower sort of people in the Town of Halifax and its vicinity, are addicted in the most shameful manner to the vice of drunkenness [sic]. That it is not uncommon, to meet, at all times of the day, people staggering in the streets, oppressed with intoxication, while others, in a still worse condition, are found lying in a manner disgraceful to the Police in any civilized country, and, however shocking it may be to Humanity, the Grand Jury declare, that to their knowledge, many persons have died in the streets, whose deaths were attributed solely to excessive drinking.

That from the testimony of the Physician and Keeper of Poor House, they find it is crowded in the Fall of the year, with sick persons, who have been cured in the preceding winter of disorders contracted by excessive drinking, and discharged in the Spring, and have, in some instances, continued a course of intoxication and debauchery during summer, and thereby become an expense to the public in winter.[14]

Dr Christopher Nicolai had been providing medical attendance to the poor house since 1 November 1783[15] and was listed as the dispensing apothecary and surgeon to the poor in July 1786.[16] Dr William J. Almon was appointed visiting physician to the sick in the poor house in April 1785.[17] Although a committee of the House was formed in July 1786 to wait on the governor and request that there be only one person to attend as dispensing physician and surgeon to the poor house, both Almon and Nicolai continued to attend the poor of that institution until the turn of the century.

In Digby, the Reverend Roger Viets petitioned King George III on 15 August 1789 "for medical and surgical assistance for the poor and distressed loyal subjects in this infant settlement." Viets recommended that Dr Peter Huggeford, a native of England but late of the province of New York, be paid for "his unselfish and largely unrewarded labour" among the poor of Digby.[18] The overseers of the poor in Truro, Windsor, and Cornwallis were also experiencing difficulty in dealing with expenses incurred by them in support of the transient poor. Petitions for reimbursement were sent to the House of Assembly from these townships. However, on 8 December 1787, the House voted that "the accounts for supplies to Transient Poor in the several Counties presented in the past and present sessions were dismissed."[19]

It appears that prior to 1800, Shelburne and possibly Liverpool were the only towns in Nova Scotia, other than Halifax, that could afford to build a poor house and workhouse.[20] Shelburne had established both as early as 1785, in September of which year Hugh Walker was recommended to be in charge of the house of correction.[21] The persons who had affixed their signatures to the recommendation wrote that Mr Walker was "formerly used to the command of various turbulent spirits." In his proposal regarding his own appointment as master of the workhouse, Walker provided a list of jobs that he would have the inmates perform and a list of the punishments that he would administer:[22] "That as Master of the House of Correction I may have authority from your Worships to set all such persons as shall be duly committed to hard Labour (provided they be able) and to punish them by putting fetters, or shackles upon them if necessary, and moderate whipping them not exceeding ten stripes, except the Warrant of Commitment shall otherwise direct, which shall be inflicted at their first coming in, and from time to time afterwards, as the case may require in respect to their being stubborn and idle."

In addition to the fifty-seven people who arrived from New York on the *Clinton* in January 1784, and the poor people and convicts who arrived in Halifax on the *Sally* in August, another shipload of destitute people arrived in April 1785: "A few days ago, 194 negroes, men, women, and children arrived here from St Augustine. They are naked and destitute of every necessary of life. I shall do the utmost in my power to provide for these wretched people and if possible without an expence."[23]

By 1787, the cost of supporting of the poor had climbed significantly in relation to the annual provincial revenue. According to the minutes of the Assembly for 6 December 1787, the accounts submitted by the overseers of the poor for the ten months from January to October 1787 totalled £1,051, whereas the provincial revenue for the fifteen-month period between March 1786 and June 1787 was £9,967. This indicates that the cost per month of caring for the poor was £105, sixteen percent of the average monthly revenue of £646.

In April 1789, the House of Assembly continued its attempt to enact legislation dealing with the poor, particularly the transient poor. The total cost of supporting the poor in Halifax from November 1787 to December 1788 was reported in the House, on 21 March 1789, to be £1,378. Major Thomas Barclay moved, on 4 April, that the treasury amount to support the transient and other poor at Halifax be limited for the year to seven hundred pounds, but his motion was defeated seventeen to fourteen. One explanation for the defeat is that, on the previous day, Mr Benjamin Belcher had moved for leave to bring in a bill, entitled an Act for the better laying a Duty on the several articles imported from the United States of America, except such as are herein after excepted. This bill was adopted by both the House and Council and received Lt Gov. Parr's assent on 9 April 1789. It read, in part, that "all monies collected are to be appropriated one-half to the informer and one-half to the poor of the County wherein the same was collected."

Andrew Rohl, a Loyalist who had found his way to Halifax after attempting unsuccessfully to settle in Shelburne County, wrote that after he fell sick in Halifax, he was admitted to the poor house and, in February 1788, was sent to London with eighteen other poor persons.[24] Whitehall objected to Parr's sending such persons to London, but he continued to do so. In December 1789, he explained to Nepean, "About 20 poor wretches have been here for some time past, mostly old and unable to earn their bread, from England, Scotland, and Ireland. The town being unable to maintain so many transient poor, they are being sent home.[25] In June 1790, Parr received a memorial from the overseers of the poor indicating that the problem of supporting the poor still existed. They asked for £350 to prevent the necessity of discharging "a large number of distressed miserable objects" out of the poor house.[26] In March 1790, the House of Assembly had introduced a Bill "to prevent Indigent Persons from coming into the Province." This action followed a committee report that the House had received concerning the state of the poor house. The committee reported that the poor house was "orderly, neat and does honor to humanity," its account books were "well kept," and the paupers appeared to be "truely [sic] poor." The committee recommended, nonetheless:

that a Law to oblige all Masters of Vessels on their arrival from Foreign Countries or from our sister Colonies to give security not to leave behind them any persons incapable of maintaining themselves, and obliging all Innkeepers and other persons keeping Lodging-Houses to make report of such persons not belonging to the Province, as shall from time to time remain at their Houses more than twenty-four hours would be very salutory. The Committee also recommends a Law ascertaining what persons shall in future be denominated transient Poor, and appointing one or more Commissioners or Overseers of such Poor in each County subject to such Regulations as may be thought necessary.[27]

The bill received first reading in the House on 13 March and second reading on 22 March, but it was not mentioned further in the 1790 session. An amended bill "for preventing Introduction of Indigent persons into this Province" was introduced in the 1791 session and read for a second time on 13 June of that year;[28] however, it, too, was mentioned no further in that session.

The House and Council did enact a poor bill in March 1790. It was entitled an Act for appointing Commissioners to superintend and direct the Maintainance and Support of certain Poor persons, known by the general Appellation of Transient Poor.[29] It received Lieutenant Governor Parr's assent on 3 April 1790 and stated that after the first of May 1790, no transient poor would be received into the poor house or the workhouse in Halifax. Commissioners were to be appointed and empowered to examine the condition of the transient poor and to decide whether they should remain in the poor house in Halifax or be boarded in various parts of the province. The commissioners were empowered, also, to apprentice out such poor persons as they saw fit. It was reported in the House, on 21 June 1791, that no commissioners had been appointed, for "His Excellency could not prevail on any persons in Halifax to take that burthen upon them."[30] On 4 July 1791, the Council agreed to another bill, entitled an Act to provide for the future Maintainance of the Poor, now maintained at the Province's Expence.[31] In this bill, which received the lieutenant governor's assent on 5 July, £1,500 was voted and applied to the town of Halifax for the transient poor, to be spent at a rate of no more than three hundred pounds per year. It is believed that this £1,500 was to cover the five-year period 1792–97, so that the transient poor could be moved back to the counties from which they had come and be supported by the local overseers of the poor. This was deemed to be absolutely necessary, for the treasurer's accounts presented to the House on 16 June 1791 indicated that, during the previous eleven months, £1,834 had been paid towards support of the transient poor.[32]

This action did not solve the problem of the transient poor, and the terrible financial burden of supporting such a large number of poor continued throughout the 1790s. On 11 July 1792, an act was passed "to Alter and Amend an Act, passed in the thirty-third year of his late Majesty's reign, entitled an Act for regulating and maintaining an House of Correction, or Work-House, within the Town of Halifax, and binding out Poor Children, and to extend certain Provisions therein, to the whole of the Province." The act stated that it would be lawful for justices of the peace to provide proper buildings, or to appropriate part of a county or district gaol, as a workhouse or house of correction. It read, in part:

that the Overseers of the Poor for the Town of Halifax shall no longer support or maintain any poor person or persons, as out pensioners, in manner hitherto practiced, but shall maintain and support the poor chargeable on said town; in that part of the Work house allotted by the Act hereby amended, for the reception of such poor, and all such poor persons, who shall refuse to accept of the provision made for their maintainance in said house, shall be entitled to receive nothing from said town of Halifax, and the Overseers of the Poor, after the publication thereof, shall not be allowed, in their account, and charge whatsoever, except what has been actually incurred for the support of the poor maintained in said House.[33]

Considering the money spent to support the poor, including the transient poor, between 1785 and 1799, and the provincial debt for the same period[34], it is clear that both amounts peaked in 1792. After that, because of the shift in responsibility for the transient poor to the counties, as well as the introduction of a capitation or poll tax in 1791, both the provincial debt and the amount spent on the poor declined dramatically.[35] By 1799, however, the expense of the poor house had increased again, to £1,600.[36] In July of that year, the inhabitants of Halifax asked to be relieved because many of the "poor persons are not properly chargeable to any part of the province."[37] Additional expense to the provincial treasury in 1799 was incurred by native Indians who were "an additional description of paupers who have encamped in very considerable numbers in the vicinity and [are] depending entirely upon the inhabitants of Halifax for their maintainance during the great part of the winter."[38]

The closure of the orphan house in 1784 added to the problems of the overseers of the poor. In October of that year, Parr was informed by Whitehall that, "because of the improved trade of Nova Scotia, the Orphan House seems no longer necessary."[39] Samuel Albro, the keeper of the orphan house, was paid £393 for the care and support of the orphan children in 1784, after which the office of keeper ceased to exist.[40] The surgeon who had been attending the orphan house since 26 April 1773, Dr John Philipps, sent a memorial to the House of Assembly on 15 November 1784 asking compensation for his last six and a half years of service to the sick there. On 16 November 1784, he was voted a payment of £130.[41]

On 23 November 1784, it was advertised in the *Nova Scotia Gazette and Weekly Chronicle* that the orphan house would be leased for a term of seven years. The lease was not taken up and four years later, on 6 August 1788, the lot and buildings of the orphan house were put up for auction.[42] Orphans now became the responsibility of the overseers of the poor, to be supported from provincial revenues, and were duly moved into the poor house. On 2 December, "a charity sermon was preached at St Paul's to raise money to cloath [*sic*] the poor children."[43] Three years later, in 1791, a bill was presented in the Assembly and adopted on 13 June 1791, establishing a charity school in the town of Halifax.[44] Significant expense was associated with the support of the orphans; moreover, in 1795, £397 was spent to care for "a number of old infirm persons in the Poor House besides orphan children."[45] In each of 1798 and 1799, about two hundred pounds were spent to support the fourteen illegitimate children who also occupied the poor house.[46]

During the 1790s, two large influxes of people into Nova Scotia added to the numbers of those who had to be provided with food, lodging, and medical attendance. France had declared war on Britain on 1 February 1793, and Lieutenant Governor John Wentworth was immediately authorized to raise a provincial regiment.[47] On 14 May, Brigadier General James Ogilvie and the 4th and 65th regiments took control of St Pierre and Miquelon, where they captured 120 French troops and 450 fishermen.[48] All in all, about six hundred of these French prisoners of war were brought to Halifax on 20 June 1793 and housed, for about a year, in the Cornwallis Barracks until they were transferred to the island of Guernsey.[49] Naval prisoners of war also were brought into Halifax and housed in the captured Spanish ship *La Feliz*. Sometime after 3 September 1797, it was converted into a prison ship.[50] Rear Admiral George Murray appointed Dr John Halliburton, the agent and principal surgeon at the naval hospital, to take care of the sick and wounded naval prisoners, and he was assisted by Dr John McEvoy.[51] Halliburton wrote Murray, on 21 August 1794, that "the sick multiply so fast upon us by the arrival of the different ships of the squadron under your command that it will become necessary for their comfort and accommodation that the whole of the Naval Hospital building and Surgeon's House be converted into a Hospital."[52] A survey was made of the naval hospital, the wards, apartments, and surgeon's house, and it was reported on 23 August that a total of 212 patients could be accommodated.[53]

On 30 August, Halliburton reported to Admiral Murray that he had hired a commodious house on the outskirts of town for the reception of still more French prisoners from St Domingo. Residents in the area complained to the lieutenant governor that these prisoners might be infected with diseases such as the fever that had broken out in Philadelphia,[54] which was said to have come from St Domingo. Halliburton, concerned that local residents might burn the house to the ground, hired two smaller houses two miles out of town for the reception of his sick and wounded prisoners.[55] These two houses were likely on Kavanagh's Island[56] in the Northwest Arm, for Admiral Murray reported that there were seventy patients in the prison hospital on the island in June 1795. In August, he wrote that Dr Halliburton had represented to him that the prison hospital on Kavanagh's Island was in constant use and that he needed an additional assistant surgeon.[57] In April 1796, sixteen soldiers of the Royal Nova Scotia Regiment were stationed on Kavanagh's. It is possible that they were guarding French sailors or soldiers imprisoned there.[58]

In August of 1796, "a fever of a malignant and infectious kind" made its appearance on the HM *Dover*, and the ship's commander sent afflicted sailors to the naval hospital. Because of the fear that patients already there would become infected, Dr Halliburton immediately asked for and received authorization to remove the sick sailors into tents erected on the Dartmouth shore. He directed Dr John McEvoy, the assistant surgeon and dispenser at the naval hospital, to provide them with medical attendance.[59]

The second large group to be brought to Nova Scotia during this period consisted at 530 Maroons, who arrived in Halifax on 22 July

1796. They were under the medical care of Dr John Oxley, formerly surgeon of the disbanded Ninety-sixth Regiment, who had taken care of them for two months prior to their departure from Jamaica.[60] He came with them to Dartmouth, where he set up for their care a small hospital and made monthly reports concerning their number and condition. His returns, which cover the period from June 1797 to April 1798, indicate that there were never at one time more than four persons sick in hospital.[61] In April 1798, Dr Oxley resigned because his income had been reduced and he immediately took passage to England.[62] His successor as surgeon to the Maroons was Dr John Fraser. In a report to Lieutenant Governor Wentworth in May 1799, Fraser wrote, "Since the beginning of April, nine [Maroons] have died."[63] On 3 August 1800, after four winters in Nova Scotia, 551 Maroons embarked in the ship *Asia* for Sierra Leone.[64] This was actually the second exodus of a large number of black people from Nova Scotia to Sierra Leone: in January 1792, some 1,190 persons, 800 of them from Shelburne, had departed from Halifax on fifteen transports for the African colony.[65]

THE LAST FIFTEEN YEARS OF THE EIGHTEENTH CENTURY in Nova Scotia were free from major epidemics. There were, however, numerous instances of putrid sore throat, scarlet fever, black scurvy, yellow fever, and smallpox. Lord Charles Montague, who had been commanding officer of the Duke of Cumberland's Regiment, died in Halifax on 3 February 1784 of putrid sore throat. Major General John Campbell reported[66] that Montague's illness was "a disorder which prevailed here for some time past and has proved fatal to many."

Simeon Perkins, in his diary entry of 17 November 1790, reported that "my daughter Nabby was taken Sick last night, a Sore throat, & Feever. Doc. Kendrick Visits her, & has given her Something of Liquid, to be taken, 2 Spoonfulls every three Hours. She breaks out towards night, in the Same manner that the other Children have done, So conclude her disorder is the Scarlet Feever." A second instance of scarlet fever occurred in Halifax in 1796, when the secretary of the Council, J.M. Freke Bulkeley, took ill on 8 November and died four days later, at the age of thirty-five.[67]

Black scurvy was brought to Sydney on 13 September 1795, when approximately four hundred soldiers of the Second Battalion of the Royal Fusiliers in three transports made there an unscheduled stop after their long Atlantic voyage. To attend the sick soldiers, an unidentified doctor was brought from Halifax. During the five weeks that the troops were in Sydney, nine died.[68]

As mentioned earlier, Jades, a passenger on the ship *Sally*, which arrived in Halifax in September 1785, indicated that he had contracted yellow fever from convicts on board; fortunately, the fever did not spread to the citizens of Halifax. Eight years later, on 9 October 1793, Lieutenant Governor Wentworth announced in Council that a contagious distemper was raging in Philadelphia and that proper steps should be taken "to prevent its reaching this Country."[69] The distemper was yellow fever, which caused the death of over four thousand of the fifty thousand people living in Philadelphia in 1793.[70] Considering the great number of ships arriving daily at Halifax in that year, it is surprising that the town escaped an outbreak of yellow fever. That it did so was probably due to two prudent measures taken by Lieutenant Governor Wentworth and the Council. A proclamation,[71] posted on 9 October, appeared in the *Royal Gazette and Nova Scotia Advertiser* on 15 October, and a health boat was appointed to watch vessels entering the harbour and to issue to the captains instructions about how to proceed.[72] Wentworth declared in the proclamation:

I do hereby strictly forbid and prohibit all vessels coming from Philadelphia aforesaid, and all other vessels coming from any other place infected with any contagious distempers, or having on board any person or persons infected therewith, from entering any of the Ports of this Province or to approach nearer to the Town of Halifax than midway between George's Island and major's[sic] beach. And I do hereby further direct vessels coming from Philadelphia aforesaid, or other place infected with such contagious Distemper to perform Quarantine below George's Island until such vessel be duly discharged

Minor epidemics of smallpox were reported in Guysborough, Lunenburg, Shelburne, Port Medway, and Liverpool in 1790 and 1791. On 1 April 1791, Drs John Hoose, William Burns, and John Perry of Shelburne were sent a circular letter ordering them to stop inoculating against smallpox, which points to the erstwhile fear that persons would contact the disease from inoculation.[73] At Liverpool, Perkins recorded on 20 June 1791 that "there is complaints of people going to the Small pox House, by which the Inhabitants may be exposed and also that Docr Kendrick is not So careful as he aught to be." On 21 June, he wrote, "Complaints are Still made that there is not Sufficient care taken to prevent Spreading the Contagion." On 22 June: "The Magistrates & Overseers of the Poor met to Consider of methods to prevent Spreading the Small Pox, and have published Advertisements, and made some Regulations to be observed with the Doctor, and other people."

Smallpox became, once again, a major scare in Halifax in May 1799. On 13 May, Lieutenant Governor Wentworth submitted to Council an application received from some physicians and other inhabitants of the town, for leave to inoculate against the disease. Council advised[74] "that there is not sufficient reason to justify the inoculating for that Distemper [*sic*] in the Town at this time, but that if there are housekeepers who are desirous of having their children or others inoculated [they] will provide either at Dartmouth or elsewhere out of the Town a suitable house or houses sufficiently remote from other habitations to prevent the spreading of the disorder ... they may be permitted to do so."

The House of Assembly appointed a committee in June 1799 to consider the several acts designed to prevent the spreading of contagious disorders and to bring in a bill to amend existing legislation by making whatever further provisions and regulations necessary to prevent yellow fever and other pestilential diseases from entering the province. The new bill, enacted by the House of Assembly on 27 June 1799 and assented to by Wentworth on 24 July, began:

Whereas the neighbouring States of America, have, for several years past, been visited by the yellow or putrid fever, or some other infectious distemper, which has raged to a most alarming degree, and proved fatal to great numbers of their inhabitants, whereby it hath become highly necessary, that the Legislature of this Province should make some provision, for obliging persons coming from infected places to perform quarantine, in such manner as may be ordered by the Governor, Lieutenant Governor, or Commander-in-Chief for the time being, and for punishing offenders in a more expeditious manner, than can be done by the ordinary course of Law.

The King's Printer, Anthony Henry, produced a one-page proclamation outlining the substance of the act. This proclamation was posted throughout the province on Lieutenant Governor Wentworth's order.[75]

A bill to regulate inoculation against smallpox was introduced into the Assembly on 6 July 1799, received third reading on 9 July, and assent on 20 July. It specified that any physician, surgeon, or person residing anywhere in the province was legally permitted to inoculate any other person, but only between the dates of 1 October and 30 April.[76]

On 14 August 1799, health officers were appointed to Halifax; Shelburne; Queens County; LaHave, Lunenburg, and Chester; Pictou; Windsor; Horton and Cornwallis; Annapolis; Digby; Yarmouth, Barrington and Argyle; and Gut of Canso, Country Harbour, and Manchester. These appointments indicate the heightened concern over smallpox, and it is therefore surprising that only three of the health officers were doctors: Dr John Bolman was appointed for LaHave, Lunenburg, and Chester; Dr John F.T. Gschwind for Halifax; and Dr George Henkell for Annapolis.[77]

The concern over epidemic diseases continued during the late summer and early fall of 1799. On 17 September, the *Royal Gazette and Nova Scotia Advertiser* reported that "the destructive yellow fever has again commenced its ravages in the ill-fated cities of Philadelphia and New York." On 26 August, it was reported that forty-two persons in Philadelphia had died of the disease in two days and that, on 25 August, ten deaths had been recorded in New York. In November, however, Council advised that, since the fever in the United States had all but disappeared, the quarantine was to be discontinued on Vessels arriving at various ports in Nova Scotia.

DURING THE PERIOD 1784 TO 1799, six doctors sat as members of the Nova Scotia House of Assembly. Both Dr John Harris and Dr John Philipps held seats in the Fifth Assembly, which ended in 1785. Dr Philipps advertised in the *Halifax Journal*, 28 October 1785, for re-election as the member for Halifax County, stating that he "has been a resident of the Province for upwards of 27 years." He was unsuccessful in retaining his seat. Dr Gurdon Dennison served in the Sixth Assembly, representing Horton Township from 1785 to 1793, and Drs William Baxter, John Bolman, and Daniel Eaton[78] sat in the Seventh Assembly, which ran from 1793 to 1799.

In addition to their participation in debates concerning the poor, the spread of contagious diseases, and similar matters touched upon thus far, these members were involved in a range of issues affecting provincial life and the conduct of government. Some, however, were noteworthy largely because of their own brushes with the law.

Both Dr Philipps and Dr Harris took an active part in the Fifth Assembly. On 3 November 1784, Dr Philipps introduced a motion,[79] which was subsequently adopted, "that in the future, when the House shall be divided, that every Member's Name, who is present, shall be entered on the Journals, distinguishing the side which each member shall take on such division." At the same meeting, Dr Philipps was named to a committee of the House "to take the State of the Revenues into consideration and to prepare such a Plan for the future support of Government." Dr John Harris brought in three bills in 1784 and, on 30 November 1784, was appointed to a committee "to confer with a Committee of Council on An Act sent down from Council entitled An Act to ascertain the Number of Representatives to be elected to serve in General Assembly for the several Townships therein mentioned." When, on 23 November 1784, the House refused to grant Governor Parr's request for a daily report of its business, Dr Philipps favoured refusal, while Dr Harris supported approval. Dr Harris had sent a unique memorial to the Assembly on 12 November 1784, in which he stated that, soon after arriving in Pictou in 1767, he had opened a road through the woods to Cobequid (Truro), a distance of thirty miles. He explained that he had kept the road open during the past fourteen years at his own expense and asked the House for relief of the cost and support in keeping the road open.[80]

Dr Gurdon Dennison was the only doctor to sit in the Sixth Assembly. According to the lists of members who voted on motions, frequently he was absent from the House. The only committee on which he sat was one asked to enquire into the circumstances that had led to construction of a bridge between Windsor and Falmouth.[81] When the Assembly voted, on 12 March 1789, concerning acceptability of results of a judges' trial, Dr Dennison voted in the affirmative; the motion passed with fifteen members for and fourteen against. When the motion supporting a charge of impeachment against Hon. Isaac Deschamps and James Brenton, assistant judges of the Supreme Court, was introduced on 10 March 1790, Dr Dennison voted against it; but the motion was adopted seventeen to ten. The two assistant judges were impeached for high crimes and misdemeanors. Two additional motions, adopted in the House on 6 April, requested that the lieutenant governor and Council suspend the two judges "until His Majesty's pleasure be known." Dr Dennison's name was not recorded in the list of members who voted on that occasion.[82]

Dr John Halliburton was the only member of the medical profession who sat on the Council between 1784 and 1799. He was a brother-in-law of James Brenton, one of the two judges impeached by the House. Halliburton and the Council supported the judges, and Halliburton wrote[83] to Nepean that the two were "much injured and insulted." He attributed the impeachment to the "Union of the two Parties which have for some time past divided the Government, each having their respective Person in view if they finally succeed in Supplanting the Judges." He named the two parties as the "Old Settlers" and the "New Settlers."

Of the three doctors in the Seventh Assembly, Dr John Bolman was the only one who took an active part in the proceedings. On 24 July 1799, he was appointed to a committee of five "to enquire for, and report to this House a suitable situation for the Erection of a Government House." Prior to his election, a number of unfortunate incidents had been associated with Dr Bolman's medical practice. On 20 April 1784, he was charged, in the Inferior Court of Common Pleas in Lunenburg, with adultery. A Mr Urban Bender had accused him of using violence and force against his wife. The incident was alleged to have taken place on 13 February 1782, when Mrs Bender visited Dr Bolman's house to pay for a tooth extraction.[84] On 24 october 1784, the same court fined Dr Bolman fifty pounds for striking Jacob Smith; on 31 October 1786, he was accused of beating another doctor, Joseph Falt, with a cane. The latter charge was withdrawn.[85]

Dr Bolman also appeared on four occasions, between 1784 and 1799, in the Supreme Court of Nova Scotia. One incident took place shortly after votes had been counted for the provincial election held in February 1793. Dr Bolman ran against Lewis Morris Wilkins, Attorney at Law, for the seat representing Lunenburg Township. After Dr Bolman's election was announced, Wilkins and four other residents of Lunenburg were alleged to have caused excessive damage to Bolman's house and apothecary shop. About 150 of the house's windowpanes, as well as window frames, doors, and furniture, were damaged. In the apothecary shop, over a hundred medicine bottles were broken, and ten gallons of medicines and one hundred pounds of drugs were destroyed. Richard John Uniacke, who represented Dr Bolman, wrote, "His said dwelling house was rendered uninhabitable, his family and himself being obliged to fly from the same and his business and trade as a Druggist and Apothecary was totally prevented, stop[p]ed and put to an end so that he the said John Bollman being obliged to shut up his said shop the windows thereof and the Drugs and Medicines as aforesaid and divers other wrongs injuries and outrages then and there committed against the peace of our Lord." Court records note Wilkins's belief that Dr Bolman had "opposed him out of spite." According to Dr Bolman, Wilkins called him "that Hessian Bug[g]er."[86]

Dr William Baxter, elected in 1793 to represent Cornwallis Township, had many visits to court. On 27 August 1792, he was charged with having assaulted John Chipman on the highway,[87] and on three occasions during the 1790s, he appeared in the Supreme Court of Nova Scotia.[88] Five of the six doctors who served as members of the House of Assembly in this period were, in fact, either plaintiffs or defendants before the Supreme Court. In all, thirty doctors, thirty-six percent of those practising during the period, were involved in a total of 161 cases brought to the high court. In six of these cases, both the plaintiff and defendant were doctors. Most of the cases involved non-payment of loans either by a doctor, or by people who had borrowed from a doctor. In twenty-one cases, doctors brought patients to court for non-payment for medicines and attendance, and in seven cases, the charge was assault.[89]

ONE OF THE MOST NOTABLE MEDICAL FIGURES in Nova Scotia at the time was Dr William Smith. He arrived in Cape Breton from London on the *Blenheim* in November 1784, after having been appointed surgeon to the garrison[90] in the newly established town of Sydney. Dr Smith is undoubtedly one of the most interesting physicians and surgeons to have resided in Nova Scotia in the eighteenth century. While information about his medical education and early career has proved elusive, it is known that Dr Smith wrote eleven books, the earliest of which, *A Dissertation upon the Nerves*, was published in London in 1768.[91] The title page of this book refers to the author as "William Smith MD." This book could have been the thesis that Dr Smith prepared for his medical degree, but I have been unable to identify the granting institution. It is clear, from the breadth of topics covered in his numerous books and from the quotations that follow, that Dr William Smith was well educated and highly regarded. It is difficult to imagine why he decided to accept an offer to become surgeon to the garrison in the as yet unestablished town of Sydney, Nova Scotia. It is known, however, that from 25 March 1776 to 10 November 1779, he provided daily medical attendance to the gaols of London, Westminister, and Southwark, at the request of Sir Charles Whitworth. Since Dr Smith received no payment whatsoever for this service, he petitioned the House of Commons for compensation and, in December 1779, was voted £1,200 by the House.[92] For some unknown reason, payment was not allowed by the House of Lords and, in July 1784, Sir Herbert Mackworth wrote[93] on Dr Smith's behalf to the Lords of Trade, but to no avail. Mackworth's letter contains comments concerning Smith which are very laudatory and, at the same time, somewhat mysterious:

He [Smith] has been in exile from home waiting with very little hopes of something being done for him. It appears to me that he would be a very useful man to my friend Major DesBarres as a Physician and Surgeon, and a man of letters, with much activity of mind, zealous in his pursuits, and of very liberal sentiments. He would be a person most completely qualified for such a station if there is to be an appointment of that sort in the Island of Cape Breton. If your Lordships recollect Dr Smith's case, you will feel it to be unparalleled in point of hardship and that there are few objects more deserving of compassion of humanity.

It can be surmised that Dr Smith's "exile" (which, according to note 90, was to America) resulted from an inability to discharge his debts, thanks to lack of payment for the medical attendance that he had provided to the gaols. In December 1791, having been then for six years a resident of Sydney, Dr Smith returned to London to plead once again for adequate compensation for his attendance at the gaols.[94] Remaining in London until 1798, and requesting constantly some form of compensation, finally he received what he thought would be satisfactory: the position of chief justice of Cape Breton. He returned[95] to Sydney in June 1798, but realized soon that his new appointment was one of many items that had polarized factions within the Council of the colony of Cape Breton. He left the colony, never to return, in September 1800.

The town of Sydney did not grow fast, and when Lieutenant William Booth arrived there on 4 August 1785, he reported[96] that he found only a dozen families and six companies of the 33rd Regiment. His watercolour of Sydney, painted in the same year, is the first such sketch of the town. The hospital, whose construction was begun sometime prior to 1 September 1785 by David Tait,[97] is quite likely one of the buildings in the sketch. As early as 3 March 1785, there was a workhouse at Point Edward, near Sydney, as well as a workhouse sawmill, but it appears from the records that the persons at the house and sawmill were labourers rather than criminals.[98]

On 5 March 1785, Dr William Smith was appointed a member of the Council of Cape Breton,[99] a position he held during most of the time that he resided in Sydney. In December 1785, he was joined in Sydney by a surgeon named Alexander Gordon,[100] who had been appointed surgeon's mate to the 33rd Regiment.[101] (One of Dr Gordon's daughters was to become a close friend of the poet Thomas Carlyle and the subject of Raymond Archibald's book, *Carlyle's First Love*.) Dr Gordon remained at the hospital in Sydney until June 1786 when the 33rd Regiment was transferred to the island of St John and replaced by the 42nd Regiment.[102] He and Dr Smith were among eleven persons in Sydney who signed a petition, undated, asking for the removal of Lieutenant Governor DesBarres.[103] Part of Dr Smith's reason for not supporting DesBarres could have been that the lieutenant governor had informed Smith that he could not hold two offices – military physician and surgeon, and member of Council – at the same time.[104] DesBarres's insistence, which applied also to three other councillors who held military appointments, was probably precipitated by his intense conflict, during the winter of 1785–86, with Colonel John Yorke, commanding officer of the Thirty-third Regiment. The conflict centred around DesBarres's position that food supplies sent to Sydney for the military, and under the control of Colonel Yorke, should be made available to the civilian settlers.[105] Shortly after DesBarres's departure and the arrival of his successor, Lieutenant Governor William Macarmick, on 10 October 1787, Dr Smith was reappointed member of Council and made a justice of the peace for the County of Sydney.[106]

The surgeon to the 42nd Regiment was Dr William Robertson, who arrived in Halifax from England on 5 September 1786 on the *Friendship*, and in Sydney probably soon afterwards.[107] He became highly regarded in the Sydney area because of his humanitarian approach in providing medical treatment following the shipwreck of the *Providence*, which, on 10 December 1788,[108] left seventy-six convicts thrown on the shore near the town. On 18 March 1789, a letter[109] from Lieutenant Governor Macarmick to Lord Sydney recorded that Doctor Robertson had taken the convicts under his care and had attended and dispensed medicines to all of the inhabitants of Sydney for two years without charging a fee. Dr William Smith was also highly regarded for his professional work, as indicated by a testimonial[110] presented to him by the citizens of Sydney prior to his departure in 1791 for London. It included this statement: "In your office of Surgeon General of this Island, the sick have found in you an able and experienced Physician and a tender hearted friend."

By 1790, there were 598 inhabitants on the island of Cape Breton who were liable for service in the militia. One hundred and twenty-five of these resided in Sydney.[111] The only permanent doctor in Sydney at the time was Dr William Smith, who had been appointed a puisne judge of the Supreme Court of Cape Breton in March 1788[112] and, in May 1791, was approved unanimously as judge of the Court of Exchequer.[113] Although Dr Smith's time was divided among his several appointments, he apparently was still esteemed for his medical attendance, as indicated by the testimonial. He was also well respected by the Reverend Ranna Cossitt, the rector of St George's Anglican Church, Sydney. Upon Smith's departure in December 1791, Cossitt wrote[114] that Dr Smith was "a true churchman and has endeavoured to propagate and establish the Church of England here but to no effect."

After Dr Smith's departure, and until the arrival of Dr William Stafford early in 1797, Sydney and the entire colony of Cape Breton were without a physician or surgeon.[115] Dr Smith was dismissed officially as surgeon to the garrison on 18 February 1796, partly because of his four-year absence from Sydney and because Prince Edward's Regiment had put into the town and found no medical attendance there.[116] Dr Stafford was appointed surgeon to the garrison at Sydney, on 20 October 1796, but did not arrive there until early 1797.[117] Dr Stafford was put in charge of the hospital, which is referred to as an "infirmary" on James Miller's 1795 plan of Sydney (Figure 23) and located near the Military Wharf in the lower left of the plan. Dr Stafford's memorial to Portland, dated 10 March 1798, indicates that he had been surgeon to the Maryland Volunteers during the revolution and upon its cessation had boarded the ill-fated *Martha*, which was bringing Loyalists to Nova Scotia. The *Martha* foundered subsequently on the rocks near Cape Sable Island, and all except a few passengers were drowned.

As mentioned earlier, Dr William Smith had been appointed chief justice of Cape Breton on 6 March 1798. His appointment was unusual in that it was a joint appointment with Ingram Ball.[118] During the next two years, Smith and Ball constantly opposed each other, each trying to have the other removed from office.[119] Smith opposed the Honourable William McKinnon's suspension as a member of Council by the Honourable David Mathews, president of HM Council, describing the suspension as "unjust, tyrannical, and oppressive," whereas Ball concluded that Mathews was perfectly correct in suspending McKinnon.[120] On 11 October 1799, Ball was dismissed and Dr Smith was appointed chief justice of Cape Breton.[121] However, Major General Despard, who arrived in June 1800, concluded that the government had been conducted by Brig. Gen. John Murray, Chief Justice William Smith, and Rev. Ranna Cossitt, and wrote, "I have witnessed an evident intention in them to mislead and misrepresent everything which respects the government and state of the Country."[122] Dr Smith left Sydney on 16 September 1800 without Despard's knowledge and permission, and returned to London.[123] During the next three years he attempted unsuccessfully to draw his salary as chief justice of Cape Breton and also asked to be appointed chief justice of Newfoundland.[124] Subsequent to the publication in 1803 of his last book. *A Caveat Against Emigration to America with the State of the Island of Cape Breton*, Dr Smith's name disappears from the state papers. It is not known where or when he died.[125]

TURNING NOW TO MEDICAL PRACTITIONERS AS A GROUP, there were a number of well-qualified medical personnel in Nova Scotia from 1784–99, but it was not until the next century that they or their successors made any concerted effort to shape themselves into a pro-

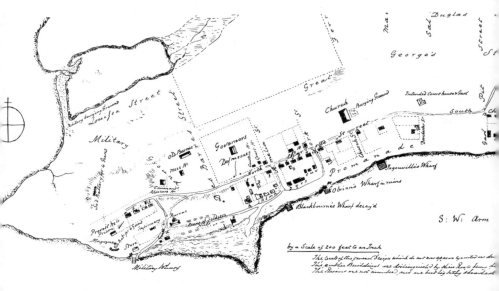

Figure 23
Plan of Sydney drawn by James Miller in 1795. The hospital, referred to as an infirmary, is located near the Military Wharf in the lower left of the plan. (National Archives of Canada, NMC 648)

fessional body. Professionalization implies that a body of people with special skill or expertise has been granted a degree of authority over themselves. Their authority manifests itself in the setting of educational and training standards to be met by everyone seeking admittance to the profession, and in having government-sanctioned responsibility for licensing and policing those admitted. Professionalization presupposes that the body has not only special expertise but, also, that it is based clearly in the public interest. It would be understood that the body had established, already, a professional society, journal, code of ethics, fee schedule, and a public perception of its expertise as both creditable and desirable. The final step is enactment of legislation granting explicit professional status.

In the last fifteen years of the eighteenth century, however, there is no indication that medical practitioners contemplated making plans to establish a medical society. There is no record of any proposal to introduce a provincial medical and surgical journal, nor any suggestion by the medical community to establish a public civilian hospital. Neither was there any representation, by the medical practitioners sitting in the House of Assembly, to enact legislation to regulate the practice of medicine and surgery. John Sargent, the member for Barrington, introduced in 1797 a bill "to regulate the Practice of Physick and Surgery." He may have been responding to lobbying by members of the medical community, but I have found no evidence of this. The bill faded away,[126] and it was not until well into the next century, in 1819, that medical doctors in Halifax petitioned[127] the Assembly for a medical act. Not until 1828 did the act become a reality.[128]

Legislation governing the practice of medicine had already been enacted in North America, as described shortly. In England, the first parliamentary enactment concerning medical matters was effected in 1512,[129] in the third year of the reign of King Henry VIII. Parliament adopted a bill that read:

Forasmuch as the Science and Cunning of Physick and Surgery (to the perfect knowledge whereof be requisite both great Learning and ripe Experience) is daily within this realm exercised by a great multitude of ignorant persons, of whom the greater part have no manner of Insight in the same, nor in any other kind of Learning; some also can no Letters on the Book [read] so far forth, that common Artificers, as Smiths, Weavers, and Women, boldly and accustomably take upon them great Cures, and things of great Difficulty, in the which they partly use Sorcary and Witchcraft, partly apply such Medicines unto the Disease as be very no[x]ious, and nothing meet therefore, to the Displeasure of God, great infamy to the Faculty, and the grievous Hurt, Damage, and Destruction of many of the King's liege People, most especially of whom that cannot discern the cunning from the uncunning.

It was enacted, therefore, that no person in the City of London or within seven miles of it should take upon himself to "exercise and occupy" as a physician or surgeon without first being examined, appointed, and admitted by the Bishop of London or the Dean of St Paul's "calling to him or them four doctors of physic and for surgery other expert persons in that faculty." Anyone who practised without being examined and admitted was to forfeit five pounds for every month, half of which was to go to the King and the other half to the informer. In 1540, some thirty years later, during the reign of Henry VIII, the act of Parliament uniting barbers and surgeons into the Company of Barber-Surgeons came into being. This arrangement continued until 1745, when, as noted earlier, the Company of Surgeons of London was instituted by act of Parliament and granted power to examine and license surgeons.

In the American colonies, the first law to provide for the examining of prospective medical practitioners was enacted in 1760 and entitled an Act to Regulate the Practice of Physick and Surgery in the City of New York.[130] In 1772, New Jersey became the first of the American colonies to adopt a law requiring prospective physicians to pass an examination for licensure; this examination was to be conducted by two judges of the Supreme Court, and a fine of five pounds was to be assessed against anyone found practising without a licence.[131] In 1781, the Massachusetts Legislature granted the newly incorporated Massachusetts Medical Society the right to regulate medical practice[132] in Massachusetts, and the State of Connecticut gave the Connecticut Medical Society the same right in 1792.

In Canada, under the French regime, Intendant François Bigot established a medical act in 1750. It forbade any surgeon coming from France or any other country to doctor without first having passed an examination before the King's Doctor at either Quebec, Montreal, or Three Rivers. The act provided for a fine of two hundred livres and confiscation of the unlicensed doctor's drugs and instruments.[133] In 1784, twenty-five years after the British had acquired Canada from the French, a Dr James Fisher addressed to the Legislative Council of Quebec a memorandum concerning the uncontrolled state of medical practice and made suggestions for reform. The number of qualified physicians practising in Lower Canada was very small, he pointed out, while that of the charlatan practitioners was immense. The harm caused to the health of the people by charlatans was incalculable, he observed. There was no law to regulate the practice of medicine; anyone who chose to practise had only to announce himself. Neither knowledge, study, nor examination was necessary. Dr Fisher suggested, to correct this untenable state of affairs, the formation of a bureau of medical examiners at the towns of Montreal and Quebec, to whom candidates for the practice of medicine would present themselves. Candidates who either passed bureau examinations or possessed other qualifications approved by it should receive a certificate permitting them to practise.

In 1786, the Legislative Council reported to Lord Dorchester, the governor:

On the subject of the population, the most efficacious method to preserve the life of His Majesty's subjects and of increasing the population is the systematic control of the practice of medicine, surgery, and obstetrics in the whole province. The representations of Mr James Fisher, Surgeon to the Garrison at Quebec, and those of Mr Charles Blake, surgeon at Montreal, appear to deserve the attention of the Legislature, seeing that they at least expound the methods which will contribute to realize this result of such capital importance to the State and of an extreme interest to humanity.

On 3 March 1787, a bill was brought before the Quebec Legislative Council "to prevent persons from practising Medicine, Surgery, or Midwifery without license." A year later, on 3 April 1788, the Council adopted a medical act[134] entitled an Ordinance to prevent persons practising Physic and Surgery within the Province of Quebec and Midwifery in the towns of Quebec and Montreal. The act stated that, from the first day of November next, no person should sell or distribute medicines for gain, or practise in any field of medicine without a licence, granted to him by the governor-in-chief, showing that the applicant had been examined for his knowledge of physic or his skill in surgery, midwifery, or pharmacy, by persons whom the governor had appointed for that purpose. Failure to comply would result in a fine of twenty pounds for the first offence, fifty pounds for the second, and, for every subsequent offence, one hundred pounds and three months' imprisonment. Since the territory that became Ontario was part of Lower Canada until 1791, this medical act applied there as well.[135]

Despite these developments, medical practitioners in Nova Scotia still made no attempt to form a society, establish a journal, or regulate their profession prior to 1800. There are several reasons for this. To begin with, there is no evidence in Nova Scotia of any

Table 6
Academic Qualifications of Civilian Doctors in Nova Scotia, 1784–99

Examining Body	Location	Diploma	Number
University	Aberdeen	MD	3
	NY (King's)	MD	1
	St Andrew's	MD	1
	Edinburgh*		4
Royal College of Physicians	London	LRCP**	1
Company of Surgeons	London		18
St George's Hospital	London		3
Guy's Hospital	London		2
College of Surgeons	Hesse-Cassell		1

Sources: For information on the doctors who qualified at Aberbeen (Richard Fletcher, William Paine, Alexander A. Peters), see Anderson, ed., Officers and Graduates; for King's College, New York (Robert Tucker), see Columbia University, Alumni Register 1754–1931; for Royal College of Physicians, London (William Paine), see Munk, The Roll of the Royal College; for the Company of Surgeons, London, see Company of Surgeons' Examination Book, 1745–1800, Royal College of Surgeons Library, London; for St George's Hospital (John Chichester, Alexander A. Peters, John Philipps Jr.), see Register of Pupils and and House Officers, 1756–1837, St George's Hospital Medical School, London; for Guy's Hospital, London (George Philipps, Edward Wyer), see Index to St Thomas's Pupils and Dressers, Pupils and Dressers 1723–1819, St Thomas's Hospital Medical School, London; for the College of Surgeons, Hesse-Cassell (J.F.T. Gschwind), see PRO WO25, 3904:143. Information on W.J. Almon's MD from St Andrew's was received from Robert N. Smart, University Library, St Andrew's (pers. com. 1985).
* According to student records, four men (George F. Boyd, Duncan Clark, George Gillespie, and Fleming Pinckston) attended lectures given by the medical faculty of Edinburgh University. As was common for the period, these students did not complete the requirements for the medical degree.
** Licentiate of the Royal College of Physicians.

concerns, such as those raised in Lower Canada, about the quality of medicine, surgery, and midwifery practised in the province. Eighteenth-century Nova Scotia newspapers[136] contain no editorials or letters describing medical and surgical attendance as inadequate or of poor quality. The minutes of both the Council and the Assembly are entirely devoid of any comments suggesting that the medical and surgical qualifications of practitioners in Nova Scotia were considered inferior or inadequate. Apparently, then, the public attitude towards the medical profession was positive, and there was no perceived need for regulation. This positive perception is attributable in part to the relatively high level of qualification among the province's medical practitioners. Table 6 shows the known academic qualifications of thirty-four of the eighty-four civilian doctors who practised in Nova Scotia during the period 1784 to 1799.

The table indicates that, during the last fifteen years of the eighteenth century, at least forty percent of practitioners in Nova Scotia held an official qualification in medicine or surgery. In contrast, Packard[137] estimates that, at the outset of the American Revolution, there were upwards of 3,500 medical practitioners in the American colonies, of whom only about 400 (eleven percent) had medical degrees. Furthermore, Marks and Beatty[138] estimate that, "of the nearly 1,200 physicians involved in the [American] War, there were not more than a hundred with medical degrees." I am unaware of any studies that attempt to provide a similar quantitative assessment for Lower Canada, although Dr James Fisher's comment on the number of charlatans practising medicine suggests that, in Lower Canada, the problem was acute. But again, public perception in Nova Scotia seems to have been that the qualifications of those who were administering medicines and performing surgery were higher than in neighbouring provinces and states, so that very few complaints, if any, were submitted to the authorities or to the newspapers in Nova Scotia. The large number of available civilian medical practitioners per capita during this period in Nova Scotia may also have had a favourable influence on public attitudes. The ratio of civilian population to civilian practitioners in Nova Scotia was 625:1 in 1784. This figure is only slightly higher than the 522:1 ratio reported for the year 1790 for Massachusetts and only slightly higher than the 1984 figure of 507:1 for Nova Scotia, as reported by Statistics Canada.

Some of the leading families in Nova Scotia during this period encouraged their sons to enter the medical profession. These young men were sent to England and Scotland for medical and surgical training, rather than to the new country to the south, The United States of America. This preference reflected, no doubt, a less than fully accepting attitude towards American institutions, but also recognition that the universities, colleges, and hospitals in Great Britain, were highly regarded for their long-established medical and surgical training programs and examination procedures. In the United States, four universities were offering medical degrees by the end of the eighteenth century. These were the medical faculties of King's College, New York (established 1767); the University of Pennsylvania (1771); Harvard Medical School (1783); and Dartmouth College (1798). Although the first person to receive a medical degree from an American medical school (Robert Tucker, MD, King's, 1770) came to Nova Scotia with the Loyalists and practised at Annapolis Royal until *circa* 1792, Nova Scotian families did not send their sons south to medical school until twenty years after the end of

Table 7
Members of Nova Scotian Families Who Studied Medicine/Surgery Abroad

Nova Scotian	Home Town	Training	Diploma
Benjamin De St Croix	Granville	London	MRCS*
Henry G. Farish	Shelburne	London	
James Geddes	Halifax	Guy's	MRCS
William Greaves	Halifax	Guy's	MRCS
John Halliburton Jr	Halifax	St George's	
Samuel Head	Halifax	St George's	MRCS
John B. Houseal	Halifax	London	
John H. McMonagle	Windsor	London	
Thomas Newell	Halifax	Aberdeen	MD
Alexander A. Peters	Halifax	Aberdeen	MD
George Philipps	Halifax	Guy's	
John Philipps Jr	Halifax	St George's	
William Philipps	Halifax	Guy's	MRCS
David Rowlands	Shelburne	Aberdeen	MD
James Simpson	Falmouth	London	

Sources: Information on De St Croix, Geddes, Greaves, Head, and W. Philipps comes from the Company of Surgeons' Examination Book, 1745–1800, and the Membership Lists of the Royal College of Surgeons, Royal College of Surgeons Library, London; for Halliburton, Head, and J. Philipps, see Register of Pupils and House Officers, 1756–1837 St George's Hospital Medical School, London; for Newell, Peters, and Rowlands, see Anderson, ed., *Officers and Graduates*; for Greaves, G. Philipps, and W. Philipps, see Index to St Thomas's Pupils and Dressers, 1723–1819, St Thomas's Hospital Medical School, which includes students who attended Guy's Hospital Medical School. Farish is mentioned in Yarmouth County Scrapbook, Scrapbook no. 91 (PANS MG9). McMonagle is mentioned in Wentworth to Prince Edward, 6 October 1798 (PANS RG1, 52:224). Simpson is mentioned in the Will of John Simpson of Halifax (PANS RG48, Reel 358).
* Member of the Royal College of Surgeons.

the American Revolution.[140] The medical faculties to the south did not attempt to lure students from Nova Scotia into enrolling until 1794, when Columbia College, the new name of King's College, New York, placed an advertisement on 23 September in the *Nova Scotia Gazette and Weekly Chronicle*.[141]

Table 7 lists the names of fifteen young men, members of well-known families residing in various parts of Nova Scotia, who are known to have gone abroad to obtain their medical and surgical training during the period 1784 to 1799. The table lists the towns they came from, the institutions or cities they were trained in, and the diplomas they received.[142] Only three of the fifteen – Henry G. Farish, Samuel Head, and John Philipps Jr – returned to Nova Scotia to pursue a career in medicine, while five others – William Greaves, John Halliburton, George Philipps, William Philipps, and David Rowlands – spent short periods in the province with the army

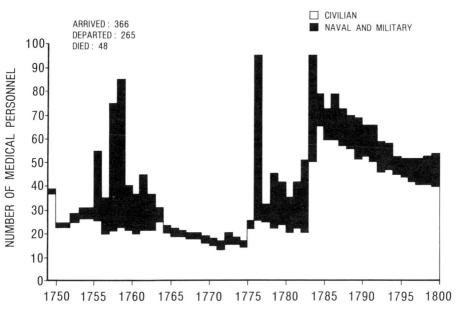

Figure 24
Civilian, naval, and military surgeons, physicians, apothecaries, chymists, and druggists in Nova Scotia, 1750–1800.

and navy. In the latter part of the eighteenth century, Nova Scotia was not an attractive place for a newly trained physician or surgeon to establish a practice. Not only were there no civilian hospital, medical society, medical journal, or medical legislation limiting practice to those who were properly qualified but the population of the province did not increase much between the end of the American Revolution and the end of the century. As Figure 24 shows, the number of civilian doctors in Nova Scotia declined from sixty-four in 1784 to thirty-nine in 1799, a decrease of forty percent.[143] Of the thirty-nine civilian doctors in Nova Scotia in 1799, eight had practised in the province prior to the revolution, twenty had arrived during or immediately after cessation of the war, either as Loyalists or with regiments, and eleven had arrived and begun practice during the fifteen-year period 1784–99.

The heterogeneous nature of the medical education of these thirty-nine practitioners, and indeed of those in the province throughout the period covered in this book, was another key factor in the failure to establish a cohesive, regulated profession before the nineteenth century. The eclectic education of medical practitioners in the province was, to some extent, a result of the vast difference in the way that medical education developed in England and Scotland during the eighteenth century. Both medical educational systems were based on the teaching of anatomy which, during the seventeenth century, was centred at the University of Leyden in Holland. By the beginning of the eighteenth century, Paris became the focus for students seeking an opportunity to learn anatomy through the dissection of cadavers. In England, during the first half of the century, the barber-surgeons' company controlled the teaching of surgeons, and the teaching of anatomy consisted of demonstrations held four times per year at Barbers' Hall in London. At these demonstration, students sat on benches and observed and were taught anatomy from prepared dissections. In spite of the restrictive control of the barber-surgeons' company and its outright suppression of private schools of anatomy in London prior to 1745, at least four London surgeons began to conduct lectures on anatomy and surgery in their own homes.[144] The first to carry out this practice was William Cheselden, surgeon at St Thomas's Hospital, who commenced private lectures and demonstrations in his home in 1710. Three other who conducted lectures in their homes were Samuel Sharp, surgeon at Guy's; William Bromfield, surgeon at St George's; and Edward Nourse, surgeon at St Bartholomew's, who gave his lectures at his home on Aldersgate Street. Nourse was the first to announce that his course of lectures would be offered at a hospital, St Bartholomew's, and this took place in 1734. In Scotland, Alexander Monro, *primus*, who had studied at Leyden and with Cheselden in London, commenced lecturing on anatomy at Edinburgh in 1720.[145]

The main development in the teaching of anatomy in England, however, took place in 1746, three years before the founding of Halifax, and one year after the surgeons separated from the barbers and formed the Company of Surgeons of London. In that year William Hunter (1718–83), began to offer the first course in anatomy in London in which the student actually carried out dissection "in the same manner as at Paris."[146] Hunter continued his lectures for over thirty years, and in 1768, established the Great Windmill Street School in Anatomy and Surgery. One of his very highly regarded contemporaries was Percival Pott (1714–88), surgeon at St Bartholomew's, who gave a course in anatomy, first in his home on Watling Street, and later at his hospital. The most highly esteemed teacher in London during the last half of the eighteenth century, however, was William Hunter's younger brother, John (1728–93). He had studied under Cheselden, Pott, and his older brother, and in 1775 offered his own course of lectures at St George's Hospital. John Hunter's course was unique because it included physiology and pathology, as well as anatomy and surgery and attracted many students, two of whom, John Abernethy (1764–1831) and Sir Astley Cooper (1768–1841), became renowned for contributions to surgery both in the classroom and in their writings. John Abernethy began to teach anatomy and surgery at St Bartholomew's in 1788 and continued teaching there for over forty years. It is interesting to note that none of the these surgeons who lectured on anatomy in London possessed degrees in medicine, except for William Hunter.

The foregoing indicates that in England, during the last half of the eighteenth century, hospitals became the purveyors of medical education. The annual lectures in anatomy that were supposed to be provided by the College of Physicians were frequently omitted. Susan Lawrence has written that "medical education between 1780 and 1820 in London was an unregulated decentralized system of private enterprise. London offered what many Universities did, without the expense and formality of degree regulations."[147] In contrast to this, the university medical schools in Scotland, particularly those of Edinburgh and Glasgow, provided the lead in medical education. The two individuals mainly responsible for the approach of providing medical education within a university environment were Alexander Monro, *primus*, and his student William Cullen. According to Fielding H. Garrison Alexander Monro and his son Alexander, *secundus*, taught anatomy to 12,800 students at Edinburgh University between 1720 and 1790. William Cullen, who was granted an MD degree by the University of Glasgow in 1740, began in 1744 to offer a course of lectures on medicine in Glasgow and in 1746 at the university. In 1747 he, along with Joseph Black, laid the foundations for the faculty of medicine at Glasgow. Cullen continued to teach chemistry, *materica medica*, and botany at Glasgow until 1755, when he moved to the University of Edinburgh to teach chemistry. He began giving clinical lectures there in 1757 and served as professor of medicine at Edinburgh from 1773 to 1790.

Although all five Scottish universities had conferred medical degrees during the period 1654 to 1726, these degrees were honorary or *in absentia* and did not necessarily require the recipient to attend classes at the university or to write examinations. In 1726, the University of Edinburgh formally established a faculty of medicine and began to confer medical degrees only after three years of study and successful completion of examinations. The Edinburgh medical degree soon became recognized by many as the superior medical qualification in Great Britain, and from 1726 to 1800, a total of 1,193 degrees were conferred. The medical faculty at the University of Glasgow was not officially established until early in the nineteenth century; however, it continued, as did Aberdeen, Marischal, and St Andrews, to confer degrees during the eighteenth century without requiring a rigorous course of study and examinations such as those at Edinburgh. Of the total of 366 surgeons, physicians, and apothecaries who were known to be in Nova Scotia during the period 1749 and 1799, not one possessed a medical degree from Edinburgh or from Glasgow. Fourteen of the 366 medical practitioners had been awarded medical degrees, but thirteen of these obtained their degrees *in absentia*, six from Marischal, five from Aberdeen, and two from St Andrews. Robert Tucker was the only doctor practising in Nova Scotia during the period 1749–99 who possessed a medical degree that he had earned by attending classes and writing examinations.

It is not surprising, therefore, that before 1800, very little had been done to regularize the practice of medicine and surgery in Nova Scotia. The great majority of physicians and surgeons who practised in the province had been trained in Great Britain, and prior to the second decade of the nineteenth century, as already noted, it did not have a medical act to regulate the profession. This lack of leadership shown by Great Britain in the area of licensing medical and surgical practitioners was an outgrowth of the long-standing rivalry between three very strong organizations: the College of Physicians, the Company of Surgeons, and the Society of Apothecaries.

John Ransom has written that the status of hospitals at any given time reflects the status of medical science and practice.[148] As pointed out in chapter 2 of this book, hospitals in eighteenth-century England and Scotland were voluntary institutions with no government regulation, and consequently patients, who were mainly the sick poor and the helpless, received treatment that was provided by medical men of varying levels of training and competence. Susan Lawrence has pointed out that there was no license required to practise medicine in England and Wales until the year 1815. She also concluded that licensing of medical men in England and Scotland in the eighteenth century was, in fact, largely irrelevant. The College of Physicians, which had been granted the power in 1518 to regulate the practice of medicine within a seven-mile radius of central London, did not police the profession during the eighteenth century. Lester King has written that, "during the entire eighteenth century, the Royal College of Physicians represented moral and ethical failure; through selfish exploitation of monopoly it revealed the defective morality of the period and of the medical profession." The College was so restrictive in its membership that by 1688 there were only 114 members (i.e., physicians) to provide medical treatment for the estimated five and one-half million people in England.[149] Thanks to this dearth of physicians, London had an estimated one thousand surgeons and apothecaries at the beginning of the eighteenth century.[150] The ratio of ten surgeons and apothecaries to every one physician continued throughout the century. Only the élite could afford the services of physicians, who in turn congregated in the cities and were tied to the purse strings of rich patients. Jewson has concluded that "for authority, status, reward, and advancement, doctors [physicians] looked not to collective professional paths to glory, but to the personal favour of grandees."[151] The medical marketplace was therefore eclectic and open and was determined chiefly by the ability to pay. As Porter has written, a medical self-help culture flourished, since the great mass of the population was too poor to employ medical men no matter whether they were physicians of quacks.[152]

The reason for the lack of leadership by the Royal College of Physicians was twofold. The College lost a court case with the apothecaries in 1704, which resulted in a judgement allowing the latter not only to prepare medicines but also to prescribe them. In addition, during most of the century, the College was involved in an internal squabble over the qualifications required for elevation to its highest grade of membership, the Fellowship. The College held that, whereas graduates of Cambridge and Oxford could become fellows of the College, graduates in medicine from Scottish universities could only qualify as licentiates. One reason for the stand taken by the College was the practice among Scottish universities, noted above, of selling their diplomas without requiring that the applicant attend classes at the university or sit examinations. It appears that the universities of Aberdeen, Marischal, and St Andrews continued this practice all throughout the eighteenth century.

Thus, it is clear that, prior to 1800, the physicians licensed by the Royal College of Physicians failed to meet the public need and the surgeon and apothecary treated the vast majority of the population of England.[153] It is not surprising, therefore, that the same situation existed in the infant British colony of Nova Scotia during the last half of the eighteenth century.

As for the hospitals in Nova Scotia, specifically in Halifax, the situation did not alter significantly between 1784 and 1799 from what it had been during the American Revolution (Appendix 8). The only hospital for civilians in Halifax continued to be the two rooms at the poor house. The naval hospital, under the direction of Dr John Halliburton and located near the Narrows (Figure 20), was overcrowded during the 1790s. In 1794, Dr Halliburton recommended that he should make available for patients the hospital wing in which he lived and rent a house nearby.[154] As noted earlier, a prison hospital had been established on Kavanagh's Island in 1794 and continued to function for at least the next two years.[155] During this period a major change occurred with respect to military hospitals. The military hospital on the corner of Grafton and Blowers Streets, in use since 1758 and under the direction of Dr Donald McIntyre since 1784, closed its doors sometime in 1797. The *Royal Gazette and Nova Scotia Advertiser* of 25 July 1797 carried a notice that the "military hospital lots" were for sale. The public was informed in the same issue that Doctor McIntyre and his son had arrived safely in Guadaloupe in June 1797, having departed recently from Halifax. In the following September, the military hospital lots were granted to James Creighton.[156]

Dr James Boggs, who had been an assistant surgeon to Dr McIntyre since 1784, was appointed garrison surgeon on 22 November 1797. As such, he was in charge of the various regimental hospitals that had been established to provide medical and surgical services to army personnel.[157] On 9 November 1797, Dr Thomas Irwin, garrison surgeon at Annapolis Royal for many years, was appointed assistant inspector of hospitals in Nova Scotia.[158] During the 1790s, it is likely that each of the twelve regiments stationed in the province had its own hospital.[159] For instance, Fort Massey, built during the American revolutionary war, was being used as a hospital in 1795 and had a resident surgeon and hospital mate.[160] Frequent mention is made of the regimental hospital of the Royal Nova Scotia Regiment in Halifax, although I have been unable to ascertain exactly where it was located.[161] Drs John Fraser and Jonathan W. Clarke were surgeon and assistant surgeon of the Royal Nova Scotia Regiment from its establishment in 1793 until the end of the century.[162]

BEFORE TURNING TO THE STATISTICS heralded at the outset of the chapter, mention should be made of the many interesting advertisements related to the practice of medicine that appeared in Nova Scotia newspapers between 1784 and 1799. At least six doctors advertised drugs and medicines, while others had for sale such items as a therapeutic electrical apparatus and cures for cancer, venereal disease,[163] coughs,[164] and hydrophobia.[165] One doctor advertised a series of lectures in chemistry as applied to medicine, another offered his services to perform inoculations, and others simply announced the fact they were setting up practice in Halifax.[166]

Two advertisements for drugs and medicines appeared in the *Nova Scotia Gazette and Weekly Chronicle* of 11 May 1784. One of these ran from February until May 1784:

To be sold by Donald M'Lean, lately arrived from New York, at the House formerly occupied by Major Alex. M'Donald, 84th Regiment, and next Door to Henry Loy's Esq. Wholesale and Retail on very low terms.

A Large and general assortment of Fresh imported Drugs and Medicines, Surgeon's Instruments, Lint and Tow, a great Variety of Genuine Patent Medicines and Perfumeries, Spices, Isinglass, Grain and Bowen's patent Sago, Preserved Tamorinds and fresh Castor Oil, spirits of Turpentine, with a Number of Articles suitable for Grocers and Distillers.

N.B. Physicians and Family Prescriptions made up with Care and Accuracy, all orders from Town and Country Practitioners put up with Care and Expedition.

The second advertisement had completely different wording and was placed in the paper by a Donald MacLean. It ran from May until November 1784. As I explain below,[167] there could very easily have been two surgeons with the names Donald M'Lean (McLean) and Donald MacLean in Halifax at the same time. However, it does represent something of a coincidence and a mystery.

The Shelburne newspapers for 1785 contained advertisements by two surgeons. On 24 January 1785, Joseph Bond, who later practised in Yarmouth from 1787 until 1830, inserted the following announcement in the *Royal American Gazette*:

JOSEPH BOND,
Surgeon,
Begs leave to inform the public, that he has entered into Partnership with Mr Francis Brinley, under the Firm of
BOND and BRINLEY
who have for sale,
a general assortment of
MEDICINES,
of the first quality, lately arrived from England; together with a quantity of the most approved PATENT MEDICINES and PERFUMERY, viz.

Turlington's Balsam	Oil of Lavender
James's Powder	Oil of Rosemary
Anderson's Pills	Lavender Water
Norton's drops	Milk of Roses
British Oil	Rose Water
Court-Plaister	

Daffy's Elixir	Tamarinds
Godfrey's Cordial	Tooth Powder
Stoughton's Bitters	Sallad Oil
Ointment for the itch	Honey
Essence of Lavender	Hartshorn Shavings
Essence of Burgamotte	Isinglass
Essence of Lemons	Spanish Liquorice
Essence of Citron	Allum, and
Essence of Peppermint	Spices of every kind.

LIKEWISE,

A few Family MEDICINE CHESTS, with printed directions for using them, from two to five guineas each, very suitable for fishing vessels, or small settlements, that have no surgeon.

All orders for medicines, family prescriptions, &c. will be attended to with the greatest care and dispatch.[168]

A second surgeon in Shelburne, John Boyd,[169] who later practised in Windsor from 1788 until 1816, advertised in the 12 May 1785 issue of the *Port Roseway Gazetteer*:

JOHN BOYD
Has for Sale

At his medicinal Store, in Water Street between John and Ann Streets, A Choice assortment of DRUGS and MEDICINES; together with a quantity of the most approved PATENT MEDICINES, viz. James's Powders, Anderson's Pills, Hooper's Female Pills, Bateman's Pectoral Drops, Maredants Antiscorbutic Drops, British Oil, Turlington's Balsam, Essence of Peppermint, Daffy's Elixir, Corn Salve, &c. – Also, Breast Pipes, compleat Tobacco Machines, Elastic Trusses, Lancets, Smelling Bottles, Sago Powder, Alum, Honey, Tamarinds, Cinnamon, Mace, Cloves, Nutmegs, Spanish Liquorice, Essence of Lemons, Essence of Bergamot, Court Plaisters, &c.

Family Prescriptions will be accurately prepared and Orders executed with fidelity and Dispatch.

Back in Halifax, Dr John Philipps, who had been there since 1758 and had first advertised drugs and medicines in the Halifax newspaper in 1774, listed for sale the following assortment of medicines in the *Nova Scotia Gazette and Weekly Advertiser*, 28 April 1789:[170]

PHILIPPS, Drugist
Has received by the *Ark*, Capt. Squires,
A general fresh Assortment of

MEDICINES, &c.

Viz.

Jesuits Bark of the first quality,

Turkey Rheubarb
Camphire and Saffron
Dr James's Antiseptic Pills
Dr James's fever Powders
Glass's Magnif—
Balsom of Honey
Sago Powder in Canisters
Pearl Sago
Salt of Lemon
Genuine Anderson's and
Hooper's Pills
Storey's worm destroying
   Cakes
Carolina Pink root for
   destroying worms
Stoughton's bitter
Essence of Peppermint.

Large and small bottles Turlington's
   Balsom,
Betton's true british Oil,
Steer's Opodeldoc
Dalby's Carminative
Squire's Elixir
Surgeon's lint and tow
Oil of Vitriol,
Salt Petre and Verdigrease
Best Russian pearl ash

Hartshorn shavings
Fine cut Isinglass
Castor Oil and Tamarinds
Fresh camom–, Sage, b——
   and Pennyroyal from
   Covent Garden.

Physicians, Surgeons, and others supplyed with the above Articles fresh
every Six Months.

The most comprehensive list of medicines and drugs advertised in
Nova Scotia newspapers during this period was that prepared by
Dr Michael Head, who operated a drug-and-medicine store first on
Hollis Street and later on Granville Street, Halifax, from 1790 until
his death in 1805. Dr Head had operated a similar store at Windsor
from 1779 until 1790. On 27 October 1795, this advertisement appeared in the *Nova Scotia Gazette and Weekly Chronicle*:

HEAD'S DRUG & MEDICINE STORE
in Granville Street
is now replenished by an extensive and general assortment of
DRUGS & MEDICINES
Received in the Ship HERO from London, and sold wholesale
and Retail by
MICHAEL HEAD

By whom the greatest attention will be paid to all orders and prescriptions
from gentlemen of the professions, of the navy and army, town and
country——. Also all family prescriptions, and Medicine chests, made up on
the shortest notice.

He has also received the following articles:

Salt Petre	Keyser's pills
Isinglass	James's pills
Sago and Salep	Wash-balls, violet, and windsor
British violet, pearl, and	soap
opiate dentrifice	Best scented French hard and
Essence of Coltsfoot	soft pomatum
Essence of Peppermint	Vermillion & carmine
Essence of Pennyroyal	Red and black lead
Essence of Bergamot	Lancets
Essence of Lavender	Syringes
Essence of Lemon	Crucibles
Darby's Carminiative	Liquorice and pearl barley
Balsam honey	Verdigris, & arnetta
Patent blue	Allum, copperas & logwood
Jesuit drops	Aniseed
Greenough's tincture	Caraway seeds
Best red pale bark	Lint
Steer's opodeldoc	Tow
Lavender & hungary waters	Best restified spirit of wine or
Cephalic snuff	alcohol, rose & orange flower
Analeptic pills	water
Anderson's pills	Horse medicines of all kinds
Hooper's pills	

Two years later, in the *Gazette* of 3 October 1797, Michael Head had expanded his advertisement to read, "Drugs, Medicines, Patent Medicines, Groceries, etc." This advertisement required an entire newspaper column. Interesting additions to his earlier list included tooth powders and brushes, pectoral lozenges, nipple glasses, and surgeons' instruments. Dr Lewis Davis (mentioned in the previous chapter as surgeon to the King's Rangers) undoubtedly was the person who inserted the following advertisement in the *Gazette*, 22 February 1785. It is presumed that the electric apparatus was for therapeutic purposes.[171]

"To be sold, An Elegent Portative electric Aparatus, compleat, the whole of which is neatly fixed in a mohogony case.

Lewis Davis, opposite Mr Boyers, Jun."

A unique and surprising advertisement appeared in the *Weekly Chronicle*, 13 July 1799. It was unique because it was the first and only notice published in an eighteenth-century Nova Scotian news-paper claiming a cure for cancer. Moreover, it was placed by a woman living in an area of the province that was newly settled and essentially isolated from established towns.[172] The advertisement read:

Cures for the Cancer,
Great Cures have been made for the Cancer by the Subscriber, who under-takes to Cure this dreadful Disease in all its various Stages, with the most tri-fling pain to the Person afflicted – She having made a great number of effected Cures for the years past, to which the most respectable persons in the Country she resides in, can testify. Applications to be made to her at Clare in the County of Annapolis.

Margaret Doucett

Accompanying the advertisement was a statement by one of her subscribers.

I The Subscriber do testify that the above mentioned Margaret Doucett, has to my knowledge cured a great number of Persons afflicted with the dread-ful disorder, the Cancer.

John Taylor

Another item reported in the *Gazette* of 13 July 1790, concerned the curing of wens on the head of a soldier:

I the subscriber having been afflicted with 6 Wens on my head for 30 years past in so much it was with great difficulty I could wear my Regimental hat, and being informed that Benjamin Green Esq., of this Town, had formerly cured one for a soldier in the 37th Regt, I made application to Mr Green who engaged to cure them all gratis — and which he hath accordingly per-formed in the most easy and effectual manner, by means of poultices, leav-ing no scars. They were all of the stealoma kind encysted tumors, stuffed with a sulty matter, two of the size of pidgeons eggs.

Robert Seaton, 4th or King's Own Regt.[173]

Another unique event in Halifax during the last decade of the eighteenth century was an announcement in December 1790 by Mr John Chichester, surgeon of the Fourth or King's American Regiment, concerning a course of lectures on the theory and prac-tice of chemistry. The use of chemical substances in medicine was to be included, and Mr Chichester's lectures were to be given from two to three o'clock, every Monday, Wednesday, and Friday after-noon.[174]

Two early advertisements by dentists are worth noting here, particularly since Gullett's *History of Dentistry in Canada*[175] states that the first such advertisement did not appear until 1814. In fact the first appeared in the *Gazette* of 27 June 1786:

DR TEMPLEMAN,

Informs the Public, that it is probable he shall be in Halifax about twenty days; part of which time he shall be able to devote to those Ladies and Gentlemen who wish to have any of the following operations performed on their Teeth viz.

Taking the tartar from them;
Curing the scurvey in the Gums;
Plumbing caries Teeth;
Substituting Ivory Teeth;
Substituting natural Teeth artificially,
with gold sockets;
Transplanting Teeth;
Separating defective Teeth;
Cleansing and Polishing the Teeth in
the most beautiful manner, &c
Advice may be had on all the various diseases

to which Human Teeth are subject, and an excellent Dentifrice, with proper Brusher and Chewsticks, by applying at Mrs Philip's.

In 1791, John Beath, the second dentist to advertise in the *Gazette*, offered cash for natural teeth and indicated that he would fix natural and artificial teeth on gold plates.[176]

Only one midwife advertised during the period 1784–99: a Mrs Smith placed an advertisement in the *Gazette* in 1787 stating that she was a "sworn midwife from London."[177] In the same year, Dr Christopher Nicolai, who, as noted earlier, had been in Halifax since 1751, advertised as a man-midwife in the *Nova Scotia Gazette and Weekly Advertiser* for 10 April 1787.

CHRISTOPHER NICHOLAI
Surgeon and Man Mid-Wife

Takes this method of acquainting the Public that he has been conversant with the Treatment of the SMALL-POCKS, both Natural and by Innoculation, for above thirty years – Intends to innoculate and attend the Patients in the Town and Suburbs of Halifax, through the whole course, with proper Medicines, at

Half a Guinea Each

Strangers, who intend to be innoculated, can be accomodated with proper

Diet, Nurse and Lodgings at his House on the Parade, at 17s 6d, each, bringing their own Bedding.[178]

Mrs James MacNeil, midwife at Shelburne (see note 177), possessed an injection device described as a "bladder and pipe," which she brought from New England to Shelburne in 1783. Lieutenant William Booth mentioned this device when he described Dr George Drummond's treatment of his wife, Hannah, and her death, on 22 February 1789, from "nervous fever" at Shelburne.[179] It is unclear whether the device was actually used in treating Mrs Booth. Lieutenant Booth's diary does include, however, a number of entries describing the types of medication that Dr Drummond administered to Lieutenant and Mrs Booth. For instance, in January 1789, Drummond ordered for Hannah some drops of spirit of lavender on sugar and some hartshorn and water, while in March, for the lieutenant's cough, he recommended liquorice root boiled in water.

An item on the use of bloodstone is found in the letters of the Reverend Mather Byles,[180] who had arrived in Halifax from Boston with General Howe in April 1776, Byles's daughter Rebecca was married to Dr William J. Almon. On 16 December 1787, the Reverend Mr Byles wrote: "Dr Allmon, the Systems-Monger came in great distress to borrow my Blood-Stone for a man who not withstanding all his scientific efforts was absolutely bleeding to death. The man put on the Blood-Stone and the bleeding stopped: but the Doctor is of opinion that this was owing to the violents stiptics [*sic*] which he had been taking for several days before, and which exactly at that instant began to operate."

During the last half of the eighteenth century, at least 11,503 deaths are known to have occurred in Nova Scotia.[181] Figure 25 shows the number of deaths each year for the period 1749 to 1799 and confirms that major epidemics occurred in 1750–51, 1755–56, 1757–58, and 1775–76. However, the large increases in the number of deaths during these years cannot be attributed solely to the epidemics, since many regiments and squadrons arrived in 1755, 1757, 1758, and 1776, as well as throughout Seven Years' and the American revolutionary wars. In addition to soldiers and sailors, who were young and probably in reasonable health, there came a large number of camp followers who, with the departure of a regiment for a war zone, were left in Halifax, destitute and probably sickly, to be supported by the local government. As already pointed out, the British government had eliminated all support for health-care facilities

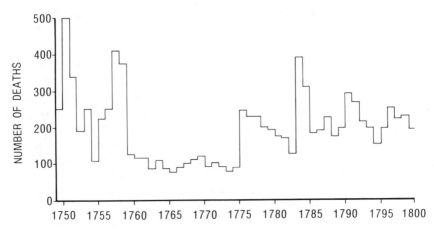

Figure 25
Deaths in Nova Scotia, 1749–99.

and medical personnel by 1760, and the burden of the poor on the local government was so great that it could not provide any medical services whatsoever, not even a civilian hospital, at any time during the eighteenth century. It is likely, therefore, that many of the deaths shown in Figure 25, particularly during and immediately after the war years, represent those of a transitory population shaped by the arrival and departure of soldiers and sailors and, to a greater extent, by camp followers and prisoners of war who remained, for the most part, in Halifax to be cared for. The minor epidemic of smallpox reported in 1790–91 in towns such as Lunenburg and Guysborough took at least seventeen lives.[182] Figure 25 shows a substantial increase in the number of deaths during these two years, and probably many more than seventeen succumbed to smallpox. The large number of deaths in 1783 and 1784 was due to the province's increased population after the arrival of the approximately thirty thousand Loyalists.

Of the 11,503 people whose deaths were recorded, the ages of only 2,824 were given in the death and burial records. The mean age of the deceased was twenty-eight years, while the median age was twenty-two. A total of 724 of the 2,824 (twenty-five percent) were infants, i.e., less than one year of age, and 1,188 (forty-two percent) were ten years old or younger. Only five percent of the 2,824 lived to the age of seventy-five or beyond. The average age at time of death of adult civilian Nova Scotians during the years 1780–99, compared with 1981, is presented in Figure 26. Age was stated in the death records of over seventy percent of adult Nova Scotians who

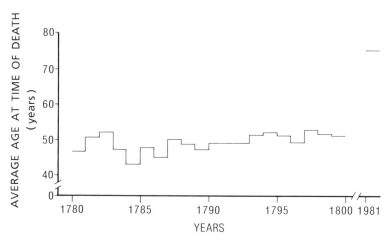

Figure 26
Mean age of civilian Nova Scotians at time of death during the period 1780–99, as compared to life expectancy at birth of Canadians in 1981.

died during this period. Very few of the recorded deaths prior to 1780 give the age of the deceased, and therefore the period 1749–79 is not included in Figure 26. This figure indicates that, whereas age at time of death during the last twenty years of the eighteenth century was approximately forty-nine years, twentieth-century Nova Scotians, particularily those living in 1981, could hope to live to the age of seventy-five. The only other studies of this type for the eighteenth century that I am aware of are those reported by T.H. Hollingsworth, A.E. Imhof, and S.J. Kunitz. Hollingsworth determined the life expectancy of aristocratic women in England during the period 1725–1800.[183] He found that, for such a select group, life expectancy ranged from thirty-six years in 1725 to forty-nine years in 1800. Arthur Imhof, in a recent paper[184] on urban mortality, shows very clearly how one can gain a great deal of information about social history from demographic data, and some of his conclusions will be presented below. S.J. Kunitz, using figures from a book by E.A. Wrigley and R.S. Schofield, entitled *The Population History of England, 1541–1871*, concluded that life expectancy at birth from 1741 to 1801 in England ranged from thirty-two to thirty-eight years.[185]

The death rate of Nova Scotians during the period 1749–84 is shown in figure 27. For many of these years, population figures for Nova Scotia are readily available. For the last fifteen years of the eighteenth century, however, such figures are not known, and that

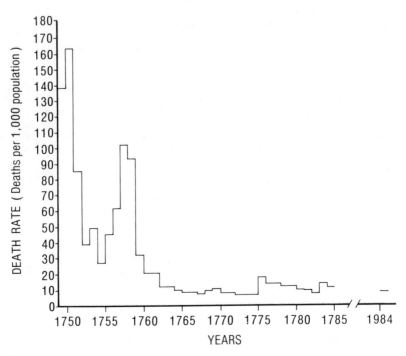

Figure 27
Death rate of civilians in Nova Scotia during the period 1749–84, as compared to 1984.

is why the period 1785–99 is not included in the figure. It should be noted that the death rates presented in Figure 27 are lower than actual rates, since, as explained in note 181, not every death that occurred between 1749 and 1784 was recorded. This explains the extremely low death rates for the years 1764–74, a decade during which a higher death rate might be expected given that Halifax was without any health-care facilities whatsoever. It is clear, however, that the rate was very high for the first ten years of settlement in Nova Scotia and also higher than normal for those years in which the four epidemics are known to have occurred, and during which large numbers of military and naval personnel and their camp followers were stationed in Halifax. In contrast to the numbers given in Figure 27, Imhof presents the mortality rates for Berlin for the period 1721 to 1980 and shows that, from 1750 to 1800, the death rate varied from a low of thirty per thousand to a high of sixty-eight.

I have been able to determine, from death and burial records, the cause of death for 1,935 Nova Scotians who died between 1749 and

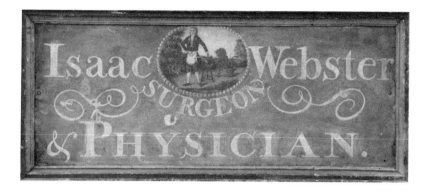

Figure 28
The shingle of Dr Isaac Webster, physician and surgeon at Cornwallis from 1791 to 1851. The original is in the possession of descendants and measures twenty-one by forty-eight inches. (Courtesy, C.R. Webster, Mississauga).

1799. The stated causes differ dramatically from those experienced by present-day citizens. The most marked difference concerns infant mortality, which represented thirty-seven percent of the deaths whose cause was given; in contrast, infant mortality in Canada in 1984, according to Statistics Canada, was less than one percent. This figure of thirty-seven percent is not much higher than that found by Imhof (32.7 percent) in his study of infant mortality in Philipsburg in the German empire for the slightly later period 1780 to 1809.

In 1984, the five leading causes of death in Nova Scotia were heart disease, cancer, accidents, stroke, and respiratory disease. The leading causes during the last fifty years of the eighteenth century were accidents, smallpox, fever, consumption, and gout. A tabulation of causes of death in eighteenth-century Nova Scotia is given in Appendix 9. Heart disease is not mentioned at all, while cancer, respiratory disease, and stroke are given as the causes of death in fewer than fifty of the 1,935 deaths.[186]

Appendices

Appendix One

PASSENGERS IN THE CORNWALLIS MESS LISTS WITH HEALTH-CARE OCCUPATIONS

Passenger	Occupation	Transport Ship	Total in Family
Alexander Abercrombie	Apothecary's mate	Roehampton	2
Daniel Brown	Surgeon's mate	Everley	1
Georgius Bruscourt*	Surgeon	Charlton	2
Archibald Campbell	Surgeon's mate	Baltimore	1
David Carnegie	Surgeon	London	2
Cochran Dickson	Surgeon	London	3
John Farrington	Chymist and Druggist	Roehampton	2
John Grant	Surgeon's mate	Everley	3
Robert Grant	Surgeon's mate	Charlton	3
William Grant	Surgeon	Alexander	1
Fenton Griffith	Surgeon's mate	Wilmington	2
James Handasyde	Surgeon	Fair Lady	1
Augustus Harbin	Assistant Surgeon	Roehampton	1
Alexander Hay	Surgeon's mate	Charlton	4
Patrick Hay	Surgeon	Beaufort	2
John Inman	Surgeon	Canning	1
Matthew Jones	Surgeon	Everley	4
Matthew Jones	Surgeon	Beaufort	5
Robert Kerr	Apothecary's mate	Wilmington	2
William Lascelles	Surgeon's mate	Alexander	2
Leonard Lockman	Major [surgeon]	Roehampton	6
Thomas Louthian	Surgeon's mate	Wilmington	1
Ann Medlicott**	Midwife	Everley	3
Henry Meriton	Surgeon's mate	Winchelsea	7
William Merry	Apothecary	Roehampton	6
Charles Paine	Surgeon	Merry Jacks	1
Harry Pitt	Surgeon	Baltimore	7
Thomas Reeve	Apothecary	Winchelsea	3
Thomas Rust***	Doctor and Surgeon	Charlton	1
Joshua Sacheverell	Surgeon	Baltimore	6

Passengers in the Cornwallis Mess Lists with Health-Care Occupations (Cont'd)

Passenger	Occupation	Transport Ship	Total in Family
John Steele	Lieutenant and Surgeon	Beaufort	4
Robert Throckmorton	Pupil Surgeon	Beaufort	2
John Wallace	Surgeon's mate	Everley	2
Robert White	Surgeon	Beaufort	1
John Wildman	Surgeon	Canning	4
Elizabeth Williams	Midwife	Wilmington	1
John Willis	Chymist and Surgeon	Winchelsea	5
Thomas Wilson	Surgeon	Wilmington	1

Source: PANS RG1, vol. 523.

* Given as G.P.W. Bruscowitz in a land sale on 13 September 1751 (o.s.) (Halifax County Deeds, vol. 2, PANS RG47) and, on 1 February 1753 (n.s.), as George Phillipps Bruscovit, MD (Ibid., 184).

** Ann Medlicot practised midwifery in Halifax according to CO217, 10: 70–1. This source indicates that she was the midwife in Halifax at least during the period August 1749 to September 1750. She was paid twelve pounds per year for her services. An Ann Medecott [sic] was buried from St Paul's Church in Halifax on 28 April 1776.

*** In the "books" referred to earlier (CO221, vol. 36), a surgeon by the name of Rust is listed but only by surname. In the mess lists (PANS RG1, vol. 523) a doctor and surgeon by the name of Rush is listed on the transport Charlton. I suggest that the person in question is Thomas Rust, who, on 8 August 1749 (o.s.), was allotted land in Ewer's Division, C5 (PANS RG1, vol. 410) and is listed, as late as 2 September 1752 (o.s.), as a "practioner [sic] of phisick [sic] and surgery" in Halifax (Halifax County Inferior Court of Common Pleas, vol. A: 196, PANS RG37).

Appendix Two

AN EXPLANATION OF
MEDICATIONS AND TREATMENTS
ADMINISTERED BY SURGEONS
IN HALIFAX DURING THE PERIOD
1750−53

As indicated in chapter 2, the court records for Halifax, in the early 1750s, contain numerous cases of surgeons charging citizens for non-payment of medical bills. These medical bills list the types and quantities of medications administered and their prices. The medications and treatments, along with an explanation of each, appears below. I have also attempted to identify the illness for which each of the medications was known to be a treatment. I have also corrected the spellings given in the court records.

In the eighteenth century, inflammation and fever were the primary indications that some disease process was present. It was the belief and teaching of the highly respected Dr Hermann Boerhaave, professor of medicine, chemistry, and botany at the University of Leyden from 1709–26, that inflammation existed whenever two conditions were present. There must be an obstruction of the small arteries and, at the same time, an increased velocity or momentum of the blood stream acting on the obstructing matter: "Boerhaave had no difficulty correlating the clinical signs of inflammation and pathogenic factors. Obstruction produced distention and redness. Distention caused pain. The solids and fluids were compacted – hence the hardness and resistance. Local heat arose from the attrition of the fluid particles and the solids against each other. Blood under increased force caused pulsations. Irritation of the various nerve fibers could induce a fever; in Boerhaave's day it was generally accepted that fever could result from pain alone."[1] The treatment of inflammation would depend upon dislodging the obstruction and there were various methods of doing this, such as administering diluents or following a mild softening diet. Bleeding was used to reduce the velocity of the blood acting on the obstruction. Both bleeding and purging were considered valuable therapeutic aids because they reduced the volume of fluids and the impetus or violence of the arterial blood. In addition to bleeding, the redistribution of blood away from the site of inflammation was considered to be important. This was done by using counter-irritants such as warm baths, cupping, and blistering and mustard plasters, in order to draw the blood away from the inflamed area.

Other approaches to treating illness and disease in the eighteenth century, in addition to blood-letting and purging, were emetics, diuretics, and sweating. The idea was to cleanse the bowels, kidneys, and stomach in order to drive out the disorder, and then to rebuild the body with tonics. Whereas blood-letting was used in pleurisy and rheumatism, purges and vomits were used to treat fevers.[2] One of the most common purgatives or cathartics was calomel, or chloride of mercury. It exerted its effect as a laxative because the mercuric ion is extremely irritating to the intestinal tract.[3] Dr Benjamin Rush (1746–1813), a graduate of Edinburgh and a student of Dr William Cullen, is remembered for his use of a mixture of calomel and jalap[4] as a purgative during the devastating yellow-fever epidemic in Philadelphia in 1793. Commonly used emetics were ipecac,[5] antimony, and salts of copper, while turpentine, potassium iodine, and balsam were used as diuretics.

The "fever" theory of disease suggested that disease was a result of irritation or excitement. Before being treated with rehabilitating tonics and stimulents, the patient was first depressed or calmed by blood-letting, followed by diuretics, purgatives, and emetics. Among the tonics used to rebuild the body were mercury,[6] iron, arsenic, quinine, and wine. Stimulents included camphor, opium, musk, and alcohol.

MEDICATIONS AND
TREATMENTS ADMINISTERED
IN HALIFAX IN
THE 1750S

Anodyne draft. A medicine used to relieve pain by diminishing sensibility. Hoffmann's anodyne contained alcohol (65 percent), ether (32 percent), and ethereal oil (3 percent). Other anodynes contained opium, and morphine.

Anti-icteric pills. Icterus is another word for jaundice, and therefore the anti-icteric pills would be administered in order to treat liver disease. The common barberry bush was traditionally used in the treatment of liver disease since it was thought that preparations made from the plant would stimulate the production of bile by the liver.

Astringent bolus. A substance such as alum or tannin that was administered to contract or bind together organic tissues, thus aiding in diminishing secretion or discharge. An astringent bolus had the opposite effect to a laxative.

Attenuating mixture. A mixture such as wine or quinine which thins, weakens, or reduces the density of body fluids. Used as a tonic or stimulent.

Balsamic Bolus. A Balsam was any fragrant ointment derived from the resin of trees and used as a diuretic.

Blooding. Another way of describing bleeding or blood-letting.

Bolus. A rounded mass of a pharmaceutical preparation which, during the eighteenth century, would be swallowed rather than given intravenously.

Camphorated spirits. Camphor is a white, volatile, translucent crystalline compound distilled from the wood and bark of the camphor tree. Used as a stimulent.

Cephalic mixture. The word cephalic pertains to the head or skull. This could have been a mixture taken to alleviate a headache.

Clysters. Another name for an enema.

Colic tincture. This refers to a solution that was administered to relieve acute abdominal pain resulting from muscular spasm. It would be very interesting to know exactly what made up the "Colic Tincture" that was administered by Dr William Merry to William Kneeland on 4 July 1751, and that cost two pounds six shillings.

Compound emetic. A mixture that caused vomiting, such as ipecac or antimony.

Cordial bolus. A medical stimulent such as anisette or benedictine that was intended to invigorate the heart. Foxglove was not discovered to be a cardiac stimulent until 1775.

Corroborating plaster. The adjective corroborating indicates that the plaster has been strengthened. A plaster consists of a viscid, hot substance spread on linen or silk and then applied to some part of the body.

Decoction. This is a solution prepared by boiling an animal or vegetable substance to create an extract.

Detergent. Having cleansing or purging qualities.

Digestive. A medicine to aid digestion.

Electuary. A medicine mixed with honey or syrup to form a paste.

Elixir. This was a sweetened, alcoholic, medicinal preparation supposed to invigorate the person. Elixir of vitriol consisted of aromatic sulfuric acid.

Emetic. A mixture that, if swallowed, caused vomiting, such as tartar emetic (antimony potassium tartrate), or ipecac.

Enema. A liquid injected into the rectum for cleansing, diagnostic, or nutritive purposes.

Fermentation. The decomposition of organic compounds induced by the action of various ferments.

Gargarism. This refers to a liquid used to gargle or rinse the throat.

Glauber salts. This salt is reported to have been used as a purgative by Dr John Redman, MD (Leiden, 1748). It consisted of sodium sulphate.

Hartshorn shavings. Also referred to as Spirit of Hartshorn. It was made by the distillation of deer horns, since the result was an ammoniacal liquor, which contained ammonium carbonate. The latter was used as smelling salts, a stimulent. A dose of one dram in a cup of wine was given for pleurisy by the American colonists in the seventeenth century.

Hysteric mixture. This consisted of opium, castor oil, saffron, and maple seed, one dram of each, in four ounces of Lisbon wine.

Isinglass. A preparation of nearly pure gelatin made from the swim bladders of certain fishes. This was used in the clearing or fining of wine or liquor.

Pectoral bolus. Pectoral drops were formulated to relieve or cure diseases of the lungs or chest.

Plaster. Mustard plasters were the most common. These were also referred to as blisters and were applied to, or near, the inflamed area using a cloth or tape. A thick, hot, drawing poultice containing mustard, turpentine, spirits of hartshorn, pepper, and/or brandy was spread on the cloth and the plaster was then placed and secured on the inflamed area. Once the blistered area had been raised or enlarged, it was snipped and allowed to discharge. After a sufficient discharge, the blistered site was reduced using poultices made from bread, milk, flax seed, or hog's lard.

Purging pills. A pill to induce the evacuation of the bowels, such as calomel.

Rhubarb bolus. A mild laxative.

Salts. Emetics to cause vomiting. Salts of copper and zinc sulphate were frequently used, since they acted directly upon the nerves of the stomach.

Salutes. Another name for salts.

Spanish liquorice. A perennial leguminous herb of southern and central Europe, the dried root of which is used as a medicine to treat headache.

Tincture. A solution, usually in alcohol, of some distinctly coloured substance used in medicine.

Appendix Three

AN ACT TO PREVENT THE SPREADING OF CONTAGIOUS DISTEMPERS*

Be it enacted by the Honorable the Commander in Chief, the Council and Assembly, That every vessel coming into the port of Halifax, having any person on board infected with any plague, small-pox, malignant fever, or other contagious distemper, shall anchor at least two miles below the Town of Halifax, towards the sea, and on her anchoring shall hoist an ensign with the union downwards at the main-top mast head; and the master thereof shall not permit any of the mariners or passengers belonging to or coming in such Vessel to land. And the said master shall be obliged, within twenty four hours after his arrival, to give notice thereof to the Governor, Lieutenant-Governor, or Commander in Chief, both for the performing quarantine, for the airing and cleansing the passengers, vessels, and goods on board, and for removing the infected and sick persons out of the said vessel.

II. And be it further Enacted, That before any such sick or infected persons be put onshore, the master of such ship or vessel shall give security for the payment of the charge of removing them on shore, and also for the necessary refreshments, medicines, and attendance, which shall be ordered and directed by the Governor, Lieutenant-Governor, or Commander in Chief.

III. And be it further enacted, That any master or masters of any vessel or vessels, who shall not conform themselves to the rule and directions prescribed by this Act, shall be liable to pay a fine not exceeding one hundred pounds, on due conviction thereof, to be recovered by bill, plaint, or information, in any of his Majesty's courts of record.

---

* 2 Geo. 3d, c.6, 1761

IV. And be it further enacted, That for the preventing any infectious distempers from being brought into, and spreading in any of the other towns within this province, any one or more Justices of the Peace, residing within or nearest to such town within this province, where any vessel infected with the small pox or infectious distempers, shall arrive, shall forthwith take care to prevent and restrain all persons belonging to or transported in such ship or vessel, from coming on shore: or if any be before on shore, to send them on board again; as also to restrain persons from going on board such ship or vessel, and to that end may make out a warrant directed to the constable of any such town, who are accordingly impowered and required to execute the same; and such Justices are forthwith to transmit the intelligence thereof, to the Governor, Lieutenant-Governor, or Commander in Chief, for their direction and order thereon.

Appendix Four

AN ACT TO PREVENT
IMPORTING IMPOTENT, LAME,
AND INFIRM PERSONS INTO THIS
PROVINCE*

Be it enacted by the Lieutenant Governor, Council, and Assembly, that every Master of any ship or other vessel, arriving in any Port within this Province, at the time of entering his Ship or Vessel, shall deliver to the Secretary of the Province if at Halifax, and if at any other Port then to his deputy to be thereunto by him appointed for that purpose, a perfect List or Certificate under his hand of the Christian and Sir Names of all Passengers, as well servants as others, brought in said Ship or Vessel, and their circumstances so far as he knows; on pain of forfeiting the sum of Five Pounds to the use of the Poor of the Town or place where such Passenger shall be landed or sent on Shore, for every Passenger that he shall omit to enter his or her Name in such List or certificate upon Conviction thereof before any two of His Majesty's Justices of The Peace, in such Towns where two Justices shall be Resident, otherwise before one Justice of the Peace for the County or place where such Passenger shall be so landed or sent on Shore. And upon Neglect or Refusal of such Offender to pay such Fine such Justice or Justices may issue his or their Warrant for levying the same by distress and sale of such Offenders Goods and chattels, and in default of such Goods or Chattels whereon to levy such Distress, may Commit such Offenders to Gaol for the space of one month.

And be it further enacted that if any Passenger so brought, shall be impotent, lame, or otherwise infirm, or likely to be a Charge to the place, it shall and may be lawful for any one or more of His Majesty's Justices of the Peace in such Town or place where such Vessel shall arrive upon Notice being given by the Secretary or his Deputy

* PANS CO 217, 25:77–9

to require a Security from such Passengers with Sufficient Surety or Sureties to become bound in the sum of Twenty Pounds to the Secretary or his Deputy for his idemnifying the Town from such charity and upon such Passenger refusing or neglecting to give such security, the Master of the Ship or Vessel inwhich such Passenger came, shall be and thereby is obliged and required to give sufficient security before such Justice or Justices and for such sum as aforesaid to indemnify and keep the Town free from all charge for the Relief or support of such impotent, lame, or infirm persons unless such person was before an Inhabitant of this Province or that such impotence, lameness, or other infirmity befell or happened to him or her during the passage: And in such case, if they be Servants their Masters shall provide for him, and others shall be relieved at the charge of the Town or place where such impotent, lame, or infirm persons shall be brought or imposed, and if any Master of any Ship or Vessel shall neglect or refuse to give such Security as aforesaid, he shall forfeit and pay the sum of Twenty Pounds to be recovered by Bill plaint or Information in any of His Majesty's Courts of Record in this Province where the said Offence shall be committed and to be applied to the use of the poor in such Town or place.

Appendix Five

LOYALIST PHYSICIANS AND SURGEONS WHO SETTLED IN NOVA SCOTIA DURING 1783

Physician or Surgeon	Birthplace and Birthdate	Former Practice	Regiment or Hospital	Place of Settlement	Years in Nova Scotia	Month of Arrival	Loyalist Claim[1]
Charles Adams[2]				Digby	1	June	
William J. Almon[3]	RI, 1755	NY	Royal Artillery	Halifax	34	May	
Peter Berton[4]		NY		Chester	3	May	
Azor Betts[5]	c.1739	NY	Queen's Rangers	Saint John	10	May	Yes
Charles Bode[6]				Shelburne	3	May	
James Boggs[7]	DE, 1740	NJ	NY General Hosp.	Halifax	47	November	Yes
Joseph N Bond[8]	England, 1758	Eng.	Regimental Hosp.	Yarmouth	47	May	
John Boyd[9]	c.1754	PA	NY General Hosp.	Windsor	32	May	Yes
Francis Brinley[10]	c.1756	MA	NY Volunteers	Shelburne	2	May	
John Brown[11]	c.1745		Captain Reed's Coy	Shelburne	6	May	
Peter Browne[12]		NJ	NY General Hosp.	Windsor	4	September	Yes
Nathaniel Bullein[13]	SC	SC	SC Refugee Hosp.	Halifax	10	July	Yes
William Burns[14]	c.1757			Shelburne	8	May	
Matthew Cahill[15]			20th Regt	Shelburne	6	May	
John Calef[16]	MA, 1726	MA		Saint John		May	Yes
Daniel Cornwall[17]			SC Royals	Country Hbr	17		
George Drummond[18]	Scotland, c.1715	PA	NY General Hosp.	Shelburne	10	May	Yes

Name	Birth	Colony	German Aux. Forces / Unit	Destination	No.	Month	
Joseph Falt[19]			German Aux. Forces	Petite Rivière	56	October	Yes
Abraham Florentine[20]	Germany, 1757	NY	Hessian Regt	Digby	3	November	Yes
Isaac Goodman[21]	Germany	RI	Regimental Hosp.	Conway	1	May	Yes
John Gould[22]	MA, 1760	MA	SC Royals	Shelburne	6		
Joseph Hatton[23]	Hessen c. 1753		Prince Carl Regt	Country Hbr			
George W. Holland[24]	Hessen c. 1752		Hessian Regt	Lunenburg	13	July	Yes
John Hoose[25]	c. 1760			Shelburne	16	May	Yes
John Huggeford[26]		NY	Loyal Amer. Regt	Shelburne	6	May	
Peter Huggeford[27]	England c. 1725	NY	60th Regt	Digby	7	May	
Ludovic Joppe[28]			Prince of Wales Regt	Manchester	37	September	
Daniel Kendrick[29]	c. 1735	NY	NY General Hosp.	Liverpool	17	May	
David Landeg[30]	Wales		NY General Hosp.	Shelburne	1	May	
John Lawrence[31]				Annapolis	10	May	
Benjamin Loring[32]			NY General Hosp.	Shelburne	1	June	
Joseph Marvin[33]			Delancey's Brigade	Digby	3	August	
Donald McIntyre[34]			43rd Regt	Halifax	14	November	
Donald McLean[35]			77th Regt	Shelburne			
Murdock McLeod[36]	Scotland, c. 1742	NC	NC Volunteers	Country Hbr	1	May	Yes
John McPherson[37]			Duke of Cumb. Regt	Manchester	48	November	
Jonathan Ogden[38]			NY General Hosp.	Halifax	1	June	
John Perry[39]		VA		Shelburne	9	June	
Alexander J. Phillips[40]				Digby			
Fleming Pinckston[41]				Weymouth	1		
Joseph Russell[42]		NY	33rd Regt	Halifax			
Andrew Seidler[43]	Germany		German Service	Clements	5	October	
John C. Sieger[44]	Saxony, c. 1753		Jager Corps	Halifax	20	June	
Johannes Skener[45]			Hessian Service	Digby		October	
Edward Smith[46]	Ireland		Tarleton's Legion	Liverpool		May	
John F.T. Stickells[47]	Germany		Hessian Regt	Guysborough	25	September	
Bartholomew Sullivan[48]	Ireland, c. 1743	NY		Shelburne			
Christian Tobias[49]		NY		Digby	17	November	Yes

Physician or Surgeon	Birthplace and Birthdate	Former Practice	Regiment or Hospital	Place of Settlement	Years in Nova Scotia	Month of Arrival	Loyalist Claim[1]
Robert Tucker[50]	NY, 1741	NC	King's American Regt	Annapolis	9		Yes
James Van Buren[51]	NJ, 1729	NJ		Granville	7		Yes
Abraham Van Buskirk[52]	c. 1735	NJ	NJ Volunteers	Shelburne	16	October	Yes
William Young[53]			NY General Hosp.	Digby	6		

1 As noted by W.B. Antliff in "Loyalist Claims, A Wealth of Information" (PANS VF, vol. 312, no. 29). "Many bundles of Memorials have been lost."

2 Annapolis County Estates, Reel 4, PANS RG48. The administration of his estate is dated 29 October 1784.

3 The Army List for 1781 includes Almon as surgeon's mate. Fourth Battalion, Royal Artillery.

4 Robertson, *The King's Bounty, A History of Early Shelburne*, 287. Dr Berton is listed as one of the grantees of Shelburne. He was a resident of Chester Township as late as September 1787 (Lunenburg County Deeds, 3:354. Reel 136!, PANS RG47) and was witness to a land sale.

5 Dr Betts appears to have moved from Saint John to Digby *circa* 1799. He died in Digby on 14 September 1809 (*Columbian Centennial*, 25 October 1809). The inscription on his gravestone records incorrectly that his death took place on 15 September 1811.

6 Robertson, *The King's Bounty, A History of Early Shelburne*, 287. Dr Bode is last recorded as being in Shelburne in 1786 (Shelburne Christ Church Baptism, 11 June 1786, PANS MG4, vol 141).

7 A letter from Dr Boggs to his wife Mary, written from Port Matoun (*sic*) and dated 3 March 1784, is printed in Boggs, *The Genealogical Record of the Boggs Family*, 83. Dr Boggs indicated that he had arrived at Port Mouton in November 1783.

8 Dr Bond resided at Shelburne from 1783 to 1787, and then removed to Yarmouth.

9 Dr Boyd moved from Shelburne to Windsor *circa* 1787. He had been assigned, in July 1783, Lot 5, Letter B, in the South Division, Town of Shelburne (PANS RG1, 372:3).

10 Shelburne Christ Church Burials, 1 July 1785, PANS MG4, vol. 141. Dr Brinley was twenty-nine years old.

11 Muster Book of Free Blacks, Port Roseway, 30 April 1784, PANS MG100, vol. 220, no. 4, includes John Brown, doctor.

12 Dr Browne was a surgeon's mate at Annapolis Royal from 1783 to 1786, and was then posted to Windsor (Muster Roll of Annapolis County, June 1784, PANS RG1 376:48).

13 Dr Bullein also resided in Horton, Shelburne, and Dartmouth, prior to leaving Nova Scotia *circa* 1793. He indicated that he had come to Nova Scotia and lived at Horton as early as August 1783 (PANS Misc. "L," AO 12, 49:224).

14 Dr Burns resided in Shelburne from 1783 to 1791 (Ledger of Stephen Skinners, PANS MG3, vol. 305).

15 Matthew Cahill does not appear to have practised medicine in Shelburne. He left the town *circa* 1789 (PANS RG1, 169: 182).

16 It is not clear whether Dr Calef came to Halifax or to Saint John in 1783; however, he did treat patients in Digby prior to 1798 (Halifax Estates, Reel 401, Estate of Henry Coggin, PANS RG48).

17 Land Grants, Book 13 (old), 91, PANS RG20 "A". Grant at Country Harbour, 13 May 1784.

18 There is a good account of George Drummond's practice in Shelburne in the Lieutenant William Booth Diary, Acadia University Archives, F1039.5, S546B6.

19 Lunenburg County Deeds, 3:104, PANS RG47. Joseph Falt was a witness to a land sale on 29 March 1784.

20 PANS Misc "L," AO13, Bundle 26:112 indicates that Dr Florentine arrived in Nova Scotia on 17 October 1783.

21 Ibid., AO12, 101:130 indicates that Dr Goodman left the township of Conway for England in May 1784.

22 Dr Gould resided in Halifax, Windsor, and Shelburne before leaving Nova Scotia *circa* 1786. He was in Halifax as early as 16 June 1783 (PANS RG37, vol. 6, file 12.7).

23 Land Grants, Book 13 (old):91, PANS RG20 A. Grant at Country Harbour, 13 May 1784, two hundred acres.

24 Robertson, *The King's Bounty, A History of Early Shelburne*, 293. He was assigned a water lot in the town of Shelburne in July 1783 (PANS RG1, 372:80).

25 *Hessische Truppen* 2. Johannes Hooses was discharged in America in September 1783.

26 Dr John Huggeford resided in Shelburne until 1789.

27 Dr Peter Huggeford returned to New York in 1790.

28 Two battalions of the Sixtieth Regiment were disbanded in Halifax on 30 October 1783 (*Nova Scotia Gazette and Weekly Chronicle*, 14 October 1783).

29 Robertson, *The King's Bounty, A History of Early Shelburne*, 294. Dr Kendrick was listed as a physician in Shelburne on 30 October 1783 (Shelburne County Deeds, Book 1:77, PANS RG47).

30 Shelburne Estate Papers, Reel 1166. PANS RG48. David Landeg made his will on 7 May 1784, and it was proved on 27 May 1784.

31 A John Lawrence is listed in the Muster Roll for Annapolis County, June 1784, as settled in Granville (PANS RG 1, 376:56). Dr Lawrence was residing in Granville as late as 1793.

32 Dr Loring's name appears in the records of Shelburne for 1784, but not thereafter (Shelburne Court of Common Pleas, March 1785, PANS RG37).

33 Dr Marvin was a resident of Digby until at least 1786 (Digby County Deeds, Book 1B:686, PANS RG47).

34 Dr McIntyre was a surgeon to the forces in Nova Scotia as late as 1797 (*An Almanack ... Calculated for the Meridian of Halifax in Nova Scotia ... by Theophrastus, Halifax, printed and sold by John Howe, 1797*).

35 I am uncertain whether the Donald (Daniel) McLean, surgeon, who arrived at Shelburne in November 1783 was the surgeon of that name with the Seventy-seventh Regiment. It is also unclear whether the Donald McLean, surgeon, who sold land there on 10 November 1789 (Shelburne County Deeds, Book 1:105, PANS RG47) is the same person.

36 A letter from Henry Duncan to W. Bridekirk, master of the *William and Ann*, dated 19 February 1784, mentions that Dr MacCloud (*sic*) and family are to board a certain ship for passage to England (Halifax Dockyard Records, Reel 4, HAL/F/1:62, PANS MG13).

37 Guysborough Christ Church Records, PANS MG4 indicate that a John McPherson died there on 19 November 1831. I am not sure whether this was Dr John McPherson.

38 CO217, 41:43. Jonathan Ogden was listed as a hospital mate at Halifax on 1 January 1784.

39 Shelburne Court of General Sessions Records, PANS RG60 list John Perry as a practitioner of physic in 1784. He returned to Virginia *circa* 1791.

40 PANS RG1, 376:42. The Muster Roll for Annapolis County, June 1784, lists Dr Phillips at Granville. On 13 February 1786, Alexander Josiah Phillips of Granville, practitioner of physic, sold land in the Township of Digby.

41 Digby County Deeds, Book 1B:10, PANS RG47. Fleming Pinkston (*sic*) was listed as a doctor of physic at Weymouth in 1784.

42 PANS RG1, 370:23. Dr Joseph Russell had his town lot at Preston surveyed on 9 February 1784.

43 PANS RG1, 376:65. The Muster Roll at Bear River, 1784 includes —————— Seidleir, surgeon, German Service. He appears to have resided and practised in Clements Township until at least 1807 (see Halifax Estate Papers, Estate of Joseph Anderson, A73, Annapolis, RG48, Reel 396). The estate administration, dated 10 August 1807, includes a debt owed to Doctor Seidler of five shillings.

44 *Hessische Truppen* 4 records that Christian Seege, assistant medical officer, commissioned in the Jager Corps in May 1778, was mustered out in Halifax in October 1783. J.C. Sieger was listed as a physician in Halifax as late as 1793 (Poll Tax for Halifax, PANS RG1, vol. 444).

45 PANS RG1, 376:6. The Muster Roll at Digby in 1784 includes John Skinner, formerly surgeon of the Hessian Service. He is probably Johannes Skener, surgeon, who was mustered at Digby, according to *Hessische Truppen* 2:361.

46 Doctor Edward Smith is mentioned by Simeon Perkins as being in Liverpool as early as 29 October 1783 (Innis et al., eds., *Diary of Simeon Perkins* 2:205).

47 *Hessische Truppen* 3. Dr Stickells was separated from service in America in June 1783. He resided in New Brunswick until 1806, when he moved to Liverpool. He moved to Guysborough in 1811.

48 Shelburne Deeds vol. 1, PANS RG47, Reel 1707. Bartholomew Sullivan witnessed the sale of land at Shelburne on 27 September 1783.

49 PANS RG1, 376:14. In the Muster Roll for Digby.

50 Ibid., 49. In the Muster Roll for Annapolis County, June 1784.

51 Ibid., 39.

52 Minutes of Council, 16 January 1784, PANS RG1, 190:4. Lieutenant Colonel (Van) Buskirk was named a justice of the peace for the district of Shelburne.

53 PANS RG1, 376:14. In the Digby Muster Roll as "Late Assistant Surgeon, General Hospital."

Appendix Six

SUMMARY OF CLAIMS FOR
PROPERTY AND LOSS OF INCOME
MADE BY LOYALIST DOCTORS
WHO CAME TO NOVA SCOTIA,
COMPARED WITH THE SUMS
ALLOWED AND THE PENSIONS
AWARDED BY THE LOYALIST
CLAIMS COMMISSIONERS

Physician or Surgeon	Place and Date of Birth	Place and Date of Death	Former Practice	Claim for Loss of Property (£)	Sum Allowed (£)	Loss of Annual Income (£)	Annual Pension (£)
Azor Betts[1]	c. 1739	Digby, 1809	NY	196	50	160	60
James Boggs[2]	DE, 1740	Halifax, 1830	NJ	562	530	112	
John Boyd[3]	c. 1754	NB, 1818	PA	336			
William Brattle[4]	MA, 1706	Halifax, 1776	MA				
Peter Browne[5]		Windsor, 1787	NJ	2,676	290	225	75
Nathaniel Bullein[6]	SC		SC	1,088	70	200	100
John Calef[7]	MA, 1726	NB, 1812	MA	9,000	1,010	200	nil
George Drummond[8]	Scotland, c. 1715	Shelburne, 1793	PA	nil	nil	nil	nil
Abraham Florentine[9]			NY	896			nil
Sylvester Gardiner[10]	RI, 1707	RI, 1786	MA	47,967			

Physician or Surgeon	Place and Date of Birth	Place and Date of Death	Former Practice	Claim for Loss of Property (£)	Sum Allowed (£)	Loss of Annual Income (£)	Annual Pension (£)
Isaac Goodman[11]	Germany		RI	50	10	nil	nil
John Gould[12]	MA, 1760	Montreal, 1800	MA	2,800*		500	
John Halliburton[13]	Scotland	Halifax, 1808	RI	2,000	nil	210	nil
John Huggeford[14]	c. 1760		NY	nil		400	160
Peter Huggeford[15]	England, c. 1725	NY, 1799	NY	3,144	900	500	160
John Jeffries[16]	MA, 1745	MA, 1819	MA	6,015	500	nil	
Murdock McLeod[17]	Scotland, c. 1742		NC	540	300	100	half pay
Peter Oliver[18]	MA, 1741	England, 1822	MA	4,528	2,200		50
William Paine[19]	MA, 1750	MA, 1833	MA	4,440	300		half pay
Nathaniel Perkins[20]		1799	MA	8,000		670	240
William Lee Perkins[21]	MA, 1737	England, 1797	MA	4,782	250	540	200
John Prince[22]	MA, 1734	MA, 1816	MA	2,272			
Christian Tobias[23]		Digby, 1800	NY	653	478	45	20
Robert Tucker[24]	NY, 1741	NY, 1792	NC	1,260	390	300	75
James Van Buren[25]	NJ, 1729	NJ, 1797	NJ	503	280	112	45
Abraham Van Buskirk[26]	c. 1735	Shelburne, 1799	NJ	1,827	1,111	112	half pay
Averages:				2,130	585	274	108

Source: Loyalist Claims, PANS Misc. "L", AO12, AO13.

* Claimed jointly with his brother and sister.

1 AO12 25:334; 109:92. AO13, Bundle 11:275; Bundle 83:31. Dr Betts appears to have resided in New Brunswick until *circa* 1799.

2 AO12, 15:11; 63:1:1; 109:92. AO13, Bundle 17:93, Bundle 83:38. Dr Boggs was not awarded a pension, for he held an appointment as surgeon's mate at the military hospital in Halifax from 1783 to 1797, in which year he was appointed garrison surgeon.

3 AO13, Bundle 90:183. Dr Boyd moved from Shelburne to Windsor in 1787, to become garrison surgeon. He replaced Dr Peter Browne, who died there on 8 April 1787. Dr Boyd removed from Windsor to Saint John *circa* 1816.

4 AO12, 83:11, Dr Bratle died in Halifax in October 1776 and his financial status is not known.

5 AO12, 15:421; 63:55; 109:92. AO13, Bundle 17:223. Dr Browne was a surgeon's mate at Annapolis Royal during 1783 to 1786 and at Windsor from 1786 to 1787.

6 AO12, 49:224; 68:47; 109:94. AO13, Bundle 138:69. Dr Bullein resided at Horton, Shelburne, and Dartmouth, in addition to Halifax. He is mentioned in the records of Nova Scotia as late as 1793.

7 AO12, 101:45; 109:100. AO13, Bundle 73:80. Dr Calef was appointed to the surgical staff of the garrison at Saint John. He retired on half pay in 1802.

8 AO12, 101:151. AO13, Bundle 71:57. George Drummond practised medicine and surgery in Shelburne.

9 AO13, Bundle 26:112. Dr Florentine appears to have left Digby in the summer of 1786.

10 AO12, 81:85; 82:54. AO13, Bundle 45:286, Bundle 73:578. Dr Gardiner was in Halifax during April to June 1776, and then went to New York with General Howe. He remained there for two years, then removed to England, where he resided until 1783, before returning to the United States.

11 AO12, 101:130. AO13, Bundle 68:289. Dr Goodman left the township of Conway in May 1784 and went to England.

12 AO12, 105:115. AO13, Bundle 50:487, Bundle 73:647. Dr Gould resided in Halifax, Windsor, and Shelburne, before leaving Nova Scotia *circa* 1786.

13 AO13, Bundle 24:241. Dr Halliburton was not awarded a pension, for he held to appointment of surgeon to the naval hospital at Halifax from 1782 to 1808.

14 AO12, 21:244; 109:166. AO13, Bundle 64:344. Dr Huggeford resided in Shelburne until 1789.

15 AO12, 21:232; 89:30; 101:261; 109:162. AO13, Bundle 64:350. Dr Huggeford left Digby for New York in 1790.

16 AO12, 81:104; 99:303; 109:176. Dr Jeffries left Halifax for England in 1779.

17 AO12, 34:422; 100:364; 109:206. Dr McLeod probably left Nova Scotia in 1784, for England, where his wife and children were living.

18 AO12, 105:142; 109:238. Dr Oliver left Halifax for England in the summer of 1776.

19 AO12, 10:413; 61:52; 82:84; 109:246. AO13, Bundle 51:292. Dr Paine resided in Halifax until 1786, when he removed to Passamaquoddy, New Brunswick. He returned to Massachusetts in 1793.

20 AO12, 105:77; 109:244. AO13, Bundle 83:300, Bundle 49:71, Bundle 75:225. Dr Perkins was in Halifax until the late summer or early fall of 1776 when he removed to England.

21 AO12, 105:78; 109:242. AO13, Bundle 83:302, Bundle 49:96. Dr Perkins was in Halifax from April to July 1776, after which he removed to England.

22 AO13, Bundle 26:362. Dr Prince resided in Halifax until 1786, when he removed to New Brunswick.

23 AO12, 109:292. AO13, Bundle 16:55; Bundle 83:698.

24 AO12, 35:86; 65:17; 109:294. AO13, Bundle 83:704; Bundle 138:198. Dr Tucker left Annapolis Royal for New York *circa* 1788.

25 AO12, 15:112; 63:11; 109:300. AO13, Bundle 19:310; Bundle 83:709. Dr Van Buren left, *circa* 1790, from Annapolis County for New Jersey.

26 AO12, 15:181; 63:23; 109:300. AO13, Bundle 19:328; Bundle 83:710.

Appendix Seven

THE INDENTURE OF
APPRENTICESHIP OF WILLIAM
JAMES ALLMON

This Indenture Witnesseth That William James Allmon hath put himself, and by these presents, with the Consent of his Father-in-Law, John Nash, of this City of New York, Shopkeeper, doth voluntarily, and of his own free Will and Accord, put himself Apprentice to Andrew Anderson, of the City of New York, Physician and Surgeon, to learn the Profession of a Physician and Surgeon, and after the manner of an Apprentice to serve from the Day of the Date hereof, for and during, and until the full End and Term of five years, 7½ months next ensuing; during all which Time, the said apprentice his said Master faithfully shall serve, his secrets keep, his lawful Commands every where readily obey: He shall do no Damage to his said Master nor see it done by others, without letting or giving Notice thereof to his said Master: He shall not waste his and his master's goods, nor lend them unlawfully to any. He shall not commit Fornication, nor contract Matrimony within the said Term: At Cards, Dice, or any other unlawful game, he shall not play, whereby his said Master may have damage With his own Goods, nor the Goods of others, without Licence from his said Master, he shall neither buy nor sell: He shall not absent himself Day or Night from his said Master's service without his leave; nor haunt Ale-houses, Taverns, or Playhouses, but in all Things behave himself as a faithful Apprentice ought to do, during the said Term. And the said Master shall use the utmost of his endeavours to teach, or cause to be taught or instructed, the said Apprentice in the Profession of Physician and Surgeon. And for the true Performance of all and singular the Covenants and Agreements aforesaid, the said Parties bind themselves, each unto the other, firmly by these Presents.

In witness whereof, the said Parties have interchangeably set their Hands and Seals hereunto. Dated the first day of January, in the eleventh year of the Reign of our Soverign Lord George the Third, King of Great Britain, etc., Annoque Domini One Thousand Seven Hundred and Seventy One.

(Signed) Andrew Anderson

Sealed and Delivered in the presence of:

Jona. Holmes
John Wiley

These are to certify that William James Allmon hath behaved himself during his apprenticeship with diligence, sobriety, honesty, and faithfulness. As witness my hand this 14 August 1776.

Andrew Anderson

The indenture was published in the *Halifax Evening Mail* of 22 December 1896. John Nash, mentioned in the indenture as Allmon's father-in-law, was actually this stepfather. Most primary sources in which William James Allmon is mentioned (i.e., baptism, marriage bond, poll tax) record his name as Allmon. His descendants were known by the surname Almon.

Appendix Eight

PHYSICIANS AND SURGEONS IN CHARGE OF HOSPITALS IN HALIFAX AND ENVIRONS, 1749–1799

CIVILIAN HOSPITALS

General Hospital, Bishop St
  Dr Matthew Jones, principal surgeon — July–October 1750
  Dr Alexander Abercrombie, surgeon — October 1750–December 1758
Hospital for the Maroons, Dartmouth
  Dr John Oxley, surgeon — July 1796–April 1798
  Dr John Fraser, surgeon — April 1798–post-1799
Orphan House, Bishop St
  Dr Alexander Abercrombie, surgeon — June 1752–March 1773
  Dr John Philipps, surgeon — April 1773–October 1784
Poor House Hospital, Spring Garden Rd
  Dr Thomas Reeve, surgeon — 1764–July 1777
  Dr Edward Wyer, surgeon — July 1777–December 1780
  Dr Malachy Salter, surgeon — December 1780–December 1782
  Dr Christopher Nicolai, surgeon — January 1783–post-1799
  Dr William J. Almon, physician — April 1785–post-1799
Roehampton Hospital Ship
  Dr Leonard Lockman, surgeon — June 1749–July 1750

MILITARY HOSPITALS

General Military Hospital, Blowers St
  Dr William Adair, surgeon — November 1758–
  Dr John Jeffries, surgeon — December 1776–November 1778
  Dr John Marshall, surgeon — November 1778–August 1783
  Dr William Paine, physician — October 1782–June 1784
  Dr Donald McIntyre, surgeon — August 1783–July 1797
Hessian Regiment's Hospital
  Dr J.C. Helmerich, surgeon — January 1781–November 1782
Quarantine Hospital, George's Island
  Dr John Jeffries, surgeon — April–June 1776
Richmond Hospital Ship
  Dr James Dickson, surgeon — April–June 1776

Royal Nova Scotia Regiment's Hospital
    Dr John Fraser, surgeon   February 1793–post-1799
Two Brothers Hospital Ship
    Dr James Dickson, surgeon   April–June 1776

NAVAL HOSPITALS

Hospital for Sick and Hurt Seamen
    Dr Robert Grant, surgeon   October 1750–February 1757
Naval Hospital, Granville St
    Dr Robert Grant, surgeon   February–September 1757
    Dr Godfrey Webb, surgeon   September 1757–November 1761
    Dr Charles White, surgeon   November 1761–July 1771
    Dr George Greaves, surgeon   July 1771–December 1775
    Dr John Philipps, surgeon   December 1775–September 1776
Naval Hospital, George's Island
    Dr James Dickson, surgeon   September 1776–May 1779
Naval Hospital, Dockyard Area
    Dr James Dickson, surgeon   May 1779–January 1782
    Dr John Handasyde, surgeon   January–March 1782
    Dr John Halliburton, surgeon   March–December 1782
Naval Hospital, Narrows
    Dr John Halliburton, surgeon   December 1782–post-1799

PRISON HOSPITALS

Kavanagh's Island, Northwest Arm
    Dr John Halliburton, surgeon   August 1794–April 1796
Prison Hospital, Dockyard Area
    Dr John Marshall, surgeon   December 1779–1783

Appendix 8

HOSPITALS IN HALIFAX AND ENVIRONS, 1749–99

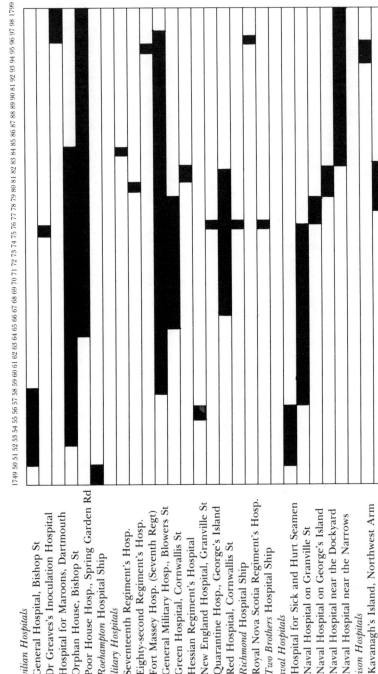

Civilian Hospitals
General Hospital, Bishop St
Dr Greaves's Inoculation Hospital
Hospital for Maroons, Dartmouth
Orphan House, Bishop St
Poor House Hosp., Spring Garden Rd
Roehampton Hospital Ship

Military Hospitals
Seventeenth Regiment's Hosp.
Eighty-second Regiment's Hosp.
Fort Massey Hosp. (Seventh Regt)
General Military Hosp., Blowers St
Green Hospital, Cornwallis St
Hessian Regiment's Hospital
New England Hospital, Granville St
Quarantine Hosp., George's Island
Red Hospital, Cornwallis St
Richmond Hospital Ship
Royal Nova Scotia Regiment's Hosp.
Two Brothers Hospital Ship

Naval Hospitals
Hospital for Sick and Hurt Seamen
Naval Hospital on Granville St
Naval Hospital on George's Island
Naval Hospital near the Dockyard
Naval Hospital near the Narrows

Prison Hospitals
Kavanagh's Island, Northwest Arm
Prison Hospital near the Dockyard

Appendix Nine

CAUSES OF DEATH OF NOVA SCOTIANS BETWEEN 1749 AND 1799

Accidental		Disease		Infant Deaths	Violent		War	Miscellaneous	
Drowned	471	Smallpox	122	724	Starvation	62	107	Decay	12
Accidents	31	Fever	58		Hanged	48		Old age	5
Perished	17	Consumption	49		Murdered	29		Mortification	3
Fire	17	Gout	30		Scalped	24		Colic	2
Childbirth	16	Bad throat	24		Suicide	21		Decline	2
Frozen	10	Dropsy	19		Shot	6		Grief	1
Falling	4	Pleurisy	10		Executed	6		Weakness	1
Scalded	4	Apoplexy	9			196			26
Suffocated	3	Cough	9						
Rupture	2	Chest	8						
Killed by a bull	1	Measles	8						
Killed by a bear	1	Stroke	7						
Lightning	1	Hectic	6						
	578	Haemorrhage	4						
		Quinsy	4						
		Cancer	3						

Causes of Death of Nova Scotians between 1749 and 1799 (cont'd)

Disease	Accidental	Infant Deaths	Violent	War	Miscellaneous
Paralytic		3			
Steckfluss		3			
Fits		3			
Asthma		2			
Convulsions		2			
Abscess		2			
Dysentry		2			
Inflammation		2			
Palsy		2			
Bad ear		1			
Bad thigh		1			
Cholera		1			
Fistula		1			
Lung disease		1			
Obstruction		1			
Putrid fever		1			
Spotted fever		1			
Stones		1			
Stomach gout		1			
Throat cancer		1			
Worms		1			
Worm fever		1			
Yellow fever		1			
		304			

Total: 1,935

Sources: See chapter 4, note 10.

Notes

ABBREVIATIONS

Adm.	Admiralty
AN	Archives Nationales, Paris
AO	Audit Office
CO	Colonial Office
GMHC	Gentleman's Magazine and Historical Chronicle
MG	Manuscript Group
NAC	National Archives of Canada
NSGWC	Nova Scotia Gazette and Weekly Chronicle
PANS	Public Archives of Nova Scotia
PRO	Public Records Office, Kew
RG	Record Group
SPGFP	Society for the Propagation of the Gospel in Foreign Parts
WO	War Office

PREFACE

1 Williams, "Poor Relief and Medicine in Nova Scotia, 1749–1783," 33–56.
2 Campbell, "Pioneers of Medicine in Nova Scotia," 16:195–210, 243–53, 519–27; 17:8–17.
3 Marble, "The History of Medicine in Nova Scotia, 1783–1854," 73–101.
4 Marble, "He Usefully Exercised the Medical Profession," 40–56.
5 Bynum, "Health, Disease, and Medical Care," 211–53.
6 McKeown, "A Sociological Approach to the History of Medicine," 342–51.

INTRODUCTION

1 Each regiment had on strength a surgeon and an assistant surgeon, and the law required each ship to have surgeon on board. Thirty-one of the thirty-eight medical personnel who came to Halifax with Governor Cornwallis in June 1749 were surgeons. All eleven of the medical personnel who arrived with the foreign Protestants in 1750, 1751, and 1752 were surgeons.

2 King, *The Medical World of the Eighteenth Century*, 4. The word surgeon, or *chirurgeon*, was derived from the two Greek words *cheir*, meaning hand, and *ergon* meaning work.

3 The Royal College of Physicians of London was established in 1518, and the Charter for the Royal College of Physicians of Edinburgh was granted in 1681. The Company of Barber-Surgeons of London came into being in 1540, while the corresponding body in Edinburgh was established in 1641. The Society of Apothecaries of London came into existence in 1617.

4 Cope, *The History of the Royal College of Surgeons of England*, 134. This apprenticeship began usually at the age of fourteen or fifteen. An indenture of apprenticeship, or contract, was drawn up between the apprentice and his mentor, a practising surgeon. The apprentice was exposed, in addition to anatomy and surgery, to materia medica, i.e., substances used as medications. It is likely that the indenture of apprenticeship of pupil-surgeons, during the latter part of the eighteenth century in England, contained the same conditions of apprenticeship at those signed in 1771 by William J. Al(l)mon, in New York. His indenture appears in Appendix 7.

5 Many hospitals in London, such as Guy's, St Bartholomew's, St George's, and St Thomas's, had their own medical schools. Edinburgh University began, in 1726, to offer a complete degree course in medicine, and Glasgow University established its Faculty of medicine in 1747. Probably the most celebrated teacher in Great Britain in the early eighteenth century was Dr Alexander Monro (1697–1767), mentioned at greater length in chapter 5. Monro taught from 1720 to 1756 at Edinburgh University. At least seven of his students went to Nova Scotia and practised there as surgeons.

6 The Examination Book of The Company of Surgeons, London, 1745–1800, indicates that many students wrote several examinations to upgrade their qualifications. For instance, John Halliburton, who was surgeon of the naval hospital at Halifax from 1782 to 1808, had written examinations at Surgeons' Hall on 18 May 1758 (second mate, third rate); 20 March 1760 (first mate, first rate); and 16 April 1761 (surgeon, fourth rate). The word mate meant hospital mate and was equivalent to assistant surgeon.

7 Dr Joseph Lister introduced antiseptic surgery in Glasgow in 1865 when he began to use carbolic acid to prevent sepsis during surgical procedures. It was not until 1876, however, that Lister was able to convince the international surgical community that the use of antiseptics during surgery was effective in reducing and, in most cases, preventing post-operative infection. A detailed account of Lister's introduction of antiseptic surgery is given in Traux, *Joseph Lister, Father of Modern Surgery,* 90 *et seq.*

8 Prior to 1846, the anaesthetics used during surgery, if any were used at all, were alcohol, opium, and, as of 1798, nitrous oxide. In 1846, Dr William Morton demonstrated in Boston that ether was an effective general anaesthetic. A year later, Dr James Simpson introduced and demonstrated, in Edinburgh, the effectiveness of chloroform as an anesthetic.

9 Blood-letting was considered necessary to eliminate symptoms of excessive rigidity or tension in the walls of blood vessels. It was believed that tension would exert excessive force on the contained liquid, thus rendering it dense and compact and predisposing the blood to clot. Clotting would lead to inflammation and thence to fever.

10 Copies of various editions of Cullen's book have been found in special collections at the Kellogg Library, Faculty of Medicine, Dalhousie University. On the title pages of these copies can be seen the autographs of three surgeons who practised in Halifax during the last two decades of the eighteenth century: Duncan Clark, Robert Hume, and John Marshall.

11 Porter, "The Gift Relation: Philanthropy and Provincial Hospitals."

12 LeFanu, "The Lost Half-Century of English Medicine, 1700–1750."

13 Risse, *Typhus Fever in 18th Century Hospitals,* 178–95.

14 Burnby, "A Study of the English Apothecary from 1660 to 1760."

15 Porter, "The Gift Relation: Philanthropy and Provincial Hospitals."

16 According to Howie, "Finance and Supply," 124–46, the total annual expenditure to operate a sixty-bed hospital in Shrewsbury in 1750 was in the order of one thousand pounds.

17 Cartwright, *Disease and History,* 117.

18 Miller, *The Adoption of Inoculation for Smallpox,* 1957.

19 Razzell, *The Conquest of Smallpox,* 128.

20 Cartwright, *Disease and History,* 121.

21 Queen Mary, wife of King William III of England, died from smallpox in 1694.

22 Hopkins, *Princes and Peasants,* 1983.

23 Levine, *Conqueror of Smallpox, Dr Edward Jenner.*

24 Razzell, *The Conquest of Smallpox,* 128.

25 King, *The Medical World of the Eighteenth Century,* 324.

26 Heagerty, *Four Centuries of Medical History in Canada,* 1928.

27 Hofstadter, *America at 1750, A Social Portrait.*
28 Potter, *Population in History.* Potter estimates that the population
of the American colonies increased from 250,000 in 1700 to 5,000,000
in 1800, a twentyfold increase.
29 Hofstadter, *America at 1750,* 16, 32.
30 PANS RG1, 186:211.

CHAPTER ONE

1 Clark, *Acadia, the Geography of Early Nova Scotia to 1760,* 211, 276,
280. Clark suggests that the total number of Acadians on mainland Nova
Scotia by the middle of the eighteenth century was about 8,300,
most of whom were residing in Annapolis Royal District (1,750); Minas,
north and west of Pisiquid and including Canard and Grand Pré
(2,500); Cobequid and the Gulf Shore (1,000); and Chignecto (1,600).
Clark estimates that the outpost population in Cape Breton (exclud-
ing Louisbourg, which, in early 1749, was still occupied by English
troops) was about 2,500 persons, residing mainly in the Arichat,
St Peters, and Ingonish areas.
2 Upton, *Micmacs and Colonists,* 32–3. Upton writes: "Ten years later
[1749] the estimates were down slightly at 1,000 Micmacs for peninsular
Nova Scotia alone." He points out that some of these figures were
not very reliable because "they were based on the numbers in either
the annual festivities at Catholic missions or at the distribution of
French presents." Upton does suggest, however, that the total Indian
population of Nova Scotia, Île St Jean, and New Brunswick was,
by mid-century, just over two thousand.
3 During the first six months of 1749, about 2,300 persons of English
origin resided in Nova Scotia: 300 at Annapolis Royal and 2,000 (mostly
military) at Louisbourg. Although Louisbourg was returned to
France by the Treaty of Aix-la-Chapelle, in October 1748, the fortress
was not turned over until 24 July 1749 (o.s.). The English garrison
at Louisbourg was transferred to Halifax, arriving there during the
three-day period 24–26 July 1749 (o.s.), according to John
Salusbury's diary (PANS Micro Biography). MacLennan, *Louisbourg From
its Foundation to its Fall 1713–1758,* 187, states that the English ships
did not sail from Louisbourg until 30 July (o.s.). Inasmuch as John
Salusbury was in Halifax at the time the ships arrived, it can be presumed that his dates are correct.
4 Most of the New England Provincial Troops who had been at
Louisbourg since June 1745 returned home in May 1746. They were
replaced by Fuller's Twenty-ninth and Warburton's Forty-fifth regiments, which were transferred to Louisbourg from Gibraltar, and by

the newly raised regiments of Sir William Pepperell (the Fifty-first) and Governor William Shirley (the Fiftieth). These four regiments appear to have defended Louisbourg until July 1749, when they were transported to Halifax; shortly afterwards, Pepperell's and Shirley's regiments were disbanded. Command of the Twenty-ninth Regiment had been handed over to Peregrine Thomas Hopson, lieutenant governor of Louisbourg, on 6 June 1748 (o.s.). Hopson was in charge of the garrison when it moved from Louisbourg to Halifax in late July 1749 (*Dictionary of Canadian Biography* 3:294–5).

5 Clark, *Acadia, the Geography of Early Nova Scotia to 1760*, 201.

6 Printed in Akins, *Selections from the Public Documents*, 495–7. This proposal was the plan of George Montagu-Dunk, Earl of Halifax, who, in the autumn of 1748, had been appointed president of the Board of Trade and Plantations.

7 The "books" referred to in the advertisement are in all likelihood "The List of Emigrants, 1748/1749" found in PANS CO221, vol. 36, in which 1,658 families (3,415 men, women, and children) are listed as having had their names entered to go to Nova Scotia between 9 March 1748/49 and 11 April 1749 (o.s.). Only the heads of families are named with their occupation. A total of forty-eight persons listed their occupation as being a member of the medical profession (i.e., surgeon, surgeon's mate, apothecary, druggist and chymist, assistant surgeon, apothecary's mate, midwife, and chymist and surgeon). Discrepancy exists in the secondary literature concerning the number of families and persons who volunteered initially to emigrate to Nova Scotia at this time. Akins, in his "History of Halifax City," 5, states that "in a short time 1176 settlers, with their families, were found to volunteer." Haliburton, in his two-volume *Historical and Statistical Account of Nova Scotia* 1:137, writes: "In a short time 3,760 adventurers, with their families, were entered for embarkation." Quite likely Haliburton meant that a total of 3,760 persons had volunteered to embark for Nova Scotia. However, he may have been led to believe that there were 3,760 individual families by an entry found in the May 1749 issue of GMHC, published by Edward Cave in London, which reads: "The number of families entered for Nova Scotia is about 3,750" (235).

8 *Dictionary of Canadian Biography* 4:168–71. Born in London on 20 February 1712/13, Cornwallis was about thirty-seven years of age in May 1749. He had been with the Twentieth Regiment since 1742 and, in 1745, was promoted to lieutenant colonel. Cornwallis served at Culloden in 1746. After leaving Halifax in October 1752, he returned to England where, in March 1753, he married Maria Townshend, niece to the late Lord Townshend (*Halifax Gazette*, 23 June

1753). Cornwallis was elected to Parliament from Westminister and held that seat until 1762. He died at Gibraltar in 1776.

9 Lords of Trade to Cornwallis, 15 May 1749 (o.s.), PANS CO218, 3:129.

10 As stated in note 7, "The List of Emigrants, 1748/1749" (PANS CO221, vol. 36) indicates that 3,415 settlers, including 1,658 families, entered their names into the books to go to Nova Scotia during the period from 9 March 1748/49 to 11 April 1749 (o.s.). Examination of these books shows that at least 1,135 of the 1,658 heads of households have an x marked beside their name. Most of the heads of households listed on two pages under the letter A are missing from PANS CO221, vol. 36; consequently the total number of families marked with an x cannot be established exactly. It is clear, however, that approximately 320 families, consisting of about 860 persons, who had entered their names in the books in London, Portsmouth, and Plymouth during the thirty-three days from 9 March 1748/49 to 11 April 1749 (o.s.) did not actually board any of the transports bound for Nova Scotia. It is possible that the 320 families decided against emigrating because the embarkation date was postponed from 20 April to 15 May. The mess lists for each of the thirteen transports, which appear in PANS RG1, vol. 523, show clearly that only 1,174 families and a total of 2,547 passengers were on the ships. Comparison of the names on the mess lists with those entered in the books and marked with an x suggests that the x was placed beside each name in the books as each person boarded one of the transports. I suggest that the mess lists were prepared after the passengers had boarded the transports. Article 24 of Cornwallis's instructions from the Lords of Trade, dated 29 April 1749 (o.s.) suggests that some of the 420 servants in the mess lists could have been black slaves (PANS CO218, 3:105). An extensive explanation of white and black servitude in eighteenth-century America is given by Hofstadter, *America at 1750, A Social Portrait*.

11 Whereas PANS CO221, vol. 36 lists a total of forty-eight persons who were in some branch of the medical profession, the mess lists (PANS RG1, vol. 523) indicate that only thirty-eight of these people actually boarded the transports and came to Chebucto. Leonard Lockman, who was the surgeon on the hospital ship *Roehampton*, is listed in RG1, vol. 523 as a major rather than surgeon.

12 LeFanu, "The Lost Half-Century," 319–48. He points out that there was more continuity in the advances in medicine and surgery during this period in France, Germany, Holland, and Scotland.

13 Porter, "Before the Fringe: 'Quackery' and the Eighteenth-Medical Market."

14 Ransom, "The Beginnings of Hospitals in the United States," 514–39.

15 King, *The Medical World of the Eighteenth Century*, xvi.

16 *Journal of the Commissioners for Trade* 8(1931):397.

17 Clark-Kennedy, *Stephen Hales: an Eighteenth Century Biography*. Hales (1677–1761) is known for having made the first quantitive measurement of blood pressure. His book, *A Description of Ventilators*, appeared in 1743. The ventilators were bellows that could be used to draw fresh air into a structure, such as a ship, and expel the foul air.

18 The Sutton air pipes and ventilators proved to be very effective, as indicated by one of the settlers in a letter from Chebucto which appeared in GMHC for September 1749, 408: "Arrived on 28 June. Not heard that any one person died on the passage or since our arrival. Our health and preservation has been in a great measure owing to the prudent measures taken by those who had the direction of this good work, in having ventilators and air pipes in all the ships and furnishing rice and fresh provisions." In fact, the same magazine indicates (August 1749, 378) that only one child died during the voyage. The expected mortality on a trans-Atlantic crossing (in which ventilators were not used) was seven to nine percent (Bell, *The Foreign Protestants*, 251).

19 The Lords of Trade who conducted the preparations for the settlement of Chebucto were George Montagu-Dunk, second earl of Halifax (1716–71); William Pitt, first earl of Chatham (1708–78); Granville Leveson-Gower, first marquis of Stafford (1721–1803); George Grenville, Lord of the Treasury, (1712–70); John Fane, seventh earl of Westmoreland (c. 1682–1762); Sir Thomas Robinson, late governor of Barbados (c. 1700–77); and Thomas Hay, Lord Dupplin (1710–87), member for Ireland.

20 *Journal of the Commissioners for Trade* 8 (1931) 404.

21 PANS RG1, 350A:4. Included in the Lords of Trade instructions to Cornwallis, 29 April 1749 (o.s.), was mention of setting up four settlements in addition to Chebucto. These were to be Menis (Minas), LaHave, Whitehead, and Bay Verte. In RG1 350A:10, the Lords of Trade outlined how the settlers should be distributed among the five settlements. A description of Whitehead, dated 14 November 1764, is given in PANS CO217, 21:103. It appears that Whitehead was located on Whitehaven Harbour in present-day Guysborough County.

22 *Journal of the Commissioners for Trade* 8 (1931) 405. The dates given beside the first seven names are the previous dates on which each surgeon had been examined.

23 Ibid., 408. The *Roehampton* was built in Boston in 1735 and registered in London on 29 April 1749 (o.s.). PANS CO221, vol. 28, which records ships and vessels that cleared the port of Halifax after 19 July 1749 (o.s.), describes the *Roehampton* as a vessel of 150 tons. The

Cornwallis passenger or mess lists (PANS RG1, vol. 523) gives the tonnage of each of the thirteen transports and lists the *Roehampton* at 230 tons. In any event, the hospital ship was the smallest of the transports and carried seventy-two passengers in addition to its medical personnel (see Appendix 1).

24 As noted earlier, Appendix 1 lists the thirty-eight medical persons who appear on the Cornwallis passenger lists. Six of the names appearing on the two lists just presented are not to be found in Appendix 1. These six (Josiah Irwin, Mark Story, Edward Turner, John Sherman, John Farquhar, and Mr Belchiss) are listed in the books referred to earlier (PANS CO221, vol. 36). None of the six has an x beside his name, which indicates (as suggested in note 10) that, after having entered their names in the books, all had changed their mind about going to Nova Scotia. PANS CO218, 3:137 records that "Mr Belchiss, one of the surgeon's mates nominated by us having declined to go to Nova Scotia ... is replaced by Mr Robert White."

25 Cornwallis to Lords of Trade, 24 July 1749 (o.s.), PANS CO217, 9:70.

26 Cornwallis, in his letter of 11 September to the Lords of Trade (PANS CO217, 9:89) refers to the new settlement as Chebucto. In his letter of 17 October 1749 (o.s.), the governor uses the name Halifax for the first time to describe his settlement. As mentioned in note 22, the original plan was to set up five settlements in Nova Scotia. Since Cornwallis could not carry out this plan immediately, the Lords of Trade wrote on 16 February 1750 (o.s.): "As the number of surgeons and apothecaries was calculated upon the supposition that five different settlements would be made and those who were appointed had notice from us that they were to be retained but for one year, we desire you will discharge from the Establishment all of them except such as you shall judge absolutely necessary for Halifax Town" (PANS RG1, vol. 129).

27 These transports were the *London, Winchelsea, Wilmington, Merry Jacks,* and *Brotherhood* (PANS CO217, 9:70).

28 PANS CO218, 3:33. On 29 April 1749 (o.s.), mention is made of the reduction of the regiments of William Shirley and William Pepperell and that the released men were to be treated like the settlers.

29 A company of soldiers consisted of approximately one hundred men and, in the eighteenth century, was commanded by a captain. A battalion consisted of three companies, and a regiment was made up of three battalions. The regiment, recognized as a distinct unit, consisted of approximately nine hundred officers and men. It was commanded by a colonel and took its name from the commanding officer. Thus, Warburton's Regiment was commanded by Col Hugh Warburton. On 1 July 1751 (o.s.), however, each regiment was given a num-

ber designation. Warburton's Regiment was assigned number forty-five and called thereafter the 45th Regiment.

30 Piers, "The Fortieth Regiment," 131.

31 Minutes of Council, 14 July 1749 (o.s.), PANS CO217, 9:77.

32 Cornwallis to Lords of Trade, 24 July 1749 (o.s.), PANS CO217, 9:71.

33 "Project for Fortifying the Town of Halifax in Nova Scotia, 1749," PANS CO217, 9:120.

34 Moses Harris and his wife arrived in Chebucto on the *Winchelsea*. He listed his occupation as sawyer. Harris's plan of the town of Halifax was published in GMHC, 23 October 1749 (o.s.), 440. "A View of Halifax Drawn from yᵉ Topmasthead" can be seen in the lower right of Figure 2. This view, drawn also by Moses Harris, was completed sometime prior to December 1749, for an advertisement announcing publication of the views presented in Figure 2 appeared in the December issue of *Gentleman's Magazine and Historical Chronicle*, 576. The advertisement read:

In a few Days will be published,
A correct Plan of HALIFAX, with the Harbour of Chebucto, and Torrington's Bay; also a perspective view of Halifax from Topmasthead. Drawn on the Spot, by Moses Harris. To which is added,
    A MAP of NOVA SCOTIA, with its boundaries and Fishingbanks; by Mons. D'Anville, Geographer to the King. N.B. Both are engravings, and will be published by Thomas Jefferys, Geographer to the Prince of Wales, at his Shop, the corner of St Martin's Lane, near Charing Cross.

The Harris plan of Halifax was published again in GMHC for February 1750. The original plan was embellished in this publication with drawings of a porcupine, two butterflies, and a beetle.

35 These blocks were 320 feet long by 120 feet deep. Each contained sixteen lots, forty feet long and sixty feet deep. The whole town was divided into five wards or divisions named, sometime before 6 December 1749 (o.s.), after the captains of the Militia: Alexander Callendar, John Galland, Robert Ewer, John Collier, and James Foreman. Each division contained enough men to supply two of the ten militia companies (PANS RG1, 186:30).

36 Minutes of Council, 14 July 1749 (o.s.), PANS CO217, 9:77.

37 Proclamation by Cornwallis, 17 July 1749 (o.s.), PANS RG1, 163/1:4.

38 It is suggested that the record of vessels clearing the port of Halifax after 21 July 1749 (o.s.) appearing in PANS CO221, vol. 28 is incomplete. Between 21 July 1749 (o.s.) and 9 July 1750 (o.s.), only three of Cornwallis's thirteen transports are listed as having left Halifax (the

London on 12 September 1749; *Roehampton* on 9 July 1750; and *Charlton* on 7 December 1749). John Salusbury records in his diary entry of 25 July 1749 (o.s.) that the *Everley* sailed that day for England. On 21 August 1749 (o.s.), he records that Hopson sailed for England in the *Brotherhood*, with the *Alexander* and the *Merry Jacks*, while the *Wilmington* and *Winchelsea* sailed for Ireland. On 12 September 1749 (o.s.), he records the departure of the *London*. As noted previously, the *London* is the only one of these ships included in the shipping records (PANS CO221, vol. 28).

39 "Diary of John Salusbury," 13 July 1749 (o.s.), PANS Micro Biography.

40 Cornwallis to Lords of Trade, 20 August 1749 (o.s.), PANS CO217, 9:82.

41 Proclamation issued by Cornwallis on 7 August 1749 (o.s.), PANS RG1, 163:7: "All heads of familys, that are settlers, are hereby required to assemble by seven in the morning, with their overseers; and single men are desired to form themselves into familys – four to a family; and every family to chuse [*sic*] one to draw for them." John Salusbury noted in his diary on 5 August 1749 (o.s.) that he has been "ordered to prepare for drawing lots." On 8 August 1749 (o.s.) he wrote, "Attended in drawing the lots and registering them"; on 9 August 1749 (o.s.), "Finished drawing the lots – the people seem satisfy'd, every one their share fairly. Ten lots remain."

42 PANS RG1, vol. 410. The 606 heads of family (or single men) could be allotted only 464 individual lots because, in numerous instances, a lot was divided between two, three, or four families (for the most part, single-member families).

43 This figure of 1,400 has been interpreted as an error by Beamish Murdoch in his *History of Nova Scotia* 2:141. He states that the number should be 2,400. However, I do not believe that the figure 1,400 is an error since, on 11 September 1749 (o.s.), Cornwallis reported (PANS CO217, 9:91) that the total population of Halifax was 1,574, and, on 7 December 1749 (o.s.), he reported (ibid., 132) a population of 1,876.

44 The records include St Paul's Anglican Church (PANS MG4); the victualling list for May and June 1750 (PANS MG1, vol. 258); probate records (PANS RG48, various volumes); and the census for July 1752 (PANS RG1, vol. 417). It is known that lots of land north of the town of Halifax had been granted prior to 14 November 1749 (o.s.). In the Council minutes of that date (PANS RG1, 186:27), one Beamsley Glazier, a settler, represented that "while he was at Minas, Sam Shipton had taken possession of his lot #25 on the north side of the Town and build a house upon it and that Mr Shipton pretended that the lot

was granted to him. The Register of the Lots being sent for, Mr Glazier's name was found registered for the lot in question." The house was being lived in, on the date indicated, by Mr Shipton and his family. The register of lots mentioned here is not the same as the Allotment Book (PANS RG1, vol. 410) mentioned previously.

45 Cornwallis to Lords of Trade, 20 August 1749 (o.s.), PANS CO217, 9:82.

46 "Diary of John Salusbury," 9 August 1749 (o.s.), PANS Micro Biography.

47 See letter from Chebucto Harbour, dated 14 August 1749 (o.s.) and published in GMHC 19:472, October 1749.

48 The Penal Laws preventing Roman Catholics from owning land, enacted in 1704 by the British Parliament, were in force in Nova Scotia until 1783 {Statute 23, George 3d, cap. 9, sections 1 and 2, 1783. An Act for the Relieving His Majesty's subjects, possessing the Popish Religion from certain Penalties and Disabilities imposed upon them by Two Acts of the General Assembly of This Province, made in the Thirty Second year of his late Majesty's Reign entitled an Act, confirming Titles to Lands and Quieting Possession (32d George 2d, cap. 2, 1758); and an Act for the Establishment of Religious Public Worship in the Province, and for Suppressing of Popery (32d George 2d, cap. 5, 1758)}. The Penal laws also applied in England's colonies prior to 1758, as indicated in Governor Shirley's letter to the Duke of Bedford (PANS RG1, vol. 29, Item 1), dated Boston, 18 February 1747/48. Shirley wrote: "That the liberty of conscience on religious worship should be extended to the Papists among the present French Inhabitants [the Acadians] for such indefinite time as His Majesty shall be pleased to determine, after which incapacities as they have in England." Of those heads of family who were in Halifax on 8 August 1749 (o.s.), but who were not granted land on that date or thereafter, a significant number were Irish in origin and probably Roman Catholic.

The directions given by the Lords of Trade to Cornwallis relating to the new settlement state, "The other mischief to be guarded against ... is the purchase of these grants [left by settlers who may desert the settlement] by Roman Catholics" (Lords of Trade to Cornwallis, 15 May 1749 o.s., PANS CO218, 3:132). At the first Council meeting held in July 1749 (o.s.) on board the *Beaufort*, the newly sworn councillors "took and subscribed [to] the Declaration mentioned in [the] Act of Parliament passed in the 25th year of the reign of King Charles the 2nd, entitled an Act for preventing dangers which may happen from Popish Recusants" (Minutes of Council, 14 July 1749 o.s., PANS RG1, 186:1). In an attempt to increase the number of Protestants, Cornwallis wrote to the Lords of Trade later that month: "Make it known through Germany, that all Husbandmen, Tradesmen, or Sailors, being Protestants, should have the same rights and privileges in this Province as were promised in His Majesty's Proclamation to his natural born subjects" (Cornwallis to Lords of Trade, 24 July 1749 o.s., PANS CO217, 9:71). In March 1750, the Lords of Trade advised Cornwallis that, "Mr Tutty having acquainted the Society for the Propagation of the Gospel that of the Germans which were sent last year, 40 turn out to be Roman Catholics. We desire that you would enquire particularly into this matter. We look upon Roman Catholics as not entitled to the privilege granted to the settlers, and if any such be found among them, we don't doubt but you will think it necessary to the Peace and Security of the Province to send them away again" (Lords of Trade to Cornwallis, 22 March 1750/51, PANS RG1, vol. 29, Item 6). In July 1751 (o.s.), Cornwallis communicated to Council that:

some Irish Roman Catholic servants in this place have entered into a combination to go over to the Indians or French. The Council hereupon, taking into consideration the great inconvenience and prejudice to this settlement that may arise from an increase in the Roman Catholics therein. It was resolved that, for the future, the masters of all vessels coming into any of the Ports of this Province, shall immediately upon their arrival make a Report in writing to the Commander-in-Chief where they arrive, of the number, names, and qualities of the passengers on board their respective vessels (Minutes of Council, 2 July 1751 o.s., PANS RG1, 186:128). The *Boston Gazette and Weekly Journal* of 30 July 1751 (o.s.) states that there were "upwards of 40 Irishmen deserted and went over to the Indian enemy. One of the Principal of them, whose name is Ryan, is taken now in Irons."

On 2 July 1751, Council adopted an act with respect to the "clandestine introduction of Roman Catholics" (An Act to Prevent Masters of vessels landing any Passengers, or Servants without Permission from the Governor or Commander in Chief of the Province, made and passed in Council at Halifax on 2 July 1751 o.s., PANS CO219, 3:51).

The first indication that there was a considerable number of Roman Catholics in Halifax appears in Rev. William Tutty's fourth letter to the Society for the Propagation of the Gospel, in October 1750 (o.s.). "He states, "I believe the members of the Church of England and the whole body of dissenters including Papists are pretty equal" ("Letters and Other Papers," 119). In his fifth letter, the Reverend Mr Tutty writes that there are "about 2,000 [dissenters] of all sorts, and many-too many-Irish Papists" (Ibid., 123). Governor Hopson, who succeeded Cornwallis in August 1752, was obligated to enforce the Parliamentary legislation discriminating against Roman Catholics. He wrote to the Lords of Trade that "no alienation [having title to] of land is allowed but by Governor's License which License is not granted before the Purchaser takes the proper oaths, and only granted to those who have improved these lands, and upon no account to Roman Catholics" (Hopson to Lords of Trade, 16 October 1752 n.s., PANS CO217, 13:309). Finally, at the Council meeting of 5 April 1753 (n.s.) it was recorded that James Monk, Esq., during a dispute with Thomas Power over a lot of land in Halifax Town, was supposed to have said that "he [Power] was not entitled to the lot as he was a Roman Catholick" (Minutes of Council, 5 April 1753, PANS RG1, 186:355). Surprisingly, Council ruled that Power should retain the land which he had been granted officially, presumably without the knowledge that he was a Roman Catholic (Allotment Book, PANS RG1, 410:50).

The foregoing indicates that Roman Catholics were in Halifax at the time the town lots were drawn, but that they did not receive any. This could explain why only 419 families on the Cornwallis passenger lists were allotted land on 8 August, when at least 606 families who came with Cornwallis appear to have been in the settlement on that day. It is likely that a large number of the approximately one thousand who left the settlement prior to 8 August were Roman Catholic, aware that the Penal Laws would be applied during the allocation of lands in the new town.

49 PANS CO217, 9:103. One of the surgeons, David Carnegie, a single man, appears to have returned to England two or three months after his arrival in Chebucto. On 10 November 1749 (o.s.) the Lords of Trade received from him in London a memorial complaining that he had not been paid for his services as a surgeon to the settlers during the crossing. I was unable to determine where the other eleven surgeons went after leaving Chebucto. They were: Archibald Campbell, surgeon's mate, single; Cochran Dickson, surgeon, married (no children); Fenton Griffith, surgeon's mate, married (no children); John Farrington, chymist and druggist, single; John Handasyde, surgeon, single; Augustus Harbin, assistant surgeon, single; Patrick Hay, surgeon, single; Matthew Jones, surgeon, single; Thomas Louthian, surgeon's mate, single; Robert Throckmorton, pupil surgeon, single; and John Wallace, surgeon's mate, married (no children).

50 Three surgeons, Henry Meriton, William Lascelles, and Robert White, and the two midwives, Ann Medlicot, and Elizabeth Williams, were not granted lots in 1749 or 1750, although they are known to have been

in Halifax during these years. The Robert White who was buried from St Paul's Church on 11 October 1749 (o.s.) probably was the surgeon mentioned above.

51 *Boston Gazette or Weekly Journal* (hereafter, *Boston Gazette*), 15 August 1749.

52 Cornwallis to Lords of Trade, 24 July 1749 (o.s.). PANS CO217, 9:72. Cornwallis writes, "This will cost money but is great oeconomy [*sic*] compared to the charge of keeping the [transport] ships."

53 Cornwallis to Lords of Trade, 20 August 1749 (o.s.), CO217, 9:81.

54 Ibid., 89. Hopson's Regiment (the 29th), which had been in Chebucto from 25 July 1749 (o.s.), left for England on 21 August 1749 (o.s.) (see Diary of John Salusbury, 21 August 1749 o.s., PANS Micro Biography). Warburton's Regiment (the 45th), which consisted probably of about 1,250 soldiers, was encamped to the south of the town as shown on "A Plan of the Harbour of Chebucto and the Town of Halifax," published in GMHC for February 1750, and shown in Figure 2. The size of regiments varied considerably from time to time. In PANS CO217, 10:18, there is an account of the distribution of 1,250 pairs of shoes sent to Warburton's Regiment in Nova Scotia on 18 July 1750 (o.s.), whereas, on 9 March 1750 (o.s.), it is recorded (PANS CO217, 33:24) that Warburton's Regiment consisted of seven hundred men.

55 This was removed during the summer of 1750 and replaced by the palisades and five forts shown on the Moses Harris plan, which appears in Figure 2 (Cornwallis to the Lords of Trade, 10 July 1750 o.s., PANS CO217, 10:8).

56 The first incident of attack that I have found in relation to the new settlement took place on 30 September 1749 o.s. (PANS RG1, 186:22). Workmen at Major Gilman's sawmill across the harbour in Dartmouth were attacked and, according to Salusbury, "five of the six people working there were butcher'd." This incident is described vividly in the *London Magazine or Gentleman's Monthly Intelligencer* (hereafter, *London Magazine*), 1749, 574. A letter from a gentleman in Halifax, dated 2 October, states "that last Saturday, as several of Gilman's workmen were hewing sticks of timber on the east side of the harbour, they were surprised by about 40 Indians, which killed 4, two of which they scalp'd and cut off the heads of the others." This was the first of numerous Indian attacks which were to keep the settlers ill at ease and within the palisades. This omnipresent fear of attack prompted Cornwallis to ask the Lords of Trade, in a letter of 7 December 1749 (o.s.), for another regiment, in addition to Warburton's, to accelerate the construction of the fortifications and defence (see PANS CO217, 9:128). Previously, at a Council meeting held on 1 October 1749 (o.s.), Cornwallis gave orders to the commanding officers at Annapolis,

Minas, and elsewhere in the province "to annoy, distress, and destroy the Indians everywhere." He further ordered that a bounty of ten guineas be promised for every Indian killed or taken prisoner (PANS RG1, 186:22). A proclamation against the Micmac Indians, dated Halifax 20 October 1749 (o.s.) and issued by Cornwallis, reads, in part: "His Majesty's Council do promise a reward of ten guineas for every Indian Micmak [*sic*] taken or killed to be paid upon producing such savage or his scalp (as is the custom in America) if killed" (PANS CO217, 9:118). On 21 June 1750 (o.s.), Cornwallis increased the bounty to an astounding fifty pounds per Indian scalp (PANS RG1, 163:41).

57 Cornwallis to Lords of Trade, 11 September 1749 (o.s.), PANS CO217, 9:91.

58 Letter from Mr Hardman to Mr Pownall dated Liverpool, 20 May 1749 (o.s.), *Journal of the Commissioners of Trade* 8(1931):417.

59 Cornwallis to Lords of Trade, 17 October 1749 (o.s.), PANS CO217, 9:110.

60 Cornwallis to Lords of Trade, 7 December 1749 (o.s.), PANS CO217, 9:132.

61 I have been unable to ascertain whether the John Day allotted Lot B13 in Callendar's Division on 8 August 1749 (o.s.) was the same person as the surgeon and druggist of that name, known to have resided in Halifax and Newport from 1755–75, except for two years (1770–72) spent in Philadelphia. Brebner, in *Neutral Yankees of Nova Scotia*. 199–200, has concluded that there were two surgeons Day, father and son, who resided at Newport and Halifax prior to 1765. Records suggest, however, that there was only one John Day in Nova Scotia during the period, who was a surgeon, druggist, and merchant (PANS RG1, 189:93). I was unable to identify any primary source that mentions the father of John Day.

62 Surgeon to Warburton's 45th Regiment of Foot, 1745–50 (see Drew, *Roll of Commissioned Officers*, vol. 1).

63 PANS RG1, 164/1:32. Commissioned to be surgeon's mate to Warburton's Forty-fifth Regiment of Foot on 11 October 1749 (o.s.).

64 William Skene is recorded (Halifax Deeds, PANS RG47, 5:291) as being a witness to a land sale which took place in Halifax on 12 October 1749 (o.s.).

65 St Paul's Anglican Church Burials, PANS MG4. The Robert White buried on 11 October 1749 (o.s.) is thought to be the surgeon who arrived on the *Beaufort*. Joshua Sacheverell, surgeon on the *Baltimore*, was buried on 28 November 1749 (o.s.).

66 The number of burials during the period probably was greater than 237. As noted by Bates, in "The Cornwallis Settlers who Didn't," 27–62, only one of the two Anglican clergymen performing burials in

Halifax at the time, Rev. William Tutty, kept records. The Reverend William Anwyl's register of burials was said by Rev. Mr Tutty, to
have been lost ("Letters and Other Papers," 113), assuming that it
ever existed.

67 This contrasts with the year 1766, the first year for which detailed
statistics were kept, during which only 137 in a total population of
13,374 in Nova Scotia died (approximately one percent). The 1766
statistics, given in PANS CO217, 22:121, are signed by Michael Francklin,
the lieutenant governor, who described the statistical report as a
"true return." Article 125 of Cornwallis's instructions from the Lords
of Trade, dated 29 April 1749 (o.s.), stated: "You shall cause an
exact account to be kept of all Persons, Born, Christened and Buried,
and send yearly fair abstracts thereof to Us" (PANS CO218, 3:106).
The same instruction was given to Hopson and Lawrence when each
was appointed governor. Unfortunately, no evidence of the where-
abouts of the "fair abstracts" can be found either at PANS or at the PRO
at Kew in Surrey, England. It is likely that the abstracts were compiled each year, since in 1761, an Act for the Registering of Marriages,
Births, and Deaths was passed by the Council and House of Assembly of Nova Scotia (George 3d, cap. 4, sections 1 and 2, no. 5).

68 Akins, "History of the Settlement of Halifax," 19. Bell, in *The Foreign Protestants* 339, questions Akins's statement: "It would seem as
strange if there should have raged a plague with quite such heavy
mortality as Akins quotes (apparently from tradition only) without any
contemporary documentary evidence of it surviving." Heagerty.
Four Centuries of Medical History 1:74, also mentions that a thousand persons died at Halifax in the fall of 1749 but gives no source for the
information and does not identify the type of disease endemic to Halifax
at the time.

69 Victualling list for May-June 1750, PANS MG1, vol. 258.

70 *The Boston Gazette.* Every issue from May 1749 to the end of 1750
inclusive were read thoroughly by the present author.

71 Cornwallis to Lords of Trade, 19 March 1749/50, PANS CO217,
30:45.

72 "A List of settlers Victuald [*sic*] at this place between the eighteenth
of May and fourth of June 1750, both days inclusive with additions for
June to ye last day," PANS RG1, 163:45. The document was signed
by Cornwallis on 28 November 1750 (o.s.) and referred to as "a true
copy." Cornwallis issued a proclamation on 11 September 1750
(o.s.) stating that the victualling of the original settlers in Halifax would
cease on 15 September 1750 (o.s.).

73 The following names, which appeared on the victualling list for May-
June 1750, probably are those of the surgeons listed in Appendix 1:

Mr Abercrombie, Daniel Brown, Dr Bruscoutz, Mr Robert Grant, John Grant, William Grant, Dr Alexander Hay, Matthew Jones, Dr Robert Kerr, Dr William Merry, Thomas Reeves, John Steel, John Wildman, John Willis, and Thomas Wilson.

As mentioned in note 64, Robert White and Joshua Sacheverell had died during the fall of 1749. William Lascelles, Leonard Lockman, Henry Meriton, and Thomas Rust were quite likely in Halifax during May-June 1750; for some reason, they were not included in the list. As pointed out in Appendix 1, Rust was in Halifax as late as September 1752, whereas, both Lockman and Meriton remained for many years in the settlement. William Lascelles is recorded as having been in Halifax as late as May 1751 (Halifax Deeds, PANS RG47, 2:47). It appears that three of the original surgeons left Halifax between 8 August 1749 (o.s.) and 18 May 1750 (o.s.): John Inman and Harry Pitt, who forfeited their lots early in 1750; and Charles Paine, who sold his lot sometime in 1749, according to the Allotment Book (PANS RG1, vol. 410). The remaining two surgeons making up the total of twenty-one mentioned previously were George Slocombe and William Catherwood, both of the Forty-fifth Regiment, which was stationed in Halifax throughout 1750.

74 "Ships and Vessels which have cleared the Port of Halifax after 19 July 1749 (o.s.)," PANS CO221, vol. 28.

75 Knowles, *Hospitals, Doctors, and the Public Interest*, 5.

76 Hoad, *Surgeons and Surgery in Île Royale*, 223–30.

77 Lords of Trade to Cornwallis, 16 February 1749/50, PANS RG1, vol. 129, Item 8.

78 Cornwallis to Lords of Trade, 30 April 1750 (o.s.), PANS CO217, 30:45.

79 Ibid., 33:24. Davidson's letter to William Merry, dated 30 April 1750 (o.s.), stated that, "the Governor being directed by the Lords of Trade to discharge surgeons and apothecaries from the establishment at the expiration of the year," Merry was discharged as of this date. The surgeons Leonard Lockman and Matthew Jones (PANS RG1, 164/1:29, 35), had been appointed as such on 1 July 1749 (o.s.). The two apothecaries were William Merry and Thomas Reeves. The surgeon's mates were probably Alexander Abercrombie and John Grant. PANS CO217, 15:279 indicates that Abercrombie was an assistant to Dr Jones prior to Jones's death on 7 October 1750 (o.s.). John Grant stated in his memorial to the Lords of Trade, dated 13 January 1755 (PANS CO217, 15:153), that he was an assistant surgeon to the settlement during its first two years. It appears also that Robert Kerr was paid as a surgeon's mate or apothecary's mate during the period 1 May 1749 (o.s.) to 26 August 1750 (o.s.). He was paid at a rate of five shillings per day (Halifax County

Wills, Book 1: 24–5, PANS RG48, Will proved on 29 August 1750 o.s.). The midwife was Ann Catherwood (see her petition in PANS CO217, 16:299).

80 Kilby to Davidson, 5 March 1759/50, PANS CO217, 9:228.

81 *Journal of the Commissioners for Trade* 9 (1932):115, entry for 8 November 1750 (o.s.).

82 Cornwallis to Lords of Trade, 16 July 1750 (o.s.), PANS CO217, 10:1. About £1,642, or two percent of the expenditures during 1749, was for health care. This amount was spent for medicines, drugs, instruments, necessaries for the hospital, and ventilators, as well as to pay the surgeons, apothecaries, and a midwife.

83 Minutes of Council, 23 August 1750 (o.s.), PANS RG1, 186:74. No passenger list is known to exist for the *Alderney*.

84 Cornwallis to Lords of Trade, 2 September 1750 (o.s.), PANS CO217, 10:95. The passenger list for the *Ann* appears in ibid., 9:276.

85 Shipping Returns, 1730–1753, PANS CO221, 28:67.

86 *Journal of the Commissioners for Trade* 9(1932):115, entry for 8 November 1750 (o.s.). Warburton's Forty-fifth, Lascelles's Forty-seventh, and Cornwallis's Fortieth regiments were stationed in Halifax, and the total population, including military, would have exceeded 5,200. Cornwallis had been appointed colonel of the 40th Regiment (formerly Philipps's) on 13 March 1749/50, and eight companies of his regiment (PANS CO217, vol. 10, 18 August 1759 o.s.), had been transferred to Halifax from Newfoundland on 1 August 1750 (o.s.), according to John Salusbury. Salusbury records also that Lascelles's Regiment arrived in Halifax from Ireland in six transports on 12 August 1750 (o.s.). It has been stated (*Northcliffe Collection*, 76) that "the Regiment consisted of ten Companies of 29 men each, 130 women, and 50 children." These regiments were deemed necessary because of the very great fear of being attacked by the French and the Indians. In fact, the *Boston Gazette* of 11 December 1750 (o.s.) includes a comment from Halifax that "we are almost at open war with the French and Indians." In late June, Mr Brown, gardener to Governor Cornwallis, was scalped, his son was killed, and four men with them went missing (*Boston Gazette*, 3 July 1750 o.s.). On 20 June 1750 (o.s.), the same newspaper records that the Indians attacked and scalped seven men at work on the other side of the harbour. On 26 August 1750, Salusbury records Francis Bartelo, a Cornwallis passenger, had been killed in a skirmish and Edward How, a member of Council, had been murdered under a French flag of truce.

87 Cornwallis to Lockman, 25 October 1750 (o.s.), PANS RG1, 163/1:47.

88 St Paul's Anglican Church Burials, PANS MG4. Alexander Aber-

crombie was appointed to take the place of Matthew Jones as one of the chief surgeons to the hospital on 18 October 1750 o.s. (see PANS RG1, 164:32).

89 Cornwallis to Lewis Hays, 5 November 1750 (o.s.), PANS RG1, 163/1:53.

90 Cornwallis to Lords of Trade, 27 November 1750 (o.s.), PANS CO217, 11:13.

91 Minutes of Council, 23 August 1750 (o.s.), PANS RG1, 186:74. The Council took into consideration the most proper way of disposing of 353 settlers who had arrived in the *Alderney*. Captain Morris, the surveyor, was asked to survey the Dartmouth side as soon as possible for a town site.

92 Dick to Hill, Secretary to the Lords of Trade, 23 February 1750 (o.s.), PANS CO217, 11:39.

93 In contrast to my own conclusions, Williams states that "there was no real epidemic until 1775" ("Poor Relief and Medicine in Nova Scotia," 33–56). It should be noted that this article was reprinted in *Medicine in Canadian Society*, edited by S.E.D. Shortt. Miss Williams married sometime between 1938 and 1981, and thus her name in *Medicine in Canadian Society* is given as Relief MacKay.

94 This could be the destructive epidemic to which Akins refers (see note 68) as having taken place during the fall and winter of 1749–50. Further evidence that the epidemic took place during 1750–51, rather than during the previous year, is found in the *Boston Gazette* of 18 July 1751 (o.s.): "We have advice from Caco [Casco Bay, on which Portland, Maine, is situated], that the epidemical fever is prevailing among them that they had at Halifax last summer and which proved too fatal to [the] multitude."

95 Risse, "Typhus Fever in the 18th Century Hospitals," 176–95.

96 A Recent paper on Sauvages is Martin, "Sauvages's Nosology: Medical Enlightenment at Montpellier."

97 William Draper, surgeon, was involved in a land sale which took place in Halifax on 5 February 1750 (o.s.) (see Halifax County Deeds, PANS RG47, 2:147).

98 Cornwallis to Lords of Trade, 30 April 1750 (o.s.), PANS CO217, 9:235. While appearing before the Lords of Trade on 9 January 1749/1750 (*Journal of the Commissioners for Trade*, vol. 58, 9 January 1749/50), Mr Kingslagh, who had been an officer at Louisbourg and went from there to Halifax, stated that "the number of settlers in Halifax increased by 7 or 800 families from New England." It is possible that he meant seven or eight hundred persons for it is doubtful that eight hundred New England families could have come to Halifax prior to 14 December 1749 (o.s.), the date on which Kingslagh

(sometimes appearing as Kinselagh, or Kingslaugh) left Halifax, when, as stated earlier by Cornwallis, the population of Halifax on 7 December 1749 (o.s.) was 1,876.

99 John Kinselagh to Lords of Trade, 6 July 1750 (o.s.), PANS CO217, 9:280.

100 Passenger list of the *Ann,* dated 29 June 1750 (o.s.), PANS CO217, 9:276.

101 Ibid., 13:230. Duckworth appears to have remained in Halifax until 24 January 1752 (o.s.). On that date, he appeared before John Hoffman, justice of the peace for Halifax County. Duckworth's petition appears in ibid., 14:17 and describes hardships he experienced as a consequence of having been a passenger on the *Nancy.*

102 Drew, *Roll of Commissioned Officers* 1:18. Arthur Price was surgeon of Lascelles's Forty-seventh Regiment of Foot from 30 September 1746 (o.s.) until July 1757.

103 PANS RG1, 164:54A. Richard Veale to be surgeon to Warburton's Regiment on 30 September 1750 (o.s.).

104 Halifax County Deeds, PANS RG47, 2:164. Nothing further is known about Edward Crafts, surgeon. He does not appear in the victualling list of May-June 1750 (PANS MG1, vol. 258), or in the 1752 census for Halifax (PANS RG1, vol. 417).

105 Wilson, *A Genuine Narrative,* 15. Wilson writes, "On 27 May, the Indians surprised Dartmouth and killed fifteen persons, wounded seven, three of whom died in the Hospital. Six men were carried away and haven't been heard of since. The soldiers who marched in after the Indians had one sergent [*sic*] shot dead." Wilson gives a vivid description of how the Indians scalped a little boy and of the treatment given by a doctor, possibly Baxter, when the boy returned to the settlement. This incident occurred quite likely on 26 March 1751 (o.s.), as recorded in Salusbury's diary for that day. Wilson's date is probably a typographical error.

106 *London Magazine* 20:341, 1751.

107 Return of the families on the *Speedwell* bound for Halifax, dated 11 May 1751 (o.s.), PANS CO217, 11:110.

108 Minutes of Council, 11 July 1751 (o.s.), PANS RG1, 186:129. "The Council were of the opinion that it would be most convenient to land them for the present at Dartmouth, and employ them in [building] pickets in the back of said Town."

109 List of Swiss on the *Gale* departing for Nova Scotia on 20 May 1751 (o.s.), PANS CO217, 12:22. Council decided, at its meeting of 31 July 1751 (o.s.), that "it will be most convenient in many respects to place them, for the present, between the Head of the Northwest Arm of the Harbour and the mouth of Bedford Bay, and to employ them ... in picketting across same" (PANS RG1, 186:133).

110 Passenger list of *Pearl*, dated 2 July 1751 (o.s.), PANS CO217, 12:70.

111 Passenger list of *Murdoch* bound for Halifax from Rotterdam, dated 23 June 1751 (o.s.), PANS CO217, 12:57.

112 Bell, *Foreign Protestants*, 251, 169, 178, 180–1. Bell records that these ships had been fitted with ventilators prior to embarkation. Also see Dick to Hill, 3 February 1750/51, PANS CO217, 11:40.

113 The eight surgeons on the four transport shps were: *(Speedwell)* Louis LeRoy, aged thirty-three, from Wurtemberg; *(Gale)* Hector Jacot, aged eighteen; Johannes Matth. Lütgens, aged twenty-six, from Lübeck; Alexandre de Rodohan, aged thirty, from Mons; *(Murdoch)* Christopher Nicolai, aged nineteen, from Darmstad; Windilinus Commeus, aged forty-one, from Northhorn; *(Pearl)* David Prins, aged twenty-six, from Amsterdam; and John Bughard Ehrhard, aged fifty-six, from Durlach.

114 Among the Cornwallis passengers of this name, the one who was most likely the surgeon was John Phillipps, purser of the *Beaufort*. The other two on the Cornwallis mess lists were John Philips, mariner, on the *Winchelsea*, and John Phillips, fisherman, on the *Canning*.

115 Cornwallis to Phillipps, 4 June 1751 (o.s.), PANS RG1, 164/1:63–4. PRO WO34, vol. 12 includes a return from Major Gorham of the two companies of Rangers serving in Nova Scotia on 29 March 1761. In this return, "Lieu^t John Philipps" is described as advanced in years (about fifty). It is also stated that "he came in [to Nova Scotia a] full Lieut. and Surgeon in 1750."

116 Minutes of Council, 28 February 1754 (n.s.), PANS RG1, 187:36.

117 William Urquhart Jr to Sir James Kempt, n.d., PANS RG1, vol. 411, Item 94.

118 Halifax County Deeds 2:313, PANS RG47.

119 Ibid., 189.

120 NSGWC, 2 October 1781.

121 Halifax County Deeds, PANS RG47, 2:51. George Winslo [*sic*] was referred to as a physician on 30 December 1751 (Halifax County Inferior Court of Common Pleas, vol. 1, PANS RG37). A document dated 3 November 1778 and entitled "30 acre lots drawn by people who left the settlement [of Lunenburg] the first year [1753–54]" indicates that George Winslow was one of a list of persons who were "married men, said dead, some left children at Halifax" (PANS RG1, vol. 221, Document 44).

122 Minutes of Council, 13 December 1751 (o.s.), PANS RG1, 186:137.

123 Lords of Trade to Cornwallis, 6 March 1751/52, PANS RG1, 29:8.

124 PANS CO217, 15:110. Mrs Wenman came to Halifax with her husband, Richard, on the *Charlton*. She was buried from St Paul's Anglican Church on 14 May 1792, aged seventy-six. Previous to the opening

of the orphan house, orphans were kept in private homes. As early as 19 March 1749/50, Cornwallis had written to the Lords of Trade (PANS RG1, vol. 35, Document 11) that "another house is erecting for a public school where I propose to put all orphans that they may be taken care till they are fit for going prentices to Fisherman." It is interesting to note that spruce beer was judged so conducive to health at that time that it was part of the diet of the orphans (PANS CO217, 15:110).

125 Ibid., 14:94, 103. From 30 October to 24 December 1752 (n.s.), there were fifty-eight in the orphan house and thirty-eight patients in the hospital.

126 Minutes of Council, 24 August 1752 (o.s.), This PANS RG1, 186:208–9. This arrangement was not feasible, however, and at the Council meeting of 25 September 1752, it was stated: "It having been represented to the Governor and Council that there will be considerable inconvenience attending the removal of sick prisoners from the gaol to the Hospital as had been by Govr and Council lately ordered, resolved that the affair be referred to further consideration and that in the meantime the justices be directed to stay further proceedings therein" (PANS RG1, 186:222).

127 The *Pearl* arrived in Halifax on 10 August 1752 (o.s.) with a total of 212 passengers, including Johann Conrad Heinrich Edmund, a surgeon, aged twenty-three, from Hamburg (PANS CO217, 13:229). The *Betty* and the *Speedwell* came into the harbour on 22 August (PANS CO221, 28:168) with 154 and 203 passengers. On 25 August, the *Sally* arrived (PANS CO217, 13:208) with 218 passengers, including Johann C. Ohme, a twenty-year-old surgeon from Saxony. The last ship, the *Gale*, with 220 foreign protestants, arrived on 6 September 1752 (CO217, 13:218), with a surgeon on board named Johann C. Degelin, aged twenty, from Wurtemberg. All of these three surgeons remained in Nova Scotia. In the minutes of Council for 24 August 1752 (o.s.), it was recorded that "they [the Germans] be placed for the coming winter, in and about the Town of Halifax and adjacent settlements and that those of them who have their passages to pay for be employed in such services, as may be of most utility to the Colony" (PANS RG1, 186:204).

128 Lords of Trade Instructions to Hopson, 23 April 1752 (o.s.), PANS CO218, 4:216.

129 Bell, *Foreign Protestants*, 251.

130 List of officers and soldiers victualled in Hopson's Regiment in Nova Scotia between 3 August and 30 August 1752 (o.s.), PANS CO217, 13:329. There were also seventy members of the Royal Regiment of Artillery in Halifax by 18 August 1752 o.s. (ibid., 13:325).

131 "A List of Families and Soldiers Victualled in Hopson's Regiment in Nova Scotia since 1749, and who, in 1752, were settlers in Halifax, its suburbs, and nearby areas," PANS RG1, vol. 417:

Census Results for Halifax and Surrounding Areas, July 1752

Location	Families	Persons
Within the Pickets of Halifax	468	2,032
Within the North Suburbs	169	765
Within the South Suburbs	151	818
Within the Town of Dartmouth	53	195
On Islands and Harbours employed in the Fishery	–	202
On the Isthmus and the Peninsula of Halifax	65	216
Totals	906	4,248

The phrase "victualled in Nova Scotia since 1749" is not meant to imply that all families were in Nova Scotia since 1749, but that some had been in Nova Scotia since that date. Not all of the families are included in the list, for the number of families above is greater, by about forty percent, than the heads of family actually named and listed.

132 Letter dated 9 November 1751 (o.s.), SPGFP, Reel 15B, 18:94.

133 Inferior Court of Common Pleas, case dated 24 September 1762. *Thomas Wood, physician of Halifax, vs. Eben. Messenger*, PANS RG37, vol. 13.

134 Minutes of Council, 16 September 1752 (n.s.), PANS RG1, 186:216. The treaty or articles of peace, found on page 240 of the minutes, are dated 22 November 1752 (n.s.). It was a treaty with the tribe of Micmac Indians inhabiting the eastern part of the province.

135 Letter dated 22 November 1752 (n.s.), Society for the Propagation of the Gospel in Foreign Parts, Reel 15B, 20:14.

136 Minutes of Council, 12 April 1753 (n.s.), PANS RG1, 186:362–3.

137 Minutes of Council, 26 March 1753 (n.s.), PANS RG1, 186:353.

138 Minutes of Council, 16 April 1753 (n.s.), PANS RG1, 186:365.

139 Hopson to Lords of Trade, 15 April 1753 (n.s.), PANS CO217, 14:151.

140 Hopson to Lords of Trade, 26 May 1753 (n.s.), PANS CO217, 14:159. "A Return of the Settlers at Lunenburg from 28 May 1753 to 22 January 1758" (PANS RG1, vol. 381) indicates that the original number of settlers at Lunenburg was 1,453.

141 Bell, *The Foreign Protestants*, 419.

CHAPTER TWO

1 Council minutes of 28 June 1759, PANS RG1, 188:79. Erad's appointment was mentioned in a memorial by John Phillipps read to Council on the above date. Erad had been "appointed one of the surgeons for the settlement of Lunenburg" prior to the departure of the settlers from Halifax in June 1753. I have found no official letter or communication either to Erad or Lockman, appointing them surgeons to the settlement of Lunenburg, but it does appear that both were paid to execute that office as described in the memorial. Erad continued to act as surgeon at Lunenburg until his death on 24 March 1757, while Lockman appears to have remained there until early in 1757 when, for health reasons, he returned to Halifax (List of people victualled at Lunenburg, January-May 1757, PANS RG1, vol. 222). Phillipps's memorial indicates that Lockman left Lunenburg in March 1757, for Phillipps wrote that he had filled the office of surgeon at Lunenburg since that date and asks to be paid for his services.

2 "A Return of the Settlers at Lunenburg from 28 May 1753 to 22 January 1758," PANS RG1, vol. 382. This document indicates that the original number of settlers at Lunenburg was 1,453. The four surgeons mentioned (Klett, Deglen, Nicolai, and Edmund) are listed in the Lunenburg Allottment Book (PANS RG47) as having been among the first settlers granted lots in the town of Lunenburg. J. Carl Deglen is given as Deglin and Degelin in some primary sources.

3 Cornwallis to Phillipps, 4 June 1751 (O.S.), PANS RG1, 164/1:64. The Independent Companies of Rangers included Gorham's Rangers (see Bates, "John Gorham, an Outline of his Activities in Nova Scotia," 27–77), and Clapham's Rangers, raised on 20 October 1749 (O.S.) by William Clapham (PANS RG1, 164:25). Each company consisted of fifty to sixty men. John Phillipps was paid two shillings and six pence per day for his services as surgeon to the Companies of Rangers (PANS CO217, 14:249).

4 St John's Anglican Marriages, Lunenburg, PANS MG4, vol. 91. John Phillipps continued to reside in Lunenburg and to offer his services as a surgeon there until 1766, when he left for England" to seek proficient medical advice" (PANS RG1, 166:11).

5 "Journal, and letters, being a day-by-day account of the founding of Lunenburg, by the Officer in Command [Charles Lawrence] of the project," *Bulletin of the Public Archives of Nova Scotia*, no. 10, Halifax, 1953.

6 According to PANS RG1, 163/2:88, detachments of Hopson's, Lascelles's, and Warburton's regiments were located at Annapolis, Fort Lawrence, and Lunenburg on 11 September 1753. It is likely that

William Skene, surgeon of Hopson's 40th Regiment, was at the Annapolis garrison, while William Catherwood (surgeon's mate of the 45th), Arthur Price (surgeon of the 47th), Richard Veale (surgeon of the 45th), and George Francheville (surgeon of Ordnance) were at Fort Lawrence. In addition to these five army surgeons, a surgeon named Ebenezer Hartshorn appears to have been at Annapolis in December 1753, where he witnessed the will of Katherine Sprainger (Halifax Wills, vol. 1, PANS RG48), and one of the surgeons who came with the foreign Protestants, Alexandre de Rodohan, was residing with the Acadians at Grand Pré in May 1754 (PANS RG1, 134:131).

7 This figure was arrived at by subtracting the 1,453 Lunenburg settlers who left Halifax in June 1753, from the number of civilians reported in the July 1752 census.

8 Hopson to Lords of Trade, 29 May 1753, PANS CO217, 33:188. Hopson wrote, "The only vessel of force here is the *Albany*, Sloop of War, Capt. Rous, Commander."

9 Lawrence to Lords of Trade, 29 December 1753, PANS CO217, 15:4. Governor Hopson had sailed for England on 1 November 1753, and Charles Lawrence was placed in command (PANS RG1, 134:1).

10 Hopson to Lords of Trade, 1 October 1753, PANS CO217, 14:302.

11 Council minutes of 27 December 1753, PANS RG1, 187:25.

12 Halifax County Supreme Court, *John Kent vs. John Grant; John Buttler vs. John Grant; Catherine Winston vs. John Grant*, PANS RG39, series "C," Box 1.

13 Halifax County Inferior Court of Common Pleas, *William Kneeland vs. William Merry*, PANS RG37, Box 2, file 22.

14 The year 1752 began on 25 March, and therefore the designation x ber 22 1752 means the tenth month following March (i.e., December). See Introduction for a detailed explanation.

15 Council minutes of 12 October 1753, PANS RG1, 186:423, and Council minutes of 28 February 1754, 186:36. Akins, "History of Halifax City," 41, indicates that a William Murray (*sic*) operated a still on Grafton Street. Prescott's was near the South Gate.

16 "Estimate of the Expense of Civil Officers, Surgeons, etc." for 1754 (PANS CO217, 14:249) includes "continuation of an allowance to Henry Meriton for his encouragement in keeping a school at Halifax."

17 PANS CO217, 15:338. John Grant states that he "is in business here [in Halifax] as a surgeon as well as in trade."

18 Lawrence to Charles Hay, 1 January 1754, PANS RG1, 163/3:27.

19 Lawrence to the Lords of Trade, 14 October 1754, PANS RG1, vol. 36, Lawrence was not officially appointed lieutenant governor of Nova Scotia until the fall of 1754. He acknowledges receipt of his commission.

20 Hopson to Lords of Trade, 23 July 1753, PANS CO217, 14:188–9.

21 John Grant's memorial to the Lords of Trade, 21 October 1754, PANS CO217, 15:162.

22 "A True and Exact State of the Expense of the Hospital at Halifax for one year, viz: from 1 July 1754 to 1 July 1755," PANS CO217, 15:289.

23 "Estimates of the Expense of Civil Officers, Surgeons, etc.," 1754, PANS CO217, 14:249.

24 Remarks on Mr Grant's representation that there is no person to inquire into the state of the hospital or the conduct of the surgeon, etc. Council minutes of 4 June 1755, PANS CO217, 15:293.

25 John Grant's memorial to Lawrence, n.d., but probably 20 September 1754, PANS CO217, 15:157.

26 John Grant's reference to Alexander Abercrombie's lack of qualifications was, in fact, completely unfounded. Abercrombie was very well educated for the time, both in the liberal arts and in physic and surgery. He had graduated in 1745 with a Bachelor of Arts degree from Marischal College, Aberdeen, Scotland and had attended, in 1746 and 1747, the lectures in anatomy given by the esteemed Dr Alexander Monro of Edinburgh University. He had worked, also, at His Majesty's Hospital in Edinburgh and served as surgeon in two military campaigns in Flanders. Marischal College, the northern university alluded to in the *Halifax Gazette* did award Abercrombie an MD *in absentia*, in July 1753, but this was (or had been) a common practice in all five of the Scottish medical colleges. See Anderson, ed., *Selections* 2:117. See also Monro's "Record Book of Scholars" at the Edinburgh University Archives. For Abercrombie's service in Flanders, see PANS CO217, 15:279. A short biography of Dr Abercrombie is included in Council minutes of 3 June 1755. The five Scottish medical colleges were Aberdeen, Edinburgh, Glasgow, Marischal, and St Andrews. Comrie (*History of Scottish Medicine to 1880*, 142–3) writes: "It was not until after the foundation of a Medical Faculty at Edinburgh in 1726, that the idea came into being in Scotland of conferring the MD on young men as the consummation of three years' medical study and to which they were entitled after successful examination." Edinburgh had granted twenty-one medical degrees prior to the establishment of its medical faculty in 1726.

27 John Grant to Lords of Trade, 13 January 1755, PANS CO217, 15:153.

28 Council minutes of 3 June 1755, PANS CO217, 15:275.

29 Ibid., 276–89.

30 "Account of the Number of Venereals treated in Hospital." Document included in Council minutes of 3 June 1755, PANS CO217, 15:281.

31 Lawrence to Lords of Trade, 28 June 1755, PANS CO217, 15:254.

32 Lords of Trade to Lawrence, 9 October 1755, PANS CO218, 5:134.

33 *Halifax Gazette*. 3 August 1754. Mrs Triggs, midwife, is mentioned as living opposite the Hospital for Sick and Hurt Seamen on Granville Street. As pointed out by Baugh, *British Naval Administration in the Age of Walpole*. 35, "The Commissioners for Sick and Wounded Seamen, commonly known as the Sick and Hurt Board, maintained the Naval Hospitals and Medical Organization," and had done so since it was first appointed in 1653. Rodger explains the naval-hospital system that existed in the early and mid-eighteenth century (*The Wooden World*, 109): "The traditional way of caring for sick men landed from ships was to put them in sick quarters, which meant rooms rented from local landladies who undertook to feed and care for their patients. A great many of those sent to sick quarters either never recovered or never returned. Consequently naval opinion by the early 1750s was unanimous in preferring a hospital. Naval hospitals were usually run by contract whereby the contractor furnished premises and non-medical staff, being paid by the number of patients he accomodated. The Sick and Hurt Board provided furniture and equipment and appointed the medical staff. This was the system on which all naval hospitals were run in 1755."

34 Letters to the Commissioners of the Sick and Hurt Board, PRO Adm. 97, vol. 85.

35 Ibid.

36 Ibid.

37 "State of the Sick left from the different Ships of Admiral Boscawen's Squadron as they now stand on the sick Books this 18 November 1755, signed by Robert Grant, surgeon," PANS Adm. 1/480:655. The *Halifax Gazette* of 6 April 1754 mentions that Robert Grant resided on Granville Street at that time.

38 Medical Department to Secretary of the Admiralty, 10 February 1757, PRO Adm. 98/6, folio 171. The letter read:

The service of His Majesty's Sick and Wounded Seamen in Nova Scotia, being before the commencement of the present War [Seven Years' War] very inconsiderable ... we appointed Mr Robert Grant, a Navy Surgeon who resided there [Halifax], to be our Surgeon and Agent at that place, and made him the usual allowances of six shil-

lings and eight pence per man per cure ... it [the allowance] remained
till the arrival of Vice Admiral Boscawan in those parts [9 July
1755], when very great numbers of sick men being sent on shore, and
the prices of medicines thereby considerably increased, he
[Boscawen] thought proper when an application [was] made to him by
the said Mr Grant, upon having referred the matter to proper
judges, to allow him eight shillings and eight pence per man per cure.

39 Minutes of Council, 27 June 1754, PANS RG1, 187:177.

40 Horseman's Fort was named for Lt Col John Horseman of Warburton's
Regiment, who had arrived in Halifax from Louisbourg on 24 July
1749 (o.s.). The fort is shown in the lower left of the Moses Harris plan
of Halifax, which appears in Figure 2. This fort was large enough
to house two companies of soldiers.

41 Lawrence to Lords of Trade, 1 June 1754, PANS CO217, 15:34.

42 *Halifax Gazette*, 2 February 1754, Merry's death notice.

43 "Total Number of Houses and Huts in the Town of Lunenburg,
16 July 1754, PANS RG1, vol. 382.

44 Minutes of Council, 10 April 1755, PANS RG1, 187:257.

45 Pownall to Lawrence, 30 November 1754, PANS CO218, 5:100.

46 Lawrence to Lords of Trade, 1 August 1754, PANS CO217, 15:85.

47 Lords of Trade to Lawrence, 29 October 1754, PANS CO218, 5:77.

48 Whitehall to Governor of Nova Scotia, 26 October 1754, PANS RG1,
vol. 29, Letter no. 29.

49 "Leave of Absence to the Hon. Lieutenant Col° Robert Monkton
[*sic*] to be on the continent for six months," dated 15 November 1754,
PANS RG1, 163/3:46.

50 Winslow, "Journal of John Winslow," 138.

51 Lawrence to Lords of Trade, 28 June 1755, PANS CO217, 15:251.

52 Thomas, "Diary," 131. Doctor March had served as an under-surgeon
of the train of Artillery sent from Massachusetts to Louisbourg in
1744 ("Louisbourg Soldiers," 377–8).

53 Winslow, "Journal of John Winslow," 232.

54 Council minutes, 18 August 1756, PANS RG1, 187:455.

55 Winslow, "Journal of Colonel John Winslow," 94. It is interesting
to note that Winslow selected Doctor Alexandre de Rodohan to deliver
the citation to the inhabitants of Grand Pré and environs, on 4 September, ordering them to congregate on the following day so that Winslow could inform them of their fate.

56 Ibid., 185. Information given in Winslow's journal indicates that 698
buildings at Gaspereau, Cannard (*sic*), Habitant, Pero (*sic*), etc.,
were burned during the period 2 November to 7 November 1755.

Prior to 2 November, 2,242 persons had been shipped from these districts.

57 Ibid., 186. The total number of Acadians expelled from Nova Scotia during the fall of 1755, as indicated by Winslow's journal (175, 177, 178, 182, 186, 188, 192), was about six thousand. The districts from which these Acadians came and the approximate dates of departure are given below:

Acadians Expelled from Nova Scotia

Deported from	Date Deported	Number Deported
Chignecto	13 October 1755	1,045
Piziquid	27 October 1755	1,100
Minas	27 October 1755	1,505
Annapolis	8 December 1755	1,664
Minas	18 December 1755	350
Grand Pré	20 December 1755	332
	Total	5,596

Colonel Winslow's journal (122) notes that a total of 2,743 Acadians were at Grand Pré, Minas, River Canard, Habitant, and environs on 15 September 1755, while the above list indicates that the number of Acadians deported from Minas and Grand Pré and environs was 2,187. The discrepency is due to the significant number of Acadians who escaped to the woods. Chief Justice Belcher wrote on 28 July 1755 to Pownall (PANS C0217, 16:26) that there were eight thousand French and three thousand English in Nova Scotia. Since the number deported was approximately six thousand, as indicated in the list, it is probable that some two thousand Acadians remained in the province after 1755. The dates of deportation given for Chignecto, Piziquid, and Minas were found in PANS Adm. 1/480:663, in a letter (22 November 1755) from Richard Spry to John Cleveland, secretary of the Admiralty. The Acadians at Cobequid deserted that settlement prior to the arrival of the English soldiers, who burned the buildings there during the period 23–29 September (Winslow, "Journal of Colonel John Winslow," 155).

58 In addition to Dr March, who was killed on 2 August 1755, and Dr Whitworth, who attended the Acadians at Minas during August, September, and October, Doctors Nye, Cast, Thomas, and Tyler remained in the Chignecto area during the fall of 1755. Nye is recorded

as being there as late as 23 August, while Dr Cast (also spelled Kast) was at Chignecto as late as 24 October 1755. Dr John Thomas (the diarist) was at Chignecto until 2 December when he went to Minas, and on 9 December, to Halifax. Dr John Tyler transferred from Shirley's Regiment to Lascelles's Regiment, which he accompanied to Halifax, where he died on 5 January 1758 (PANS Micro Misc A, Armies – Colonial).

59 *Dictionary of Canadian Biography* 3:70–1. Edward Boscawen (1711–61) was later chosen to command the naval forces at the siege of Louisbourg in 1758. Boscawen's Fleet in 1755 consisted of twenty-two ships of war, the names of which are listed in PANS Adm. 1/480:640. Boscawen's decision to put into Halifax because of sickness is recorded in his letter to John Cleveland, Secretary of the Admiralty, dated 4 July 1755 (PANS Adm. 1/481:41).

60 Drucour and Prevost to the Minister, Louisbourg, 2 June 1755, AN, Colonies, C"B, vol. 35, folios 19–22.

61 "State and Condition of HM Ships under Vice Admiral Boscawen at Halifax, 12 July 1755," PANS Adm. 1/481:46.

62 Boscawen to Cleveland, 16 July 1755, PANS Adm. 1/481:47.

63 Willard, "Journal," entry for 23 September, 3–75.

64 Winslow, "Journal of Colonel John Winslow," 147–8.

65 "State of the Sick left from the different Ships of Admiral Boscawen's Squadron as they now stand on the sick Books, 18 November 1755," PANS Adm. 1/480:655. Robert Grant's book indicate that forty-nine seamen had died during the last twelve days of October, and twenty-seven had died during the first eighteen days of November.

66 Williams, "Poor Relief and Medicine in Nova Scotia, 1749–1783," 33–56.

67 The number of burials for the period January 1755 to August 1756 was taken, for the most part, from St Paul's Anglican Church Records (PANS MG4). A small number of deaths that occurred in Halifax during that period, which are not recorded in St Paul's burials, was taken from four additional sources: The *Halifax Gazette*: St Paul's Cemetery Inscriptions (PANS MG5); St George's Cemetery Inscriptions (PANS MG5); and "An Account of the Number of Children in the Orphan House at Halifax" PANS CO217, 18:218).

68 Halifax Wills, Book 1:88, PANS RG48. William Urquhart, surgeon of Halifax, made his will on 18 July 1755, and it was proved on 4 August 1755. The burial recorded in St Paul's Anglican Church indicates that he was buried in August 1755.

69 Halifax Supreme Court Records, PANS RG39, series C, Box 2.

70 PANS Adm. 1/481:86.

71 Memorial of John Day, 22 March 1768, PANS RG1, 189:93.

72 William Best's Account Book, PANS MG3, 141:103, 141.

73 "State and Condition of HM Ships under the Command of Capt. Richard Spry at Halifax, 26 January 1756," PANS Adm. 1/480:684.

74 "Report of the State of the Orphan House, 1752–1761," PANS CO217, 18:218–25. In a letter to Governor Francis Legge (1 January 1776), Lt Col Henry Denny Denson indicates that Michael Head had served at Halifax as a surgeon's mate to the Fortieth Regiment (PANS Micro Biography, Earl of Dartmouth Papers, Reel 1, 479–81). Since the Fortieth Regiment left Halifax in June 1759, it would be expected that Dr Michael Head was in Halifax prior to that date. He could also have been the Dr Head mentioned in the Best Account Book in 1754 and 1755.

75 Marble, "He Usefully Exercised the Medical Profession," 40–71.

76 Boscawen to Cleveland, 15 November 1755, on board the *Torbay*, PANS Adm. 1/481:67. "By certain accounts the French intended to have attacked Halifax last Spring from Louisbourg, they having a Garrison of 2,500, the English Garrison at Halifax, not exceeding 400." He continues that he has captured "a Plan of Halifax with a scheme of attacking it from Canada taken out of a wash ball that was in a French Officer's Chest going to Louisbourg. This Plan, I apprehend to be the Invention of Monsr Vaudreuil, Governor of the Three Rivers, he was taken in the *Alcide*, is brother to the Vice Admiral of that name, the Governor of Canada, and the Governor of St Domingo, but is almost a Fool." The *Alcide*, a French man-of-war, was captured off Louisbourg on 8 June 1755 (Journal of Admiral Edward Boscawen NAC Adm. 50, no. 3:20) and brought into Halifax (Ibid., 27). The plan (figure 7) shows three batteries on the beach in front of Halifax. Lawrence, writing to the Lords of Trade on 28 June 1755 (PANS CO217, 15:256), states that he "sends plan of the three batteries upon the beach before the town of Halifax, of which a description follows." Lawrence indicated that the batteries were not yet completed. Since I was unable to view the plan to which Lawrence referred, it has not been possible to determine whether the plan which appears in Figure 7 is the same as that sent by the governor. It is possible that the plan was stolen by the French officer mentioned above, and that he added the numbers as well as the French writing in the upper left of the plan. Lawrence describes the batteries as "12′ high above the high water, 240′ long, and 65′ in breadth." He mentions "that fifteen guns are already mounted, in a few days the work will be ready for five guns more, and in a very short time the whole will be completed."

77 Winslow, "Journal of Colonel John Winslow," 190.

78 Thomas, "Diary," 139.

79 PANS MG3, 141:84, entry of 27 February 1756 reads: "to trucking ½ cordwood to New Eng^d Hosp^1 – 1 shilling."

80 Forman's Division, Lot B5, according to the Allotment Book (PANS RG1, vol. 410). In William Best's Account Book (PANS MG3, 141:88), there is a list of dealings that Best had with one John Solomon, wheelwright. The first was on 19 January 1756: "to 50 large bricks, ½ bushel of lime, to repare [sic] his hous [sic] Hospital, 4s, 6p." The next day, an entry for John Solomon reads, "repairing 2 chamber fireplaces at the Hospital House." This hospital appears to have operated as such until at least 18 March 1757; it is mentioned in Best's Account Book on that date.

81 Council minutes of 8 March 1756, PANS RG1, 187:409.

82 Spry to Cleveland, 18 April 1756, PANS Adm. 1/480:702.

83 Distribution of the Several corps in Nova Scotia, 21 June 1756, PANS Micro Misc. A, Armies – Colonial, Army Returns, 1757–1817.

84 Spry to Cleveland, 18 April 1756, PANS Adm. 1/480:702.

85 Whitehall to Lawrence, 17 May 1756, PANS RG1, vol. 30, Letter no. 4.

86 Returns of the regiments for 29 November 1756, PANS Micro Misc. A, Armies – Colonial, Army Returns, 1757–1817.

87 Whitehall to Lawrence, 4 February 1757, PANS RG1, vol. 30, Letter no. 11.

88 Doughty, ed., An Historical Journal 1:22. The regiments that arrived in Halifax with Admiral Holburne on 9 July 1757, were the 1st, 17th, 27th, 28th, 43rd, 46th, and 55th.

89 Hardy to Secretary of Admiralty, 1 July 1757, PANS Adm. 1/481:516.

90 London Magazine 26:457, 1757. Letters received by the Magazine on 30 August 1757 from Lord Loudoun [sic] and Admiral Holbourne [sic]. The regiments that accompanied Lord Loudon to Halifax were the Twenty-second, Forty-second, Forty-eighth, and Sixtieth, according to Doughty, ed., An Historical Journal 1:32. Lord Loudon, the fourth earl of Loudon, was known as John Campbell before he inherited the title from the third earl and took his seat in the House of Lords.

91 This included 1,239 men in Hopson's, Warburton's, and Lascelles's regiments stationed at Halifax; 5,990 soldiers and 7,135 seamen brought by Admiral Holburne; 951 men with Sir Charles Hardy; and about 5,000 soldiers and an unspecified number of seamen brought to Halifax from New York by Lord Loudon.

92 Medical Department to Secretary of the Admiralty, 10 February 1757, PRO Adm. 98/6, folio 173.

93 Fowke, Colville, and others, to Secretary of the Admiralty, 2 September 1757, PRO Adm. 98/6, folio 457. Godfrey Webb had been examined by the Company of Surgeons in London on 1 July 1756 (Company of Surgeons' Examination Book, 1745–1800, London.).

94 Medical Department to Secretary of the Admiralty, 3 February 1758, PRO Adm. 98/7, folio 113. In this letter, mention is made that "an under assistant surgeon at Nova Scotia upon the reduced Establishment [ordered on 14 September 1757, ibid., folio 107], being lately dead, Mr John Flacke is going out to succeed him." John Grant's will having been proved on 5 September 1757 Halifax County Wills, Book 1:141, PANS RG48, it is possible that he was the deceased under assistant surgeon.

95 Medical Department to Secretary of the Admiralty, 13 October 1758, PRO Adm. 98/7, folio 272. "Mr McCormick, who was sometime surgeon at His Majesty's Hospital at Nova Scotia," petitioned the board for pay for his services. He was probably the Mr John McCormick listed as a surgeon in the *Navy Lists* for 1758.

96 Minutes of Council, 16 July 1757, PANS RG1, 187:526. The Lords of Trade had recommended that Lawrence be appointed governor on 18 December 1755 (Lords of Trade to the King, 18 December 1755, PANS CO218, 5:139.)

97 "Register of the Receipts of Provisions, with the Number of men and nurses included victualled in the Naval Hospital in the years 1757–1761," PANS MG13, no. 7a. This is the earliest record referring to the Hospital for Sick and Hurt Seamen as the naval hospital. The information in Figure 9 is taken from the same source.

98 Medical Department to Secretary of the Admiralty, 6 June 1760, PRO Adm. 98/8, folio 206. Robert Grant had been sworn in as a member of Council on 15 June 1756 (PANS RG1, 187:430). He was replaced on 16 August 1759 (PANS RG1, 188:93) against his will, for the reason that he was no longer a resident of Nova Scotia.

99 Medical Department to Secretary of the Admiralty, 21 April 1759, PRO Adm. 98/7, folio 419. "The Rt Hon. Edward Boscawen, Esq., then Commander-in-Chief of His Majesties Ships and Vessels in North America did by Warrant, 27 July 1758, appoint David Thomas Karr, Surgeon for the Sick and Wounded Prisoners of War at that place [Louisbourg], that on 4 September 1758, the day Mr Karr quitted the Hospital there were then remaining 730 of those people who were delivered to the care of Mr John Baxter, our Agent for the Sick and Wounded in Halifax."

100 Monckton to Baxter, 28 April 1758, PANS RG1, 163:118.

101 Holburne to Cleveland, 4 August 1757, from Halifax Harbour, PANS Adm. 1/481:338.

102 Doughty, ed., *An Historical Journal* 1:65.

103 *London Magazine* 26:514, 1757. A letter, dated 16 October 1757, written aboard the sloop *Hunter* lately arrived from North America and published in this magazine stated that "we have only 15 Sail of the Line ... whereas the enemy have 17 Ships of the Line." It appears that ships with more than fifty guns on board were referred to as ships of the line and represented the real strength of a naval fleet or squadron. Admiral Holburne had fifteen ships of the line, while Sir Charles Hardy was reported to have six. Three of Hardy's ships carried between five hundred and six hundred men, while the other three ships have over four hundred men. Why Hardy's ships are not included in the total reported in the letter is unknown.

104 NAC WO1/102. Troops under Lord Loudon's immediate command on 24 July 1757 included sixteen regiments with 13,513 rank and file fit for duty and 716 sick. Only ten of these regiments were with Loudon in Halifax. There is quite a difference, in the secondary-source material, concerning the number of ships that the English had stationed in Halifax in July 1757. In *An Historical and Statistical Account of Nova Scotia* 1:201, Haliburton indicates that there were thirty-three ships and 10,200 seamen in Admiral Holburne's Squadron; however, only fifteen of these ships carried fifty or more guns. Akins, in his "History of Halifax City," 54, gives the naval force as ten thousand men on thirteen ships of the line. Akins states also that the land forces totalled twelve thousand men and that the total English military and naval force was twenty-two thousand. Neither Akins nor Haliburton mention Hardy's six ships of war as being in Halifax as part of the English naval force.

105 GMHC 27:432, 1757. A letter written by an anonymous French officer after the siege of Louisbourg provides another comment on the cancellation: "The eyes of all Europe are fixed on this formidable armament; they have assembled an army of 22,000 men ... with a large train of artillery and munitions of war, 22 line of battle-ships and 200 transports. Yet Admiral Holburn [*sic*], who appeared off Louisburg [*sic*] with 22 sail of men-of-war, took it into his head that our numbers were equal to his own, and has made his way back to Halifax. They will ask him there, why did you run away? Oh! says he, a superior force *venit, vedit, fugit*." This letter is printed in Akins's "History of Halifax City," 245.

106 *London Magazine* 26:514–5, 1757. Extract of a Letter from on board the *Hunter* sloop, lately arrived from North America. Plymouth, 16 October.

107 Lawrence to Lords of Trade, 9 November 1757, PANS CO217, 16:181.

108 Council minutes, 26 September 1757, PANS RG1, 188:5.

109 Family Bible of Johann Michael Schmitt of LaHave, 16, PANS MG100, vol. 218, no. 3. There appears an entry that "the smallpox raged in Halifax in 1757 so that whole families died out."

110 The *Halifax Gazette* of 30 March 1752 reported that a "Gentleman of the Faculty" in Boston had introduced a new method of performing inoculation. The article also mentions that there was an outbreak of smallpox in Boston. Inoculation was also common in Halifax from its establishment.

111 Doughty, ed., *An Historical Journal* 1:41. Knox also notes (ibid., 65) that the *Alderney* returned to England with Admiral Holburne's Fleet in November of 1757 (PANS Adm. 1/481:455).

112 John Grant, surgeon, of Halifax, made his will on 25 August 1757, and the will was proved on 5 September 1757 (Halifax County Wills, Book 1:141, PANS RG48).

113 PANS RG1, vol. 284, Document 8, 6. Document dated 14 March 1757.

114 Ibid., Document 13, n.d., 22.

115 Monckton to Lords of Trade, 13 October 1757, PANS CO217, 16:160.

116 Lawrence to Lords of Trade, 9 November 1757, PANS CO217, 16:181.

117 Holburne to Secretary of Admiralty, 4 November 1757, PANS Adm. 1/481:456.

118 Hardy to Secretary of Admiralty, 22 March 1758, PANS Adm. 1/481:533.

119 Ibid.

120 "State and Condition of HM Ships in Halifax Harbour, 22 March 1758," PANS Adm. 1/481:535.

121 Boscawen to Cleveland, 10 May 1758, PANS Adm. 1/481:108.

122 "State and Condition of HM Ships under the Command of Admiral Boscawen, 10 May 1758," PANS Adm. 1/481:111. A list of these ships, with the number of guns on each, can be found in the journal kept by William Augustus Gordon, one of the officers engaged in the siege of Louisbourg under Boscawen and Amherst (Gordon, "Journal," 99).

123 PANS Adm. 1/481:112.

124 Doughty, ed., *An Historical Journal* 3:1.

125 Webster, ed., *Journal of William Amherst*, 11.

126 The thirteen regiments in Halifax under Amherst's command are listed in Gordon, "Journal," 99. Four of these regiments (the 1st, 40th, 45th, and 47th) had wintered in Halifax, while the 28th Regiment had wintered at Chignecto. The 17th, 35th, 48th, 58th, and 60th Regiments, which had returned to New York with Lord Loudon in August 1757, came back to Halifax in mid-May 1758. It appears that the 15th, 22nd, and 78th regiments came with General Amherst and Admiral Boscawen from England (Ross to Haldimand, 21 May 1758, PANS RG1, vol. 366, Letter no. 7).

127 Doughty, ed., *An Historical Journal* 3:1.

128 Council minutes of 2 June 1758, PANS RG1, 188:25.

129 Doughty, ed., *An Historical Journal* 1:210.

130 Ibid., 35.

131 Lawrence to Adair, 2 November 1758, PANS RG1, 163/3:139.

132 PANS Map v6/240 of Halifax in 1784 shows a general hospital located on Blowers Street. Piers, *Evolution of the Halifax Fortress, 1749–1928*, 31, writes, "The New Hospital on Citadel Hill replaced the old one on the south side of Blowers Street between Argyle and Barrington."

133 Stubbing, "Dockyard Memoranda, 1894," 103, states that on 7 February 1759, Governor Lawrence signed a deed which read, "We have given granted and confirmed to Admiral Phillip Durell, Joseph Gerrish, and William Nesbitt Esqrs. in trust for uses hereinafter mentioned two lots or parcels of ground situate lying and being in the north suburbs of Halifax at or near the place commonly known by the name of Gorham's Point." Richard Short's engraving (Figure 11), one of six that he did showing different views of Halifax, depicts the King's Naval Yard jutting into the harbour in the far left.

134 Two assistant surgeons sent out for the naval hospital in Nova Scotia in early 1758 were John Philips (*sic*) and Robert Kennedy, "who have passed examinations at Surgeons' Hall and have been found qualified for their employment" (PRO Adm. 98/7, folio 113, 3 February 1758).

135 Doughty, ed., *An Historical Journal* 1:35. "Experience having discovered that ginger and sugar mixed with the water of America, prevent the ill effects of it [scurvy], and preserve the men from fevers and fluxes that anything else yet found out. Brig. Gen. Lawrence does, therefore, in the strongest manner, recommend the use of the discovery to the troops."

136 Knap, *Diary*. This was probably a second English hospital built specifically for smallpox victims. General Amherst gave orders on 3 June,

a day after the English force arrived at Louisbourg, that "there will be a Hospital, and in time its hoped there will be fresh meat for the sick and wounded men" Gordon, "Journal," 107.

137 Doughty, ed., *An Historical Journal* 3:11.

138 Boscawen to Cleveland, 13 September 1758, PANS Adm. 1/481:141.

139 Lawrence to William Adair, 2 November 1758, PANS RG1, 163/3:137.

140 PANS RG1, 165:18. In her petition (PANS CO217, 16:299) dated 18 December 1758, Ann Catherwood stated that she had been midwife in Halifax since 1749. She indicated also that her training as a mid-wive had been approved by Doctor Smelley. Mrs Catherwood added, "I have instructed a woman in my business who has performed with good success for this three years and will offishait [*sic*] for me till I return." William Smellie (1697–1763) was a pioneer of modern obstetrics and the most eminent man-midwife of his period (Medvei and Thornton, eds., *The Royal Hospital*, 327).

141 PANS RG1, 165:18. The certificate read:

> "These are to certify that Mrs Ann Catherwood appointed by their Lordships of the Board of Trade Midwife of the Colony of Nova Scotia hath at all times discharged her duty as such faith-fully and diligently and so as to give general satisfaction to the set-tlement from the time of her arrival to the date hereof and her health being now so much impaired as to render her incapable of further service, she is hereby humbly recommended to the fa-vour and protection of their Lordships."

> Given under my Hand and Seal at Halifax in the Province aforesaid this fourth day of October 1759.
> S^d Chas Lawrence

142 Belcher to Lords of Trade, 11 January 1762, Letter Book of Chief Justice Jonathan Belcher, 82, PANS Micro Biography. Belcher indicates in this letter that he received his commission as lieutenant gover-nor on 21 November 1761.

143 Belcher to Lords of Trade, 26 October 1760, PANS CO217, 18:48.

144 Belcher to Lords of Trade, 10 April 1761, PANS CO217, 18:134.

145 The name Trigg first appears in Halifax in 1749, when a Mr Trigg purchased Lot B5 in Forman's Division (Halifax Allotment Book, PANS RG1, vol. 410.). A Darius Trigg bought Lot C, no. 11 in the town of Halifax on 12 February 1753 (Halifax County Deeds, PANS RG47), and Dorcas Trigg of Halifax, widow, bought land in the South Suburbs (Lot D, no. 14) from William Foye on 6 September 1753 (Hal-

ifax County Deeds, PANS RG47). This same Dorcas Trigg(s) was
buried from St Paul's on 20 June 1761. The midwife referred to as
Mrs Triggs by Governor Belcher, in his letter of 10 April 1761,
probably was Dorcas Triggs, widow of Darius Trigg(s). If so,
Mrs Triggs died two months after having been appointed one of
the two midwives referred to by Governor Belcher.

146 Lords of Trade to Lawrence, 14 February 1759, PANS RG1, vol. 30,
Letter no. 28. The figures for the annual grant from Whitehall for
the province of Nova Scotia are taken from Papers Relating to
Nova Scotia, 1745–1817, in the George Chalmers Collection, Chalmers, George, 29, PANS Micro Biography. The figures used to construct the remaining three graphs were taken from the annual
estimates that the governor sent to the Lords of Trade: for 1753,
PANS RG1, vol. 344, Document 3; for 1754, PANS CO217, 14:249–56;
1755, ibid., 5:87–106; 1756, ibid., 15:370–6; 1757, ibid.,
16:105–21; 1758, ibid., 183–200; 1759, ibid., 278–88; 170, ibid.,
346–55; ibid., 18:61–6; 1762, ibid., 188–93; 1763, ibid.,
19:143–53.

147 Lawrence to Lords of Trade, 26 September 1758, PANS CO217,
16:278.

148 Lawrence to Lords of Trade, 20 September 1759, PANS CO217,
16:346.

149 Lords of Trade to Lawrence, 14 December 1759, PANS CO217,
5:377.

150 Proclamation by Hon. Michael Francklin, 19 November 1767,
PANS RG1, 166:42; and Council minutes of 13 November 1767, 189:81.

151 Lawrence's address to the House of Assembly, 24 December 1759;
PANS CO217, 17:21.

152 "State and Condition of HM Ships and Vessels in North America.
Signed by Phillip Durell on 5 January 1759 at Halifax," PANS Adm.
1/481:597. Akins ("History of Halifax City," 59) writes that Admiral Durell arrived in Halifax in April with four ships of the line,
whereas Admiralty records indicate that he was commander-in-
chief in Halifax during the winter of 1758–59.

153 Saunders to Secretary of Admiralty, 6 June 1759, PANS Adm.
1/482:43. Letter written on the *Neptune* off Scatari Island. The convoy
included thirty-four English transports, sixty-eight American
transports, and thirteen Ordnance ships. Admiral Saunders had arrived in Halifax with his squadron from England on 1 May 1759
(Saunders to Cleveland, on board *Neptune*, in Halifax Harbour, 2 May
1759, PANS Adm. 1/482:39).

154 "Present State of Louisbourg Grand Battery Hospital, 29 October
1759," PANS Adm. 1/482:108. According to John Baxter, the sur-

geon in attendance, fifteen seamen and six marines were suffering from fevers and fluxes. This hospital, it seems, continued to exist after the Grand Battery was demolished on 26 October 1760: on that date, Colonel John Bastide wrote to General Amherst that "the works of the Grand Battery are almost down and the Naval Hospital is Preserved" (PRO WO34, 14:16).

155 Gordon, "Journal," 107. Orders given by General Amherst on 3 June read: "There will be a Hospital, and in time its hoped there will be fresh meat for the sick and wounded men."

156 Knap, *Diary*, entries for 24 July, 27 August, and 3 September 1758.

157 Saunders to Cleveland, 8 February 1759, PANS Adm. 1/482:21.

158 "State and Condition of HM Ships in Halifax Harbour under my command, 7 November 1759. Signed Colville," PANS Adm. 1/482:94.

159 Ibid., 115.

160 Ibid., 100. "Weekly Account of Sick and Wounded Seamen, dated 5 December 1759. Signed by John Baxter."

161 Council minutes, 28 June 1759, PANS RG1, 188:79.

162 "A Return of Births and Cradles in the different Barracks at Lunenburg, 23 May 1759," PANS RG1, vol. 382. Bell *(The Foreign Protestants)* does not mention a hospital at Lunenburg in his section on health and medical Services, 1756–60 (531–3).

163 The three previous emigrant groups were: the Cornwallis passengers of June 1749, totalling 2,547 persons; the New Englanders from Louisbourg and directly from New England, during the first year of the settlement of Halifax, estimated at 1,000 persons; and a total of 2,247 foreign Protestants, who arrived in Halifax in 1750, 1751, and 1752. In contrast, the New England Planter emigration during 1760, 1761, and 1762 numbered approximately 4,500 persons.

   Another ethnic group which came into Halifax during the 1750s, but which has remained somewhat opaque to historians, was the Irish. As Punch has pointed out in "The Irish Catholics," 23–40, about one-third of the population of Halifax in 1760 came from the southern counties of Ireland. Since the Irish emigrants did not come in one distinct group, or at one time, their arrival in the province has almost remained unnoted.

164 Lords of Trade to Lawrence, 29 October 1754, PANS CO218, 5:77.

165 Lawrence to Lords of Trade, 26 December 1758, PANS CO217, 16:311.

166 Ibid., 315. The second version of the Proclamation for Lands in Western Nova Scotia was dated 11 January 1759.

167 Lawrence to Lords of Trade, 26 December 1758, PANS CO217, 16:305.

168 Ibid., 334. Grant of the Township was dated 22 May 1759. The
     Horton grantees are named in PANS RG1, vol. 222, Document 3, dated
     22 May, 1759. It should be understood, however, that many of the
     people listed in the grant never came to Nova Scotia.

169 "An Abstract of the Grants of the Several Townships lately erected
     showing the Tracts of Land, Number of Grantees to each Tract, and
     Time of Settlement" (Lawrence to Lords of Trade, 20 September
     1759, PANS CO217, 16:345). The first settlers were scheduled to arrive
     in Horton, Cornwallis, Falmouth, Granville, and Annapolis town-
     ships in May 1760, whereas grantees for the remaining eight townships
     (Onslow, Cumberland, Amherst, Sackville, Tinmouth, Liverpool,
     Barrington, and Yarmouth) were scheduled to arrive in September
     1760.

170 Lawrence to Lords of Trade, 11 May 1760, PANS CO217, 17:58.

171 Lawrence to Lords of Trade, 16 June 1760, PANS CO217, 18:2–3.

172 Ibid., 89. "State of the New England Settlements in Nova Scotia, 12 De-
     cember 1760." This record indicates that approximately 250
     houses had been built by the New Englanders. The number of families
     settling in Horton Township is not given, but it is recorded that
     the number of persons settled there on 12 December 1760 was 622.
     Assuming that there were four persons per family, the number
     of individual families in Horton on that date would have been approx-
     imately 155. Rev. John Breynton, in a letter to Rev. Thomas Wood
     on 13 December 1760 (SPGFP, Reel 15, B25, Letter 12), states that he
     proposes to solicit the Society for more missionaries for the out
     settlements, whose population number five thousand. He writes: "Al-
     though most of the settlers are dissenters, they would soon be rec-
     onciled to the Church of England." His figure of five thousand was
     some two and a half times the population recorded by Belcher in
     his report of 12 December 1760.

173 Samuel Willoughby was married in Cornwallis Township on
     28 August 1760 (Cornwallis Township Book, PANS MG4, vol. 18). He
     was the member of the House of Assembly representing Cornwal-
     lis Township from 1761–62 and 1770–76. Dr Willoughby died at
     Cornwallis early in 1785 (King's County Wills, vol. 1, PANS RG48.
     Will proved on 12 April 1785). Jonathan Woodbury came to Yarmouth
     circa 1760, moved to Granville about 1770 (Census for Granville
     Township for 1770, PANS RG22) and to Wilmot in 1790. He died at
     Wilmot on 3 March 1830, aged ninety-three years (*Acadian Re-
     corder*, 20 March 1830).

174 Richard Sears was not included in the list of Horton grantees pub-
     lished on 22 May 1759 (PANS RG1, vol. 222, Document 3). He was in
     Horton prior to 28 August 1761, since on that date he witnessed

a land sale in the township (King's County Deeds, PANS RG47, 1:36). Dr Sears made his will on 20 December 1761, and it was proved on 2 June 1762 (Hants County Wills, PANS RG48, no. 4).

175 PANS CO217, 19:134. Doctor Samuel Oats was listed as having seven persons in his family in the return for Cape Forchu dated 21 June 1762.

176 Council minutes, 18 October 1762, PANS RG1, 204:71. It was recommended that "Mr Samuel Oats should be added to the Committee for admitting settlers into the Township of Yarmouth."

177 A Samuel Oats arrived at Horton prior to 1 August 1761, on which date he applied for land in Cumberland Township (PANS RG1, 165:168). Simeon Perkins records in Innis et al., eds., *Diary of Simeon Perkins* 1:4.) that a Samuel Oates was commissioned as a justice at Liverpool in 1764. No additional evidence has been found to suggest that these were, in fact, the same person.

178 Duncanson, *Falmouth, A New England Township in Nova Scotia*. 411. Benoni Sweet was referred to as a yeoman in a land transaction in 1765 (Hants County Deeds, 3:44, PANS RG47).

179 *Dictionary of Canadian Biography* 4:593–4.

180 Nova Scotia, *Journal*, 10, 12, and 13 March 1760.

181 Belcher to the Lords of Trade, 24 December 1760, PANS CO217, 18:108.

182 Council minutes of 11 December 1760, PANS RG1, 188:170.

183 Lords of Trade to Belcher, 12 March 1761, PANS CO218, 6:69.

184 Nova Scotia, *Journal* 25 July 1761. The bill received assent on 13 August 1761. The complete wording of the act (Nova Scotia, *Laws, 1758–1804*, 68–9, Geo. 3d, cap. 6), appears in Appendix 3.

185 "State and Condition of Halifax Hospital, 14 April 1760. Signed by John Baxter," PANS Adm. 1/482:112.

186 "State and condition of Louisbourg Hospital, 11 August 1760. Signed by John Baxter," PANS Adm. 1/482:136.

187 "Disposition of HM Ships under the Command of Lord Colville, 6 October 1760," PANS Adm. 1/482:143.

188 Colville to Secretary of Admiralty, 10 April 1761, PANS Adm. 1/482:146.

189 Ibid., 151.

190 Instructions to Judge Belcher on his appointment to the presidency of the Council of Nova Scotia, 3 March 1761, PANS RG1, vol. 284, Document 15.

191 This meant that Dr Alexander Abercrombie was out of a job. Exactly when Abercrombie ceased being paid for his services as surgeon in unknown. On 28 March 1761, Council asked Doctors Abercrombie and Reeve to recommend what should be done with the cargo

on a vessel that had arrived carrying a person with smallpox. The doctors recommended that the cargo be landed at Mauger's Beach and left there to air for a few days (Council minutes, 28 March 1761, PANS RG1, 188:208).

192 Belcher to Lords of Trade, 3 November 1761, PANS CO217, 18:201. Belcher stated that 275 children were cared for in the orphan house during the first nine years of its establishment (Ibid., 218–25). Close examination of the list of orphans indicates that it represented only 243 individuals, for a number of the children entered the orphan house on two, three, or more occasions. It should be noted that the mortality rate in the orphan house during this period was just above thirty percent.

193 Information in Figure 13 was obtained from PANS CO217, 18:218–25.

194 Memorial of Colonel Alexander McNutt to the Lords of Trade, 17 April 1766, PANS CO217, 21:158–65.

195 *Dictionary of Canadian Biography* 5:555–7. For an earlier and more detailed biographical sketch of Colonel Alexander McNutt, see Raymond's paper, "Colonel Alexander McNutt and the Pre-Loyalist Settlements," 27–34, 60–102.

196 Council minutes of 10 October 1761, PANS RG1, 188:282.

197 Belcher to Lords of Trade, 3 November 1761, PANS CO217, 18:202. Colonel Alexander McNutt attended the Council meeting of 10 October 1761 (PANS RG1, 188:281), where he stated that he had arrived on the previous day, with upwards of three hundred settlers from Ireland.

198 PANS CO217, 34:182. The total number of Acadians reported as being resident in Nova Scotia during the winter of 1761–62 was 685, representing 150 families.

199 "State and Condition of HM Ships in Halifax Harbour, 26 November 1761," PANS Adm. 1/482:174. This included four ships and 1,617 men, of whom fourteen were sick on board, and thirty-eight sick on shore. The report was signed by Colville. The naval hospital was being attended by Charles White, surgeon, who reported that he had 104 patients: eighty-one seamen, sixteen marines, and seven French prisoners.

200 The number of soldiers in Halifax during the spring of 1762 was probably about one thousand. The 40th Regiment left Nova Scotia in 1760 as part of the force which captured Montreal. The 47th Regiment left Canada after the fall of Montreal. Warburton's 45th Regiment returned to Nova Scotia after the siege of Montreal and remained until 1766 (Chichester and Burges-Short, *Records and Badges*).

201 "Description of the State of Nova Scotia, 9 January 1762," PANS CO217, 18:245. Rev. Robert Vincent of Lunenburg records, in a letter (12 January 1763) to the Society for the Propagation of the Gospel in Foreign Parts, that there were about three hundred families at Lunenburg. The figures given for Horton, Cornwallis, and Falmouth are probably somewhat higher than the actual population: the Reverend Mr Bennett, the first person sent by the Church of England to minister to these four townships, wrote to the SPGFP on 4 June 1763 that the number of persons in the respective townships were: Horton, 670 persons; Cornwallis, 518 persons; Falmouth, 278 persons; and Newport, 251 persons (Records of the SPGFP, Reel 15, B25, Letter no. 21).

202 PANS CO217, 18:245.

203 *Journal of the Commissioners for Trade* 9(1932):4. Mr Kingslaugh appeared before the Board of Trade on 9 January 1749/1750.

204 The doctors of physic, surgeons, and apothecaries in Halifax during the year 1762 and the year in which each of them arrived are as follows: Alexander Abercrombie, 1749; William Adelheit, ca.1757; Thomas Ainslie, ca.1758; William Catherwood, 1749; John Cochran, 1758; John Day, 1755; John Dolhonde, 1758; George Francheville, 1751; George Greaves, 1761; Leonard Lockman, 1749; Johann M. Lutgens, 1751; John McColme, 1758; Christopher A. Nicolai, 1751; Johannes C. Ohme, 1752; John Philipps, 1758; Jonathan Prescott, 1751; Thomas Reeve, 1749; Charles White, 1761; and Thomas Wood, 1752. See 61, chapter 1, for an explanation of the uncertainty concerning the date of John Day's arrival in Nova Scotia.

205 Inferior Court of Common Pleas for Halifax County, volumes 17 and 18, PANS RG37.

206 "A General Return of the Inhabitants and Stock in the Several Townships settled at Cape Sable, July 1762," PANS CO217, 19:140.

207 Council minutes, 5 November 1762, PANS RG1, 188:362.

208 "State and Condition of HM Ships in Halifax Harbour, 18 May 1762" (PANS Adm. 1/482:201) lists two ships carrying 675 men. Lord Colville, writing to the Secretary of the Admiralty from Halifax on 6 August 1762 (ibid., 212), mentions that "there are in this Province and at Louisbourg about 1,500 regulars and Provincials," the latter referring to Troops from New England.

209 Ibid., 212. Lord Colville writes: "The Indians are said to be 1,500 men, women, and children, dispersed in the different parts of Nova Scotia and Cape Breton ... There are 915 Acadians in all now at Halifax, and about 300 more in the country." On 18 August, seven transports with over six hundred Acadians on board (PANS CO217,

19:194) were sent from Halifax to Boston. The House of Representatives of Massachusetts Bay voted not to allow the Acadians to be landed in Boston, so they were returned to Halifax (ibid., 183).

210   The number of naval surgeons was estimated by presuming that each ship of war carried at least one surgeon. Admiralty records (PANS Adm. 1/480-2) indicate that a total of thirty-five different ships of war arrived in Halifax during the years 1755, 1757, and 1758. Four additional naval surgeons were stationed at the naval hospital during these years, giving a total of thirty-nine naval surgeons.

The number of military surgeons in Nova Scotia during the period was estimated by noting that the three regiments stationed in Halifax since 1750 (the 40th, 45th, and 47th) had a total of five surgeons on establishment, and that six surgeons came to Nova Scotia from New England with the two battalions of Shirley's Regiment. Each of the regiments that arrived in Halifax in 1757 and 1758 (fourteen in all) were allocated one surgeon and two surgeon's mates on their establishment. In addition to the total of fifty-three military surgeons mentioned above, William Adair, the director of the military hospital in Halifax in 1758, brings to fifty-four the total for the ten-year period.

211   Memorial of Revd Jno Breynton, 27 September 1765, PANS CO217, vol. 37, Document 44 ½.

212   Tunis, "Dr John Latham (c. 1734–1799): Pioneer Inoculator in Canada," 1–12.

CHAPTER THREE

1   Gordon, "Journal," 99.

2   "The State and Condition of HM Ships in Halifax Harbour on 18 May 1762" (PANS Adm. 1/481:201) indicates that 675 seamen were stationed at Halifax. The number of soldiers in the province on 6 August 1762 was reported to be 1,500, according to Admiral Alexander Colville who wrote to the Secretary of the Admiralty on that date (ibid., 482: 212).

3   Belcher to Lords of Trade, 3 November 1761, PANS CO217, 18:201. Belcher was appointed lieutenant governor on 21 November 1761.

4   Northcliffe Collection, 76.

5   Breynton to Society for the Propagation of the Gospel in Foreign Parts, 16 January 1769, SPGFP, Letter no. 135. The Reverend Mr Breynton describes the state of Halifax in 1768.

6   Campbell to Bruce, April 1771, PANS RG1, 136:153.

7   PANS RG1, 163:45. Cornwallis issued a proclamation on 11 September 1750 (o.s.) stating that the victualling of the original settlers (in Halifax) would cease on 15 September 1750.

8 PANS RG1, vol. 523. None of the 420 servants was identified by name in the mess lists.

9 Minutes of Council, 24 February 1749/50, PANS RG1, 186:48. Murdoch, *History of Nova Scotia* 2:623, indicates that between 3 July and 1 December 1749 (o.s.), eighteen persons were granted licenses to sell liquor in Halifax, subject to a payment of a poor tax of one guinea a month. It is not clear whether this tax was actually collected.

10 Minutes of Council, 9 October 1750 (o.s.), PANS RG1, 186:87.

11 Minutes of Council, 11 October 1750 (o.s.), Ibid., 89.

12 *Halifax Gazette*, 2 December 1752. The *Gazette* of 16 December 1752 indicated that "a handsome collection was made for the Poor."

13 Minutes of Council, 22 December 1752, PANS RG1, vol. 186. The five justices of the peace who signed the memorial were Charles Morris, John Duport, William Bourn, James Monk, and Joseph Scott. Bridewell takes its name after St Bride's Well, which was located near a prison in London. Oakum – hemp fibre obtained by untwisting and picking out the fibres of old rope – was used for caulking seams in various seagoing vessels.

14 Minutes of Council, 26 March 1753, PANS RG1, 186:351. The corporal punishment referred to consisted of being "publickly whipt at the common whipping post in the said Town [Halifax], any number of stripes not exceeding forty." The gaol, in a stone building purchased from Lt Col John Horsman in February 1752 (ibid., 155), was located on the north side of the first block of Spring Garden Road when travelling west from Barrington Street.

15 Estimates for 1754, PANS CO217, 14:259–66. The reference to the "Black Hole" indicated that a cell for solitary confinement was to be constructed in the foundation of the workhouse.

16 "Observations on the Estimate for the year 1754 with the sums allowed and disallowed, 27 July 1754," PANS RG1, vol. 29, Document 24.

17 Minutes of Council, 27 June 1754, PANS RG1, 187:76. Richard Wenman had been using this building to store rope, fishing lines, and oakum, some of which was manufactured by the orphans in the orphan house located nearby. Wenman's advertisement for these items appeared in the *Halifax Gazette* of 29 June 1754.

18 Lawrence to Lords of Trade, 1 August 1754, PANS RG1, vol. 36, Document 7.

19 "Abstract of the account of Duties and Bounties at Nova Scotia from the Commencement thereof to 25 September 1756," PANS CO217, 16:101.

20 Minutes of Council, 21 June 1758, PANS RG1, 188:27. Josiah Marshall had been in Halifax since as early as 1 July 1752 (o.s.), on which date his lot in the South Suburbs was registered (PANS CO217, 13:340).

21 Minutes of Council, 31 July 1751 (o.s.), PANS RG1, 186:130. It was decided that a duty of three pence per gallon was to be paid on all rum and other distilled spirituous liquors imported into the province after 14 August 1751. This applied to all such products except those manufactured in Great Britain and in His Majesty's West India Plantations. The amount collected during the period 23 June 1751 to 12 October 1758 was £7,045, of which £2,204 was remaining in the hands of the provincial treasurer on the latter date, according to Nova Scotia, *Journal*, minutes of 13 October 1758.

22 Estimate Disallowances, dated 26 July 1755, PANS RG1, vol. 29, Document 40.

23 Lawrence to Lords of Trade, 26 December 1758, PANS RG1, vol. 36, Document 39. Lawrence had asked the members of the House, when he addressed them at their first Assembly meeting on 2 October 1758, for "Unanimity and dispatch in the Confirmation of such Acts and Resolutions of a Legislative nature as the Governor and Council under His Majesty's Royal Instructions have found expedient."

24 Nova Scotia, *Journal*, minutes of 13 October 1758.

25 Nova Scotia, *Journal*, minutes of 20 October 1758.

26 Ibid., 13 and 14 December 1758. The actual act appears in Nova Scotia Statutes, 1758–1759, cap. 9, PANS RG5, series s, vol. 1.

27 Nova Scotia, *Journal*, minutes of 27 October 1758.

28 Ibid., 2 November 1758.

29 PANS Vertical Map Case, Town of Halifax, v6/240. Traced from the original located in the Crown Land Office in December 1931. The original spelling (i.e., Lott, and Franklin) has been retained. I have added several modern street names to the 1762 plan (Blowers, Queen, Spring Garden, Bishop, and Hollis), and shown the location of the civilian and military hospitals, the orphan house, and the workhouse. The spelling of the name of Lieutenant Colonel Horsman is found to differ in primary sources as compared to secondary. PANS RG1, 186:155 gives the name as Horsman, while both Akins, "History of Halifax City," 32, and Piers, *The Evolution of the Halifax Fortress, 1749–1928*, 2, spell the name as Horseman.

30 Nova Scotia, *Journal*, minutes of 19 December 1759.

31 Ibid., 13 August 1759. As indicated earlier in this chapter, Council had been providing for the poor in a very minimal way through money raised from duties and fines. They had also paid Dr John Baxter for medicines which he had expended upon the poor at Halifax in 1753 and 1754 (PANS CO217, 14:255). The governor and Council had previously paid out £130, during the period August 1749 to September 1750, "to sundry persons in distress" (ibid., 10:70).

32 PANS RG5, series s, vol. 1, 14. The Act for Preventing Trepasses

was passed in the House of Assembly on 2 March 1759 and, on 22 March 1759, passed in Council and given the governor's assent.

33 Nova Scotia, *Journal,* 11 April, 1759. The persons appointed on that date were William Nesbitt, Henry Newton, Henry Ferguson, and John Burbidge. A document listing the overseers of the poor, dated 1759 (PANS RG1, vol. 411, Document 1), refers probably to those gentlemen who were appointed to assume office in April 1760. The four persons listed in this document were William Schwartz, Richard Gibbons, John Fillis, and Richard Wenman. Overseers of the poor would be, presumably, leading citizens of Halifax known to have a benevolent attitude towards the poor. I have not found a published list of overseers of the poor for the town of Halifax for the period 1759–75.

34 A letter signed by Hopson on 22 September 1752 (o.s.), PANS RG1, 163/2:17.

35 A variation of Bethlehem, and derived from the Hospital of St Mary of Bethlehem, London, for care of the insane.

36 Instructions to Cornwallis, dated 29 April 1749 (o.s.), PANS CO218, 3:119; Instructions to Hopson, 23 April 1752 (o.s.), ibid., 4:177–326; Instructions to Lawrence, 2 March 1756, ibid., 5:150–271.

37 Nova Scotia, *Journal,* minutes of 19 January 1760.

38 Ibid., 18 March 1760.

39 Ibid., 17 March 1760.

40 Minutes of Council, 19 April 1760, PANS RG1, 188:146.

41 Nova Scotia, *Journal,* minutes of 24 September 1760. One of the suppliers of materials for construction of the workhouse was William Best, who was paid £300 "on account of the Workhouse."

42 PANS RG1, vol. 284, Document 15. According to information contained in the "State of the Orphan House at Halifax, 1752–1760" (PANS CO217, 18:218–25), a total of 184 (seventy percent) of the children who entered the orphan house during the period were listed as orphans. Thirty-three of the remaining children were obviously not orphans, since they were later discharged to their parents.

43 Belcher to Lords of Trade, 3 November 1761, PANS CO217, 18:201.

44 "State of the Orphan House at Halifax," PANS CO217, 15:110. In this description, the Reverend John Breynton wrote: "The Boys are bound out if possible to Fishermen or some laborious trades and employments, and are free at the age of twenty-one. The girls are placed in sober creditable familys as servants till they are full 17 years old."

45 Nova Scotia, *Journal,* minutes of 17 July 1761.

46 Ibid., 10 September 1761.

47 PANS CO218, 6:84. Lords of Trade to Belcher, 21 April 1761.

48 Nova Scotia, *Journal*, minutes of 17 April 1762.

49 Ibid., 28 August 1762.

50 Ibid., 25 April 1763.

51 Ibid., 7 May 1763.

52 Ibid., 26 November 1763.

53 Jonathan Harris had been a passenger on the *Winchelsea*, which arrived in Chebucto during the last week of June 1749. He was granted Lot E10 in Collier's Division on 8 August 1749 (o.s.) and was listed in the 1752 census for Halifax. He died in March 1768 (*Nova Scotia Gazette*, 24 March 1768) and his will was proved on 5 August 1768 (Halifax County Wills, Book 1:336, PANS RG48).

54 Belcher to Green, 10 February and 31 July 1762, PANS RG1, 166A:42, 60.

55 Nova Scotia, *Journal*, minutes of 25 October 1763.

56 Nova Scotia, *Laws*, 96. George 3d, cap.9. An Act in Addition to an Act, entitled, an Act for regulating and maintaining an House of Correction or Workhouse, within the Town of Halifax, and for binding out poor Children.

57 Nova Scotia, *Journal*, minutes of 24 November 1763.

58 PANS RG1, vol. 30, Letter no. 28. On 14 February 1759, the Lords of Trade informed Governor Lawrence that they were omitting the item in the estimate for 1759 of the projected expense of the hospital. This instruction "was expressly ordered by His Majesty [George II] to be defrayed by the Commander-in-Chief of the Military and should not therefore be inserted in your estimate." Is is likely that by 1760, the hospital building was no longer in use; in the estimate for 1761, although an item was included for wood to heat the governor's house, public offices, and the orphan house, the hospital was not included as it had been in previous years (PANS CO217, 18:62; Lawrence to Lords of Trade, 26 September 1758, PANS RG1, vol. 36, Document 38). The location of the civilian hospital referred to here, opposite the orphan house on Bishop Street, is shown in Figure 15.

59 Instructions to Judge Jonathan Belcher on his appointment to the Presidency of the Council of Nova Scotia, 3 March 1761, PANS RG1, vol. 284, Document 15.

60 PANS Adm. 1/482:174, 201, 314, 366, 441, 510; ibid. 1/483: 264, 392.

61 Ibid. 1/484:146.

62 Ibid., 155.

63 Ibid 1/485:15.

64 Doughty, ed., *An Historical Journal* 1:210.

65 The 40th Regiment, which had arrived in Halifax in 1749, was stationed in the town almost continuously until 1765 (Secretary of State to Wilmot, 23 March 1765, PANS CO217, vol. 43, Document 263), when it was replaced by the 14th and 29th regiments. These two reg-

iments remained in Halifax until July 1769 (*Nova Scotia Chronicle and Weekly Advertizer* [hereafter, *Nova Scotia Chronicle*], 11 July 1769). The 59th Regiment began a six-year posting in Halifax in 1768 (*Nova Scotia Gazette*, 4 August 1768) and, in 1769, was joined by the 64th and 65th Regiments (*Nova Scotia Chronicle*, 25 July and 26 September 1769). These last two regiments remained in Halifax until 1771 and 1773, respectively. Throughout the eleven-year period 1763–74, at least one company of Royal Artillery was stationed in Halifax. The Fifty-ninth Regiment, prior to its arrival in Halifax in 1768, had been stationed at Louisbourg where, in 1765, it relieved part of the 45th Regiment. A memorial of subaltern officers of the Garrison of Halifax to Lt Col Otto Hamilton, commanding HM Troops in Nova Scotia (PANS RG1, vol. 366, Haldimand Collection, Letter no. 39, undated, but probably 1772) was signed by five surgeons of the above-mentioned regiments: George Francheville, surgeon, Artillery; William Fletcher, surgeon, 65th Regiment; Trotter Hill, surgeon, 59th Regiment; Ambr[ose] Sharman, surgeon's mate, 59th Regiment; and William Faries, surgeon's mate, 65th Regiment.

66 Moreau to the Society for the Propagation of the Gospel in Foreign Parts, 29 March 1762, SPGFP, Reel 73, 44.

67 Wilmot to Lords of Trade, 6 May 1766, PANS RG1, vol. 37, document 48.

68 St Paul's Anglican Church, Halifax, PANS MG4, burial on 27 May 1766.

69 Francklin's Letter of Recommendation, 20 September 1766, PANS RG1, vol. 166.

70 Wilmot to Lords of Trade, 24 June 1764, PANS CO217, 21:192.

71 Wilmot's Instructions upon being appointed Governor of Nova Scotia, dated 6 March 1764, PANS CO218, 6:279.

72 Nova Scotia, *Journal*, minutes of 24 June 1766. In a memorial to the House, Dr Reeve states, without specifying the date, that he had been appointed as surgeon to the workhouse by Governor Wilmot.

73 Ibid., 30 June 1766.

74 Ibid., 30 July 1767.

75 Ibid., 1 July 1768.

76 Ibid., 28 June 1770.

77 Ibid., 17 October 1774.

78 NSGWC, 10 October 1775. This issue published a eulogy by Chief Justice Jonathan Belcher.

79 Nova Scotia, *Journal*, minutes of 4 July 1768.

80 NSGWC, 6 April 1773.

81 PANS RG1, 170:100. The Dr John Philipps mentioned in this appointment was not the Dr John Phillipps who had been a surgeon at Lunenburg from 1757 to 1766 and for health reasons returned to En-

gland. The Dr Philipps appointed surgeon to the orphan house in 1773 arrived in Halifax in 1758 (PRO Adm. 98/6, folio 113, February 1758) as an assistant surgeon to the naval hospital, after having successfully completed an examination at Surgeon's Hall in London.

82 "Province of Nova Scotia Accounts of Supplies to Indians," 31 December 1767, PANS CO217, 25:42.

83 Ibid., 43.

84 Francklin to Abercrombie, 26 September 1766, PANS RG1, 167:18–9.

85 Nova Scotia, *Journal*, minutes of 14 June 1765.

86 Minutes of Council, 2 July 1765, PANS RG1, 188:551.

87 Green to Lords of Trade, 26 August 1766, PANS CO217, 44:18.

88 Nova Scotia, *Journal*, minutes of 31 October 1766.

89 Minutes of Council, 3 January 1767, PANS RG1, 189:37.

90 Nova Scotia, *Journal*, minutes of 31 July 1767.

91 Minutes of Council, 13 November 1767, PANS RG1, 189:81.

92 Francklin to Bulkeley, 19 November 1767, PANS RG1, 166:42.

93 Nova Scotia, *Journal*, minutes of 19 June 1768. The number of poor in Halifax had increased significantly in April, due to what was described as the worst storm ever experienced there. Admiral Hood wrote, "We had the most heavy gale of wind that ever was felt in this place ... The damage done in the Town is still great, above fifty schooners, sloops, and shallops, are either sunk at the wharfs or beat to pieces, and not a single wharf, but is in a great measure destroyed. This is truly deplorable in so poor a place as Halifax. Many families are totally ruined" (Hood to Stephens, Halifax, 4 April 1768, PRO Adm. 1/483:73).

94 Francklin to Hillsborough, 5 August 1768, PANS CO217, 22:186.

95 Campbell to Hillsborough, 3 January 1769, PANS CO217, 25:75.

96 Copy of an Order of the King in Council, dated 3 May 1767, disapproving a bill passed in Nova Scotia, PANS CO217, 26:130.

97 Nova Scotia, *Journal*, minutes of 9 November 1768.

98 Minutes of Council, 20 July 1763, PANS RG1, 188:389.

99 Campbell to Bulkeley, 6 October 1770, PANS RG1, 181:95.

100 Nova Scotia, *Journal*, minutes of 28 June 1771.

101 Minutes of Council, 2 April 1770, PANS RG1, 189:133.

102 Lords of Trade to the King, 11 April 1769, PANS CO218, 7:249.

103 Nova Scotia, *Journal*, minutes of 7 June 1770.

104 Campbell to Green, several dates, PANS RG1, 181:62–111.

105 PANS RG1, 189:153. An advertisement notifying the inhabitants of Halifax who had neglected or refused to pay the Poor Tax that they would be prosecuted appeared in the *Nova Scotia Gazette* of 24 March 1768 and was repeated in the *Nova Scotia Chronicle* of 19 June 1770. Among those who refused to pay (2 shillings per year) were William Howard Smith and Richard Gibbons Jr, who were former

overseers of the poor, as well as Thomas Fitzpatrick, a former keeper of the workhouse.

106 PANS RG34, series A, vol. 1. The case involved Richard Gibbons Jr, who objected to ten different features of the assessment, including the circumstance that "the whole of the Rateable Inhabitants in the said Town are not mentioned or assessed." Gibbons lost his case.

107 The Memorial of John Woodin, Master of the Workhouse at Halifax, 15 October 1773, PANS RG1, vol. 411, Document 2.

108 NSGWC, 20 and 27 April 1773.

109 Ibid., 2 November 1773.

110 Nova Scotia, *Laws*, 14 Geo. 3d, cap.5.

111 Lords of Trade to Wilmot, 20 March 1764, PANS RG1, vol. 31, Document 29.

112 Breynton to Wilmot, 22 June 1764, PANS CO217, 21:205.

113 Legge to Dartmouth, 12 July 1774, PANS RG1, vol. 44, Document 39.

114 Minutes of Council, 19 april 1774, PANS RG1, 189:215.

115 Legge to Dartmouth, 18 November 1774, PANS RG1, vol. 44, Document 52:10.

116 Wilmot to Lords of Trade, 24 June 1764, PANS RG1, 39:24.

117 These two midwives were, in 1764, Maria Moser and Maria Tattray (PANS RG1, vol. 382 Item 38). On 9 February 1766, in a letter from Francklin to Zouberchuler (*sic*), the former indicates that he has allowed ten pounds for midwives, which the Board of Trade had ordered struck off the estimate. Later in the same letter, Francklin indicated that Green had informed him that the midwives were dead (PANS RG1, 136:85). The only other midwive outside of Halifax that I am aware of in the 1760s was Barbary Cuffey (also spelled Cuffy), a black woman who described herself as a midwife in a Queen's County deed on 4 March 1769 (PANS RG47, Reel 606, Book 1:258). She was listed as one of the Proprietors of the Township of Liverpool on 20 November 1764.

118 Nova Scotia, *Journal*, minutes of 2 November 1769, Notice of this petition appeared also in the NSGWC, 14 November 1769.

119 Halifax County Estates, PANS RG48. Estate administered on 9 March 1772.

120 The Doctor Hill referred to here was probably Dr Trotter Hill, who is known to have been in Halifax in 1774 (Scott, ed., *The Journal of the Reverend Jonathan Scott*, 51).

121 *Halifax Gazette*, 21 July 1753.

122 The Memorial of John Grant of Halifax, surgeon, CO217, 15:153.

123 Minutes of Council, 28 June 1759, PANS RG1, 188:80.

124 Donnison, *Midwives and Medical Men*.

125 Laufe, *Obstetric Forceps*.

126 Spencer, *The History of British Midwifery from 1650 to 1800.*
127 Green to Lords of Trade, 24 August 1766, PANS CO217, 44:18.
128 Lords of Trade to Campbell, 29 July 1772, PANS RG1, vol. 32, Document 11.
129 Instructions to Governor Francis Legge, 10 June 1773, PANS CO218, 7:339.
130 Minutes of Council, 15 June 1756, PANS RG1, 187:430.
131 Minutes of Council, 21 June 1758, PANS RG1, 188:27.
132 Minutes of Council, 16 August 1759, PANS RG1, 188:93.
133 Members of Council to Lords of Trade, 12 March 1757, PANS CO217, 16:150.
134 Nova Scotia, *Journal*, minutes of 21 June 1762.
135 PANS MG1, vol. 182. 133–220.
136 Nova Scotia, *Journal*, minutes of 31 May 1765.
137 Ibid., 9 June 1766.
138 Ibid., 16 October 1769. Henry Denny Denson was returned as the member for Newport Township and took his seat on 16 October 1769. As Brebner has observed in his excellent book *The Neutral Yankees of Nova Scotia*, 182, the minutes of the Nova Scotia House of Assembly are extremely brief and it is therefore very difficult to determine when members attended meetings and who took part in debates. Just exactly when John Day ceased to attend the meetings of the House of Assembly is not known.
139 Halifax County Deeds, Book 10:138; Book 11:81, PANS RG47.
140 NSGWC, 6 August 1774.
141 Earl of Dartmouth 1:200–3, PANS Micro Biography.
142 "The *Jupiter*, full of hay, was set on hire by lightning in Boston Bay on the 29th inst and entirely consumed. His Majesty's Ship *Mercury* happened to be near and saved all the people except Col Day, a gentleman of Nova Scotia, a firm friend to Government, who was drowned." Admiral Graves to Stephens, Boston, 30 November 1775, Clark, Morgan, eds., *Naval Documents* 2:1202. Day's company in Halifax had contracted to supply the British army in Boston on 28 July 1775 and had written that "they have three vessels to sail with hay and refreshments for the Army at Boston but need a convoy for protection." Day and Scott to Shirreff, Deputy Quarter Master of the British Army, ibid., 1:993.
143 Petition of Mrs Henrietta Day, dated 1810, PANS RG20, series A. Also PANS AO13, bundle 92 of "Loyalist Claims."
144 Halifax County Estates, PANS RG48.
145 *Halifax Gazette*, 9 December 1758.
146 *Nova Scotia Gazette*, 27 March 1768. Fletcher also advised a number of medical books for sale in the NSGWC of 22 September 1772. The

medical books included: Barry, Edward, *A Treatise on a Consumption of the Lungs* (Dublin, 1726); Brookes, Richard, *The General Practice of Physic* (London, 1771); Culpeper, Nicholas, *The English Physician enlarged: with three hundred, sixty, and nine medicines, made of English herbs* ... (London, 1656); Huxham, John, *An Essay on Fevers. To which is now added, a Dissertation on the Malignant Ulcerous Sore Throat* (London, 1769); LeClerc, Daniel, *A Natural and Medicinal History of Worms, Bred in the Bodies of Men and other Animals* ... (London, 1721); Lind, James, *A Treatise of the Scurvy* ... (Edinburgh, 1753); and Shaw, Peter, *A New Practice of Physic* ... (London, 1738).

With respect to Lind's book on scurvy, R.L. Walford, in *The 120-Year Diet*, 163–4, writes: "As early as 1740, James Lind, conducting nutrition experiments on sailors in the British Royal Navy, showed that scurvy could be prevented by a daily ration of fresh lime, lemon, or orange juice. Although his results were published in 1753, it was not until 1795 – after 42 years of Royal Navy red tape and the loss of about 100,000 sailormen's lives due to scurvy – that Lind's simple preventive measure became an official regulation for "men-of-war" sailors. Being then the first nation to have warships on long voyages with crews free of scurvy, Britannia began to 'rule the waves.'" The first advertisement for citrus juice for sale in a Halifax newspaper appeared in the NSGWC, 23 May 1780: "Lemon Juice for sale – Imported, 4 shillings per bottle."

147 *Nova Scotia Chronicle*, 28 March 1769.
148 Ibid., 14 September 1773.
149 Ibid., 1 November 1774.
150 NSGWC, 1 November 1774.
151 Minutes of Council, 30 June 1763, PANS RG1, 188:382.
152 PANS Vertical File, vol. 160, no. 29. The original is at Brown University in Providence, Rhode Island.
153 Brebner, *The Neutral Yankees of Nova Scotia*, 233.
154 Yorkshire passenger lists, PANS MG100, vol. 214, no. 20. Six ships' passengers lists are given here, four of which indicate occupations. PANS RG1, vol. 44, Document 37 provides the number of Yorkshire passengers on nine different ships that arrived in Halifax between 6 May and 21 June 1774. This latter document includes five of the ships named in the former. An eleventh ship, the *Jenny*, brought Yorkshire settlers to Nova Scotia on 21 May 1775 (NSGWC, 23 May 1775), and a list of its passengers, complete with occupations, was presented by Milner, "Records of Chignecto," 43–4.
155 Ibid., Passenger list of the *Prince George* includes the name of —— Stapleton, physician, aged thirty years.
156 Chaplin, *Medicine in England during the Reign of George III*.

157 Porter, *A Social History of Madness*. 167
158 Dr Philippe Pinel (1745–1826) became director of Bicêtre, the
     Paris asylum for men, in 1793 and astonished everyone by removing
     the chains from mentally ill patients. Some of the patients were
     said to have been restrained with chains for upwards of forty years.
     He began a movement which was based on the concept of treating
     the mentally ill with kindness and humane methods.

CHAPTER FOUR

1 The colonial militiamen, or armed citizens, who pledged themselves
   to be ready for combat on a minute's notice.
2 "Abstract of the Number of Families settled in Nova Scotia, August
   1775," Earl of Dartmouth 1:349–52, PANS Micro Biography.
3 "State of the Troops now Actually in Garrison of 65th Regiment, Halifax, 14 June 1775. Signed by Francis Marsh, Capt. 65th Regt.,
   Commanding Officer," Earl of Dartmouth 1:293, PANS Micro Biography. The three companies contained five officers, fifteen non-
   commissioned officers, and fifty-seven privates. Captain Marsh
   indicated that only thirty-six of the privates were available for
   mounting a guard. Only two of the seventy-seven personnel were listed
   as being sick.
4 Legge to Dartmouth, 31 July 1775, PANS RG1, vol. 44, Document 71.
   The fire in the Navy Yard took place on the night of 8 July, and
   the following notice appeared in the NSGWC on 15 August 1775:
   "Whereas it is suggested that His Majesty's Careening Yard was wil-
   fully set on fire by some malicious person or persons on the night of
   the eighth day of July last; whoever will give information so that
   he, or they, may be brought to Justice and convicted shall be entitled
   to the sum of £100." The notice was placed by Richard Williams,
   storekeeper of the Halifax Careening Yard.
5 Minutes of Council, 14 ans 24 July 1775, PANS RG1, 189:324, 330.
6 Gage to Lt Col Allan Maclean, 12 June 1775, Sir Guy Carleton, Carleton
   Papers, Document 15, PANS Micro Biography. Order for Maclean
   to enlist two battalions of ten companies, two surgeons, and two surgeon's mates.
7 McDonald, "Letter Book." Captain Alexander McDonald was sent to
   Halifax to recruit for the Royal Highland Emigrants. Since his first
   entry (page 208) in the letter book is dated 1 September 1775, it is presumed that he arrived in Halifax from New York shortly before
   that date.
8 It is clear from the figures given in the "State of His Majesty's Forces
   at Halifax on 21 October 1775," signed by Joseph Gorham, Command-

ing Officer (Earl of Dartmouth 1:417, PANS Micro Biography), that recruiting for both regiments progressed very slowly. By that date, Gorham's Royal Fencible Americans numbered 135 men, including one surgeon and a surgeon's mate, while the Royal Highland Emigrants had only sixty-five soldiers in its ranks. A fencible was a soldier who enlisted for home service only.

9 Rev. John Breynton to the Society for the Propagation of the Gospel in Foreign Parts, 2 January 1776, SPGFP, Reel 73, 597, Letter no. 202.

10 I would alert readers to the fact that Figure 19 represents all the known deaths and burials that occurred in Nova Scotia during 1775 and 1776. It might be expected that there were additional deaths in Nova Scotia during these two years, but I have concluded that Figure 19 represents the majority of the deaths. Rev. John Breynton reported to the SPGFP (Letter no. 202, 2 January 1776) that he had buried 157 people in Halifax during the year 1775. I have a record of 170 Halifax deaths in 1775 which was used to construct Figure 19. The number of smallpox deaths shown in the figure is probably low, since records of death and burial frequently do not state the cause of death. The sources of death and burial records include the following: O'Brien Family Papers, Windsor, 1738–1818, PANS MG1, vol. 731A; Chester Township Book, PANS MG4, vol. 13; Cornwallis Township Book, PANS MG4, vol. 18; Falmouth Township Book, PANS MG4, vol. 31; Horton Township Book, PANS MG4, vol. 74; Lunenburg Dutch Reformed Church Burials, PANS MG4, vol. 86; Lunenburg Zion Lutheran Church Burials (in German), PANS MG4, vol. 88; St John's Anglican Church Burials, Lunenburg, PANS MG4, vol. 91; Onslow Township Book, PANS MG4, vol. 122; Truro Township Book, PANS MG4, vol. 150; Liverpool Township Book, PANS MG4, vol. 180; Granville Township Book (new), PANS MG4, vol. 185; Fort Lawrence Township Book, PANS MG4; Granville Township Book (old), PANS MG4; St Paul's Anglican Church Burials, PANS MG4; St Paul's Cemetery Inscriptions, Halifax, PANS MG5; St George's Cemetery Inscriptions, Halifax, PANS MG5, vol. 14; Chipman Corner Cemetery, Kings County, PANS MG5, vol. 8; Chebogue Cemetery Inscriptions, Yarmouth, PANS MG5; Falmouth Centre Cemetery Inscriptions, Hants County, PANS MG5; Akin Family Burial Ground, Falmouth, Hants County, PANS MG5; Old Parish Burying Ground, Windsor, PANS MG5, vol. 7; Arbuthnot to Germain, 20 November 1776, PANS RG1, vol. 45, Document 30; Wills, Estates, and Administrations, PANS RG48; and *Nova Scotia Chronicle*, various issues. Rev. Peter de la Roche to the Society for the Propagation of the Gospel in Foreign Parts, 22 August 1776 (SPGFP, series B, vol. 25, Letter no. 207), notes that "there was a ter-

rible outbreak of smallpox last autumn and about 80 died [in Lunen-
burg]." In preparing Figure 19, I have assumed that twenty persons
died in Lunenburg in each of the months of September, October, November, and December 1775.

11 An Act [16 Geo. 3d, cap.2, 1775] in addition to an Act made in the first
year of His Majesty's Reign Intitled an Act to Prevent the Spreading
of Contagious Distempers, passed in the House of Assembly, 11 November 1775; passed in Council, 13 November 1775; and assented
to by Gov. Legge on 17 November 1775, PANS RG5, series S, vol. 5.

12 NSGWC, 1 August 1775.

13 Ibid., 8 August 1775, Dr John Philipps had been in Halifax since 1758,
the year that he was appointed an assistant surgeon at the naval hospital (PRO Adm. 98, vol. 3, folio 113, 3 February 1758). William Faries
had taken classes in anatomy at the University of Edinburgh during
1762–63 (Matriculation Records for Students in the Faculty of Medicine, Edinburgh University Archives). He first appeared in Nova
Scotia in March 1772, when he was brought for debt before the Supreme Court in Halifax. He was described in the court records as
a surgeon's mate of the Sixty-fifth Regiment of Foot (Halifax Supreme
Court Records, 1772, PANS RG39, series C, Box 11). Faries was an
assistant surgeon to the naval hospital at Halifax in February 1781, at
the time of his death (*Nova Scotia Royal Gazette and Weekly Chronicle*,
13 February 1781).

14 Rev. Peter de la Roche to the Society for the Propagation of the
Gospel in Foreign Parts, 26 August 1776, SPGFP, no. 207.

15 Memorial of Michael Head, Surg^n, Windsor, 5 June 1777, PANS
RG1, vol. 301, Document 94. Rev. Joseph Bennett of Windsor, wrote
to the SPGFP on 15 November 1775 that smallpox had broken out
in his family (SPGFP, series B, vol. 25, letter no. 201).

16 Bulkeley to Deschamps, 29 August 1775, PANS RG1, 136:220.

17 *American Archives*, 4th series, vol. 3, 1775, 90, Washington, 1840. Colonel
Thompson's proposal was not dated.

18 Legge to Dartmouth, 17 October 1775, PANS RG1, vol. 44, Document
78.

19 Suffolk to Legge, 16 October 1775, PANS RG1, vol. 32, Document 32.

20 "State of His Majesty's Forces at Halifax, 21 October 1775. Joseph
Gorham, Commanding Officer," Earl of Dartmouth 1:417, PANS Micro
Biography. The Fourteenth Regiment numbered 77 men; the
Sixty-fifth, 113 men including one surgeon's mate; Gorham's Regiment,
135 men including one surgeon and one surgeon's mate; and
Maclean's Regiment, 65 men.

21 Legge to Dartmouth, 19 August 1775, PANS RG1, vol. 44
Document 76. Legge writes, "I cannot depend on the militia here."

22 Minutes of Council, 2 August 1775, PANS RG1, 189:333. Lt Col John Butler, commanding officer of the Halifax Militia, stated that the sickness in the town together with the daily labour of the inhabitants made it very difficult to muster enough men for the town guard. At the Council meeting of 30 September 1775, it was announced that four hundred militia from the country would soon arrive in Halifax to reinforce the town (PANS RG1, 189:364).

23 Statement made by Joshua Snow on 13 December 1775, Earl of Dartmouth 1:433–5, PANS Micro Biography.

24 Legge to Dartmouth, 20 December 1775, PANS RG1, vol. 44, Document 85.

25 Howe to Dartmouth, 13 December 1775, NAC CO5, 93:11.

26 Minutes of Council, 30 November 1775, PANS RG1, 189:376.

27 Howe to Legge, 18 December 1775, Earl of Dartmouth 1:439–40, PANS Micro Biography. According to Captain Alexander McDonald ("Letter Book," entry of 3 December 1775, Brigadier General Massey and the 27th Regiment arrived in Halifax on that date. The 27th was one of five regiments that embarked in the early fall of 1775 from Cork for North America. The others were the 17th, 28th, 46th, and 55th (Rochford to the Lord Lieutenant of Ireland, 21 September 1775, Sir Guy Carleton, Carleton Papers, Letter no. 47, PANS Micro Biography). The other four regiments continued on to Quebec and later, in April of 1776, the 17th, and 55th arrived in Halifax with General Sir William Howe ("State of the Regiments, Officers included, Boston, 17 March 1776," NAC CO5, 93:94).

In the letter of 3 December 1775, Captain McDonald also informed Lieutenant Colonel John Small, "Since I began to write this letter who should appear but Mr Quin, your surgeon's mate that deserted. I have ordered him to the blackhole and to be hand cufft."

28 Drew, *Roll of Commissioned Officers* 1:43. The will of Christian Wagner of Halifax, proved on 18 April 1775 (PANS RG48, Reel 424), included a payment to Dr Fletcher of £13s. 4d. on 18 May 1775, for medicines and attendance he had rendered Mr Wagner.

29 Halifax Supreme Court Records, PANS RG39, series C, Box 11. William Faries of Halifax, surgeon's mate of the 65th Regiment of Foot, was in court at Halifax on 24 March 1772.

30 "A Return of the Officers of the Loyal Nova Scotia Volunteers," Halifax, 23 May 1778, PANS CO217, 54:48.

31 NSGWC, 23 January 1781.

32 Estate of Christian Wagner, PANS RG48, Reel 424. Doctor Dundon (or Dondon) was paid £6 15s. on 16 November 1775 for attending Wagner's family.

33 Drew, *Roll of Commissioned Officers* 1:48. The 52nd Regiment was

one of the nineteen regiments that arrived in Halifax with General Howe on 2 April 1776 after the evacuation of Boston "State of the Regiments, Officers included, Boston, 17 March 1776," NAC CO5, 93:94).

34 Legge to Dartmouth, 12 May 1775, PANS RG1, vol. 44, Document 66. Legge wrote, "Several vessels are already arrived with some of the families that could escape and many other families [are] to follow them." The earl of Dartmouth, responding to Legge in a letter dated 1 July 1775, referred to Nova Scotia as "a happy asylum to many unfortunate Families" (PANS RG1, vol. 32, Document 31).

35 Claim signed at Halifax on 14 December 1785, PANS AO13, Loyalist Claims, Reel 21:362.

36 Minutes of Council, 20 May 1775, PANS RG1, 189:303.

37 Minutes of Council, 4 August 1775, ibid. 334.

38 Bartlet, *The Frontier Missionary*, 168.

39 Legge to Green, 8 April 1775, PANS RG1, 181:217. He was paid, on 8 April 1775, thirty pounds for one and a half years service and medicines.

40 NSGWC, 8 August 1775. He was officially appointed surgeon to the naval hospital on 12 December 1775 (Graves to Arbuthnot, 12 December 1775, Clark, Morgan, eds., *Naval Documents of the American Revolution* 3:63).

41 "Return of Officers of HM Provincial Regiment of Loyal Nova Scotia Volunteers, 23 February 1776, Earl of Dartmouth 1:546–7, PANS Micro Biography.

42 "Annual Account of the Orphans House for the year ending 1775, signed by John Fenton," ibid., 3:2,863–4.

43 The medical personnel who were in Halifax in 1775, and who had arrived in Halifax prior to 1758, included George Francheville (1751), Christopher Nicolai (1751), Thomas Reeve (1749), Thomas Wood (1752), and John Day (1755). As mentioned earlier, this could have been the same John Day who was allotted Lot B13 in Callendar's Division on 8 August 1749 (o.s.). Day, the surgeon, drowned in Boston Harbour on 29 November 1775 (Clark, Morgan, eds., *Naval Documents of the American Revolution* 2:1202).

44 Arbuthnot to Howe, 15 January 1776, PANS Adm. 1/484:376. On the preceding date, Mariot Arbuthnot was commander of the Naval Yard at Halifax; however, on 20 April 1776, he received his mandamus as lieutenant governor of Nova Scotia (*Dictionary of Canadian Biography* 4:29–30). The "State of HM Troops in Nova Scotia, 18 December 1775" (PANS CO217, 51:39) shows that there were in total 986 men in the province, with 156 sick in quarters. The recently arrived 27th Regiment (referred to as Enniskillens) contained 384 men,

of whom eighty-three were sick. That regiment had one surgeon and one surgeon's mate on its establishment.

45 General Washington to President of Congress, Cambridge, 30 January 1776, *American Archives* 4th series, 4:893, Washington, 1843. Capt. Alexander McDonald wrote to Captain MacLeod on 26 February 1776 that there were three hundred men in his regiment (the Second Battalion, Royal Highland Emigrants). He stated further that the 27th Regiment was in Halifax, along with part of the 65th and part of the 14th regiments, a company of Artillery and Colonel Gorham's Regiment. The 14th and 65th regiments were sent back to England in April 1776 (Barrington to Howe, 20 April 1776, Sir Guy Carleton, Carleton Papers, Letter no. 161, PANS Micro Biography).

46 Letter and Petition from Nova Scotia to General Washington, Cumberland, Nova Scotia, 8 February 1776, *American Archives*, 4th series, 5:936–8. It is likely that this petition was prepared by the same inhabitants who signed the letter that followed it (ibid., 938–9). These were Abijah Ayer, Nathaniel Reynolds, Amasa Killam, Jesse Bent, William Maxwell, George Forster, John Allan, William Lawrence, Simon Newcomb, Robert Foster, and Simeon Chester.

47 Legge to Dartmouth, 11 January 1776, PANS RG1, vol. 45, Document 4. Included with Legge's letter were three petitions from the inhabitants of northern Nova Scotia. The first was from 246 inhabitants of the townships of Amherst, Cumberland, and Sackville, dated 23 December 1775; the second was from fifty-six inhabitants in the township of Onslow, dated 3 January 1776; and the third was from sixty-four inhabitants in the township of Truro, dated 3 January 1776.

48 An Act in addition to the several Acts of this province made for Regulating the Militia, and more particularly an Act made in the 2[d] year of His present Majesty's Reign Intitled an act for the better Regulating the militia on actual service in time of war, PANS RG5, series s, vol. 5. Passed in the Assembly, 4 November; in Council, 13 November; and assented to by Governor Legge, 17 November 1775.

49 An Act for raising a Tax on the Inhabitants of this Province for defraying the Expence of maintaining and supporting the militia of the said province and for the defence of the same, PANS RG5, series s, vol. 5. Passed in Assembly, 9 November; in Council, 13 November; and assented to by Governor Legge on 17 November, 1775.

50 To the King's most Excellent Majesty the Petition of the Principal Gentlemen and Inhabitants of your Majesty's faithful and Loyal [subjects] of Nova Scotia, Halifax, 2 January 1776, PANS CO217, 27:218–23.

51 Howe to Dartmouth, 21 March 1776, NAC CO5, 93:86–8.

52 Ibid., 94. The nineteen regiments included the following: 4th, 5th, 10th, 17th, 22nd, 23rd, 35th, 38th, 40th, 43rd, 44th, 45th, 47th, 49th, 52nd, 55th, 63rd, 64th, and 65th.

53 Ibid., 152–73. List of Persons who removed from Boston to Halifax with His Majesty's troops in the month of March 1776 with the number of their respective families: governor and Council, 85 persons; commissioners and clerks, 74; Custom House officers, 47; Episcopal clergy, 18; refugees from the country, 105; farmers, traders, etc., 382; merchants of Boston, 213; others, 200 – a total of 1,124 people. "Others" referred to "those who have not returned their names." Of the eight physicians included in the list, six (Oliver, Coffin, Gardiner, Jeffries, and the two Perkinses) were among the 306 men banished under the Banishment Act of the State of Massachusetts, enacted in September 1778 (Stark, *The Loyalists of Massachusetts*. 137–40). One additional physician, Dr William Paine, who came to Nova Scotia in 1782, also was banished by the act, which was entitled An Act to prevent the return to this state of certain persons therein named, and others who have left this state or either of the United States, and joined the enemies thereof.

54 Minutes of Council, 3 June 1776, PANS RG1, 189:407. "A considerable number of women and children amounting to 2,030 persons are to be left in Halifax on the embarkation of the Army."

55 Distribution of Transports and Embarkation of the Troops at Boston, 17 March 1776, NAC CO5, 93:95.

56 Shuldham to Stephens, 17 March 1776, PANS Adm. 1/484:480. On page 542, James Dickson was referred to as surgeon and agent on board the *Richmond* hospital ship on 14 April 1776. On page 621, James Dickson signed a letter at Halifax on 28 May 1776 as surgeon and agent for sick and hurt seamen on the hospital ship *Two Brothers*.

57 Shuldham to Stephens, 16 April 1776, PANS Adm. 1/484:506. Admiral Shuldham reported that he had ten ships at Halifax, one at Liverpool, one at Cape Sable, and two at Annapolis.

58 Harris, *An Account of Some of the Descendants of Capt. Thomas Brattle*, 32. William Brattle was born in Cambridge, Massachusetts, on 18 April 1706, and graduated in Arts from Harvard in 1722. He became a physician and, in 1736, was elected to the House of Assembly of Massachusetts Bay. William Brattle served as the attorney general of that province. In 1776, at the age of 70, he left Cambridge with General Howe and moved to Halifax. He was buried from St Paul's Church in Halifax on 26 October 1776.

59 Jeffries, *Jeffries of Massachusetts, 1658–1914*, 11–13. Dr Jeffries was born in Boston on 5 February 1745, obtained an AM from Harvard in 1766, and was the first native-born American to be awarded (1769)

an MD from the University of Aberdeen, Scotland. He served as surgeon and, from April 1776 until February 1779, as purveyor to the general military hospital in Halifax.

60 "List of His Majesty's Council and other late Inhabitants of the Province of Massachusetts Bay in New England who embarked at Halifax on 12 May 1776 bound for Great Britain," NAC CO5, 93:164. Howe to Germain, 7 May 1776, ibid, 154, notes that "Lt Governor Oliver and five of the Council of Massachusetts Bay and some of the Inhabitants of Boston go to Britain at this time." Massey to Germain, 27 June 1776 (PANS CO217, vol. 52, Document 233) gives a return of twenty-two refugees' names who are said to be from Boston and now sent to England.

61 Howe to Germain, Halifax, 25 April 1776, in Clark, Morgan, eds., *Naval Documents of the American Revolution* 4:1247.

62 The Reverend Byles to the Society for the Propagation of the Gospel in Foreign Parts, 4 May 1776, SPGFP, B series, 22:92.

63 Legge to Germain, 10 April 1776, PANS RG1, vol. 45, Document 10. "On the 30th March arrived fifty sail of transports in the Harbour on board those inhabitants of Boston who have remained steady in their duty and allegiance to the crown." In a letter to the Secretary of the Admiralty, dated 16 April 1776 (PANS Adm. 1/484:506), Admiral Shuldham wrote: "The whole fleet arrived in Halifax on 2 April 1776."

64 General Orders, Thomas Gage [as well as William Howe], entry for 18 May 1776, PANS MG12, HQ, vol. Oa.

65 Ibid., entry for 24 May 1776. Since the first name of Mr Goldthwaite is not known, he is difficult to identify precisely. A Dr Goldwright was buried from St Paul's on 10 October 1776; also a Michael B. Goldthwaite, hospital mate at the general hospital in New York during the revolution, could have been in Halifax during April and May of 1776.

66 Mr Morehead's identity is uncertain. Simeon Perkins mentions a Dr Morehead letting blood in Liverpool on 11 January 1781 (Innis et al., eds., *The Diary of Simeon Perkins*, vol. 2, 63). This doctor appears to have remained in Liverpool until at least 16 February 1782 and was mentioned often by Perkins (ibid., 86, 88, 100, 116).

67 Dickson et al. to Shuldham, Halifax Harbour, 14 April 1776, PANS Adm. 1/484:542.

68 Ibid., 540. Charles White had been surgeon of the naval hospital at Boston (ibid., 546) and, by 12 May 1776, had returned to England (ibid., 563).

69 James Dickson, George Rutherford, John Philipps, and Robert Whyte, to Shuldham, 29 May 1776, PANS Adm. 1/484:621; Dickson et al. to Shuldham, 7 June 1776, ibid., 641.

70 Arbuthnot to Howe, 30 June 1776, Clark, Morgan, eds., *Naval Documents of the American Revolution* 5:834.

71 *The New England Chronicle*, 4 July 1776, stated that General Howe had left Halifax on 13 June 1776 with 140 sail of men-of-war, transports, etc. It is recorded, however, in Order Book, Thomas Gage [and William Howe] (PANS MG12, HQ, vol. Oa) that seventeen of the regiments that had evacuated from Boston on 17 March 1776 accompanied Howe to New York on 10 June 1776. These were the 4th, 5th, 10th, 17th, 22nd, 23rd, 35th, 38th, 40th, 43rd, 44th, 45th, 49th, 52nd, 55th, 63rd, and 64th. The 47th Regiment had left Halifax for Quebec on 20 April 1776 (Howe to Germain, 25 April 1776, NAC CO5, 93:138), while the 65th Regiment had been sent back to England (Barrington to Howe, 20 April 1776, Sir Guy Carleton, Carleton Papers, Letter no. 161, PANS Micro Biography). In addition to the seventeen regiments listed, the 42nd and the 71st, both Highland regiments, arrived in Halifax harbour on 8 June 1776 (Howe to Germain, 8 June 1776, NAC CO5, 93:212). These, along with part of Massey's 27th Regiment, were part of Howe's army as it embarked for New York on 10 June 1776, a total of twenty regiments.

72 Tillenghast to Washington, Providence, 29 June 1776, *American Archives*, 4th series, 6:1137. Howe arrived in New York on 29 June 1776 (Howe to Germain, Staten Island, 7 July 1776, NAC CO5, 93:214).

73 Clark, Morgan, eds., *Naval Documents of the American Revolution* 6:1513.

74 Howe to Germain, Staten Island, 15 August 1776, NAC CO5, 93:247.

75 Original Manuscript Journal by Admiral Sir George Collier, in Clark, Morgan, eds., *Naval Documents of the American Revolution* 6:1516, Appendix C.

76 Minutes of Council, 3 June 1776, PANS RG1, 189:407.

77 Massey to Germain, 27 June 1776, PANS CO217, vol. 52, Document 233.

78 Massey to Germain, 6 October 1776, ibid., Document 308.

79 Nova Scotia, *Journal*, minutes of 26 June 1776. A memorial was presented from John Woodin, master and keeper of the poor house, with his account for maintaining several poor, sick, lame, blind, and "lunatick" persons who had no settlement in the province. He was paid £123 out of the monies arising from the duties of Impost and Excise. The overseers of the poor for Halifax in June 1776 were William Mott, James Wakefield, Robert Killo, and Richard Tritten Jr (Minutes of 27 June 1776, *Journal of the House of Assembly*).

80 Ibid. Dr Thomas Reeve was paid sixty-four pounds out of the duties for "attendance and medicines to the poor, sick, and hurt persons of the Province from 18 June 1775 to 17 June 1776."

81 Studholme to Massey, Windsor, 6 November 1776, Sir Guy Carleton, Carleton Papers, Letter no. 310, PANS Micro Biography.

82 Drew, *Roll of Commissioned Officers* 1:25. It should be noted here that
Robert Drew has combined in one biographical sketch the careers of
two separate people named George Frederick Boyd. The Dr Boyd
who was appointed surgeon to the Second Battalion, Royal Highland
Emigrants, on 8 May 1776, died on 2 March 1789 at the age of forty
years (NSGWC, 3 March 1789), indicating that he was born *circa* 1749.
Drew's biographical sketch indicates that George Frederick Boyd
was surgeon of the 20th Foot in 1756, and died at Basingstoke, England,
in 1801.

83 Innis et al., eds., *The Diary of Simeon Perkins, 1766–1780* 1:116. This
fear of inoculation was also prevalent in other centres and, for instance, resulted in a resolution being passed at a meeting of the New
York Provincial Congress on 13 December 1775 (*American Archives,*
4th series, 4:406): "Ordered that no person whatsoever do inoculate
for the smallpox in this colony, until the further order of this Congress."

84 PANS MG1, vol. 183, no. 1, Chipman Collection.

85 John Jeffries to Richard Bulkeley, 16 December 1776, PANS RG1,
vol. 342, Document 77. It appears that Michael Head had been appointed chief surgeon of the general (military) hospital at Halifax by
General Massey, but General Howe had countermanded the appointment (Head to Pernette, 20 June 1777, PANS MG100, vol. 205,
no. 15d).

86 Graves to Arbuthnot, 12 December 1775, in Clark, Morgan, eds., *Naval
Documents of the American Revolution* 3:63.

87 Ibid., 6:1525. Collier suggests in his journal that the naval hospital incident, decribed in the text which follows, happened about four
months after his arrival in Halifax in late September 1776. Since Collier
did not actually write his journal until 1779, his recollection of the
incident's having taken place in January or February 1777 could have
been in error by a number of months. According to a statement
made by John Scott, assistant surgeon of the naval hospital, the sick
patients were turned out of the hospital on George's Island on
15 May 1777 (NSGWC, 6 October 1778).

88 Dickson to Admiralty Medical Department, 25 July 1777, PRO
Adm. 98, vol. 11, Letter no. 122. Also, James Dickson, surgeon and
agent for the Sick and Hurt Seamen and Marines in Nova Scotia,
advertised in the NSGWC on 6 October 1778 that two hundred cords
of wood were to be landed on George's Island for the use of His
Majesty's Naval Hospital.

89 Halifax County Wills, PANS RG48, Book 2:228–9. John Scott signed
as a witness on 9 December 1777, the day Andrew Ackman made his
will. Scott was referred to as surgeon, Halifax Naval Hospital.

90 Clark, Morgan, eds., *Naval Documents of the American Revolution* 6:1525.

91 Arbuthnot to Barclay, 13 August 1776, PANS RG1, 136:239.

92 Germain to Arbuthnot, 11 December 1777, PANS CO217, vol. 53, Document 247.

93 Halifax County Wills, PANS RG48, Book 2:222. Dr Reeve made his will on 20 June 1777, and it was proved on 26 July of that year.

94 Davidson to Reeve, 30 April 1750 (o.s.), PANS RG1, 163/1:38. Also Minutes of Council, 4 June 1755, PANS CO217, 15:285.

95 Nova Scotia, *Journal*, minutes of 24 June 1766. In a memorial to the House, Dr Reeve stated, without specifying the date, that Governor Wilmot had appointed him as surgeon to the workhouse.

96 Memorial of Thomas Reeve, 21 June 1777, PANS RG1, vol. 301, Document 21.

97 Cumberland County Deeds, PANS RG47, series B, 137. Parker Clark of Cumberland, physician, sold land to Jonathan Eddy on 15 May 1770.

98 Journal of Lt Col Joseph Gorham describing the attempted capture of Fort Cumberland and covering the period 4 November to 2 December 1776, PANS RG1, vol. 365, Documents 4 and 5.

99 Arbuthnot to Germain, 11 October 1777, PANS RG1, vol. 45, document 46. On the latter date, there were 170 grenadiers at Fort Cumberland. According to Arbuthnot, the additional forces in Nova Scotia were five companies of Marines at Halifax and Major Small's Highland Emigrants, two companies of which were stationed at Windsor. On 31 December 1776, Arbuthnot wrote to Germain, "The *Vulture* arrived alone near Fort Cumberland and landed Major [Thomas] Batt at the head of the Marines on the 26th of November past. On the 28th the major marched out of the fort before daylight in hopes of surprising those Banditti [*sic*], but they were too nimble and fled into the woods."

100 "Trials for Treason, 1776–1777." 112–13, 116.

101 Milner, "Records of Chignecto," 50.

102 *Columbian Centennial*, 20 October 1798. The *Ipswich Vital Records* indicates that he died of "numb palsy."

103 Raymond, "Roll of Officers of the British American or Loyalist Corps," 231.

104 Massey to Germain, 20 December 1776, PANS CO217, vol. 53, Document 113.

105 Massey to Howe, 12 January 1778, Sir Guy Carleton, Carleton Papers, Letter no. 857, PANS Micro Biography. Dr Cullen is reported as being in Windsor, Nova Scotia, on 11 February 1778 (George Deschamps diary for 1778 written on blank pages in the *Nova Scotia Calendar or, an Almanack*, printed by A. Henry, Halifax, 1778, entry dated 11 February 1778, PANS MG1, no. 258A).

106 James Silver was probably one of the surgeons in the two battalions of Marines that accompanied General William Howe to Halifax on 2 April 1776 (Howe to Dartmouth, 21 March 1776, NAC CO5, 93:94). The Marines remained in Halifax after Howe moved his headquarters to New York on 10 June 1776 (McDonald, "Letter Book," 15).

107 Halifax County Estates, Reel 425, PANS RG48. Estate of Samuel Wethered, 1777.

108 Arbuthnot to Germain, 23 December 1777, PANS RG1 45:48. John Bolman (1751–1833), one of the surgeons who was with General Burgoyne at Saratoga, was wounded in the battle and taken prisoner. After the war, he practised in Lunenburg for over fifty years (Letter to the Queen [Victoria] from Anne and Mary Bolman, Lunenburg, 27 May 1842, Canon Harris Genealogies, vol. 94, no. 16, PANS MG4).

109 Massey to Howe, 26 November 1777, Sir Guy Carleton, Carleton Papers, Letter no. 765, PANS Micro Biography.

110 McDonald, "Letter Book," letter to Mr McKenzie dated 6 May 1777.

111 Poole, *Annals*, 93–4.

112 Jeffries Family Papers, vols. 30 and 31, Massachusetts Historical Society, Boston.

113 Innis et al., eds., *The Diary of Simeon Perkins, 1766–1780* 1:163.

114 McDonald, "Letter Book," Letter to Donald McLean, 11 June 1777.

115 St Paul's Church, Halifax, PANS MG4, marriage of 15 December 1763.

116 George Deschamps diary for 1776, entries for 24 January and 12 February 1776, PANS MG1, no. 258A. Since there were a number of Harris families in Horton in 1776, it is difficult to identify the Christian name of Mrs Harris, midwife.

117 *Dictionary of Canadian Biography* 4:593–4.

118 Germain to Arbuthnot, 26 February 1778, PANS RG1, vol. 32, Document 42.

119 Barrington to Germain, 18 February 1778, NAC CO5, 170:17–18.

120 Whitehall to Clinton, 21 March 1778, NAC CO5, 95:97.

121 Barrington to Germain, 16 April 1778, NAC CO5, 170:49–50.

122 Knox to Stephens, 17 April 1778, NAC CO5, 128:123–4.

123 Massey to Clinton, 20 August 1778, Sir Guy Carleton, Carleton Papers, Letter no. 1303, PANS Micro Biography.

124 Massey to Clinton, 13 June 1778, ibid., Letter no. 1234.

125 McLean to Whitehall, 18 August 1778, PANS CO217, 54:87.

126 Establishment of the General Hospital at Halifax, 24 November 1778, Dorchester Papers, PANS RG1, vol. 368, Document 58.

127 Clinton to McLean, 19 January 1779, Sir Guy Carleton, Carleton Papers, Letter no. 1688, PANS Micro Biography. McLean had informed Clinton that John Jeffries, the purveyor, had been appointed to that position by Major General Eyre Massey (McLean to Clinton, 24 October 1778, ibid., Letter no. 9807). Brig. Gen. Francis McLean had replaced Major General Massey as officer commanding the army in Halifax in September 1778 (Clinton to McLean, 24 September 1778, ibid., Letter no. 1393). Massey left Halifax for England on 5 October 1778 (McLean to Clinton, 24 October 1778, ibid., Letter no. 9807).

128 Barrington to Germain, 5 November 1778, NAC CO5, 170:133–6.

129 "Return of Prisoners remaining sick and wounded in His Majesty's Hospital at Halifax, 9 January 1778, J. Jeffries, surgeon," PANS RG1, vol. 368, Document 12. The names of the fifty-one prisoners appear in the return. It would appear that, like the regular British soldiers, they were in the general military hospital, but held under guard and treated in a separate room, or rooms.

130 See also Byron to Stephens, 27 August 1778, PANS Adm. 1/486:118. Admiral Byron stated, "I found no ship here [in Halifax] of force except the *Culloden* and she is in a very sickly condition." The *Culloden* had arrived in Halifax on 16 August, and could have been the source of the illness that eventually broke out among the rebel prisoners.

131 Germain to Hughes and McLean, 11 November 1778, PANS CO217, 54:127.

132 Barrington to McLean, 5 November 1778, in Davies, ed., *Documents of the American Revolution, 1770–1783*, vol. 13.

133 Lewis to deGrey, 10 November 1778, NAC CO5, 170:142–7.

134 McLean to Clinton, 28 December 1778, Sir Guy Carleton, Carleton Papers, Letter no. 1634, PANS Micro Biography. Baron de Seitz (Fritz Carl Erdman) was colonel and chief of the Hessian Regiment of Foot.

135 Innis et al., eds., *The Diary of Simeon Perkins, 1766–1780* 1:225, entry of 13 December 1778. The detachment, which consisted of fifty-eight officers and men, arrived at Liverpool on 13 December.

136 "Return of the British and Brunswick Troops ordered to Lunenburg under the command of Lt Col Von Specht, Halifax, October 1778," PANS RG1, vol. 367 ½, Document 17. One of these surgeons could have been Dr John Bolman, for he is known to have been a surgeon in General Von Riedesal's Brunswick Regiment as early as 1777 (Land Grant Petition of John Bolman, 1809 PANS RG20, A) and to have been in Lunenburg as early as 25 November 1779 (Petition of Dr John Bolman, Nova Scotia, *Journal*, 1802, 25).

137 Minutes of Council, 18 November 1778, PANS RG1, 189:446.

138 Nova Scotia, *Journal*, minutes of 19 June 1778. Dr Philipps was paid fifty pounds, presumably for providing medical services during the preceding year.

139 Dr Edward Wyer was born in England *circa* 1752, attended lectures given by William Cullen and William Hunter in Edinburgh in 1771 and 1772, and entered Guy's Hospital Medical School in London in February 1776 (Burrage, *A History of the Massachusetts Medical Society*, 53, 351, 393). Dr Wyer remained in Halifax until June 1785 (NSGWC, 28 June 1785) and then removed to Boston, where he died on 16 September 1788 (*Massachusetts Centinel*, 20 September 1788).

140 Nova Scotia, *Journal*, minutes of 16 June 1778. There were thirty-four persons in the poor house in June 1778, including seventeen women (Memorial of John Woodin, late Master of the Poor House at Halifax, June 1778, PANS RG1, vol. 411, Document 8).

141 Halifax Inferior Court of Common Pleas, 24 September 1762, PANS RG37, vol. 13. Thomas Wood was referred to as a physician of Halifax. Thomas Wood had advertised at Brunswick, New Jersey, a month-long course on osteology and myology, to be succeeded by a course in angiology and neurology, if interest warranted. The advertisement appeared in the *New York Weekly Post-Boy* on 27 January 1752, and the text of the advertisement is printed in Gordon, *Aesculapius Comes to the Colonies*, 356–7. The Reverend Thomas Wood's Estate Papers (Halifax Estates, Reel 426, PANS RG48) show that, at the time of his death, he had in his library twenty-seven books on physic and surgery; unfortunately, none are identified by title.

142 Letters to the Honourable Judges of the Inferior Court and General Sessions of the Peace at Horton from Robert Kinsman (26 May 1778), and Jonathan Rockwell Jr (1 June 1778), PANS MG1, vol. 183, nos. 134, 135.

143 McLean to Campbell, 7 May 1779, Dorchester Papers, PANS RG1, vol. 368, Document 154. It is likely that the commendation dated 27 May 1783 to Dr John Philipps, surgeon of the Royal Regiment of Nova Scotia Volunteers, for having "discharged great attention and regularity in the disposal of the Hospital on George's Island in Halifax Harbour," referred to the removal of the hospital in May 1779 (PANS MG12, HQ1:4). By July 1781, there were forty-seven guns in the battery on George's Island, and it was stated that 221 men and six officers would be necessary to manage the battery in case of attack (Return of the Number of Officers and Men exclusive of the Royal Artillery that would be necessary for the management of the cannon in the several batteries in the Garrison of Halifax, 14 July 1781, Dorchester Papers, PANS RG1, vol. 368, Document 29).

144 Hamond to Commissioners for Sick and Hurt Seamen, 6 August 1781, Andrew S. Hamond, Reel 2, Section 7, PANS Micro Biography.

145 McLean to Clinton, 28 May 1779, Sir Guy Carleton, Carleton Papers, Letter no. 2024, PANS Micro Biography. McLean was first alerted on 11 February 1779 to the concern about a possible attack on Nova Scotia (ibid., Letter no. 1740).

146 Ibid., The grenadiers and light infantry companies of the 70th, 74th, and 82nd regiments had embarked from Halifax for New York in early March 1779 (NSGWC, 9 March 1779). However, the remaining companies in each regiment had remained in Halifax. Sir George Collier commanded the several transports which carried the troops to New York (ibid., 16 March 1779).

147 Hughes to Germain, 21 November 1779, PANS RG1, vol. 45, Document 83. The naval force in Halifax on that date consisted of a frigate (twenty-eight guns), a sloop (eighteen guns), and two schooners (one of fourteen guns, and another of ten guns).

148 NSGWC, 18 May 1779.

149 As early as 1712, patents were granted in England for compound medicines. They soon found their way to America and, through the medium of the newspaper, became well known. They were used by many citizens who preferred a home remedy either because it was less expensive or because of unfortunate experiences with quacks (Young, *The Toadstool Millionaires*).

150 Innis et al., eds., *The Diary of Simeon Perkins, 1766–1780* 1:236; Ellis, *A Genealogical Register of Edmund Rice Descendants*, 129. Dr Jesse Rice was born in Marlboro, Massachusetts, on 25 May 1761, received his Bachelor of Arts at Harvard in 1772, and came to Yarmouth *circa* 1778 (Memorial of Sundry Settlers in the Township of Yarmouth, 30 June 1783, PANS RG1, vol. 223, Document 5). After practising in Yarmouth and vicinity for about seventeen years, he removed to Bakersfield, Maine, where he died in 1816.

151 *Acadian Recorder*, 6 October 1821. Drake, in his article entitled "The Wet Nurse in France in the 18th Century," points out that about eighty percent of infants in Paris were cared for by wet nurses (*Bulletin of the History of Medicine* 8:934–48, 1940). Fildes *(Wet Nursing: A History from Antiquity to the Present)* indicates that the eighteenth century was the most significant period in the history of wet nursing.

152 NSGWC 14 October 1800.

153 Cope, *The History of the Royal College of Surgeons of England*, 6. William Cheselden was a member of the Company of Barber-Surgeons of London, which existed from 1540 to 1745. He was a well-known surgeon and teacher of anatomy in London and, along with John

Ranby, was responsible for the separation between the barbers and the surgeons, which took place on 2 May 1745.

154 It is likely that the thermometer, advertised in the *Gazette*, was used for clinical purposes, for the other two items included in the advertisement were newly invented elastic trusses for ruptures in adults and children and Maredant Drops. It is also possible, however, that the device in the advertisement was an instrument for making meteorological measurements.

155 Garrison, *An Introduction to the History of Medicine*, 296, 691.

156 *Boston News-Letter*, 4 October 1708.

157 Young, *The Toadstool Millionaires*, 5, 13. Galenicals were remedies thought to restore the harmonious relationship of the humours – blood, phlegm, choler, and melancholy – the four liquids of the body according to Galen (c. 130–c. 200). The chymicals mentioned by Young refer to the remedies proposed first by Paracelsus (c. 1490–1541), who felt that abnormal separation of the three elements in man ("salt," "sulphur," and "mercury") were the cause of sickness. Paracelsus introduced mineral baths; added opium, mercury, lead, sulphur, iron, arsenic, and copper sulphate to the pharmacopoeia; and popularized tinctures and alcoholic extracts.

158 Some of these patent medicines were advertised by George Greaves, surgeon of Halifax, while the remainder were sold by the printer of the *Gazette*, A. Henry. A number of the descriptive terms that are now uncommon require an explanation. Pectoral drops were formulated to relieve or to cure diseases of the lungs or chest. An elixir was a sweetened, alcoholic, medicinal preparation supposedly able to prolong life indefinitely. A cordial was a medical stimulant supposed to invigorate the heart. A balsam was any fragrant ointment, sometimes derived from the resin of trees, used for medicinal purposes. A tincture was a solution, usually in alcohol, of some distinctly coloured substance used in medicine. A nostrum was a medicine of one's own invention or preparation.

159 Young, *The Toadstool Millionaires*, 5, 13.

160 NSGWC, 11 January 1780.

161 Ibid., 3 October 1780. The first school of veterinary medicine had been founded in Lyon in 1762, and was moved to Alfort near Paris, in 1766. By 1775, over one thousand students had graduated (Hannaway, "Veterinary Medicine and Rural Health," 431–77).

162 Lind, *A Treatise of the Scurvy*.

163 Memorial of Nathaniel Russell, Keeper of the Poor House in Halifax and his Accounts, 10 October 1780, PANS RG1, vol. 411, Document 10 1/2.

164 PANS RG1, vol. 286, Document 130. In Nova Scotia, *Journal*, minutes for 8 June 1779, Nathaniel Russell was called the keeper of the workhouse and poor house.

165 Minutes of Council, 21 December 1779, PANS RG1, 189:464. The monthly return for September 1780 indicates that, during that month, twenty-one men and one woman became inmates of the poor house. The minutes of Council record that the overseers of the poor for the town had represented to Council "that on the arrival of the last cartel from Boston, many persons who had been put on shore were sickly and naked, and they were obliged to send twenty-two of them to the Poor House for cure, and to purchase necessary cloathing for them."

166 Nova Scotia, *Journal*, minutes of 9 June 1779. Dr Wyer was surgeon to the poor house until 31 December 1780, when he was succeeded by Dr Malachy Salter (PANS RG1, vol. 298, Document 87, General Court of Quarter Sessions, 14 December). Dr Salter, the first native-born Nova Scotian to become a surgeon, was baptized at St Paul's on 18 December 1757. He was the son of Malachy Salter Sr, who had come to Halifax from New England in the early 1750s. Malachy Jr entered Guy's Hospital medical school in London on 1 May 1778 and, after completing his medical training, returned to Halifax in November 1780 (NSGWC, 14 November 1780). He continued as surgeon to the poor house and operated a drug and medicine store opposite the Market House on Granville Street, until his death on 4 December 1782 (*Gazette*, 28 August 1781, and 10 December 1782). His gravestone bears the inscription, "He died in the bloomus vigor of Life."

167 Nova Scotia, *Journal*, minutes of 17 June 1779.

168 McLean to Clinton, 23 November 1778, Sir Guy Carleton, Letter no. 1634, PANS Micro Biography.

169 Piers, *The Evolution of the Halifax Fortress, 1749–1928*. Publication no. 7 of the Public Archives of Nova Scotia, 20, 5–6. Albemarle Street is known now as Market Street.

170 Johan Christian Helmerich was an assistant medical officer in the Regiment von Stein during 1778 and 1779 (von Eelking, *The German Allied Troops*, 318) and in the Regiment von Seitz during 1780–83 (Hospital Staff Surgeons and Regimental Surgeons to A. Finucane, 17 January 1782, PANS RG1, vol. 368, Document 36). He is known to have been in Halifax during 1781, 1782, and 1783. Helmerich could have been the surgeon referred to by Baroness von Riedesel in her journal (*Baronness von Riedesel and the American Revolution*, 114–15):

On this voyage [July 1781] we touched Halifax, in Nova Scotia, and even went ashore ... Since I suffered so the whole time there from my toothache, I decided to have one of my teeth drawn. In order to spare my husband and children all care and unrest, I arose at five in the morning, sent for our surgeon, who was considered a skilful man at this kind of operation, went into a room somewhat apart from the rest, where he had me sit on the floor, and with a nasty, blunt instrument he gave me such a jerk, that I thought the deed was done and asked for my tooth. "Just be patient another moment," he said, going at in again and giving me another jerk. Now, I thought, I was at last freed of it. But not at all. He had, on the contrary, taken hold of and pulled at a good tooth, without completely extracting it, I was extremely angry at this, and although he advised pulling this one now as well as the bad tooth, I neither could nor would put myself in his hands again. I have had reason to regret this attempt for a long time, for this tooth which was now out of place prevented me for more than two years from closing my teeth together. Moreover, this experience was so dreadful, that I was never able again to bring myself to undergo such an operation.

171 John Frederick Traugott Gschwind was appointed an assistant surgeon to a Hessian regiment on 2 March 1776 and, in the same year, came to America to serve with General Howe (PRO WO25, 3904:143). He was in Halifax as early as 2 February 1781 (Halifax Supreme Court Records for 1782, PANS RG39, series c).

172 Marshall to McLean, 8 May 1780, Dorchester Papers, PANS RG1, vol. 368, document 119.

173 Germain to Hughes and McLean, 11 November 1778, PANS CO217, 54:127.

174 Report of the Hospital Staff and Regimental Surgeons to A. Finucane, 17 January 1782, Sir Guy Carleton, Carleton Papers, Letter no. 4057, PANS Micro Biography. A temporary prison hospital was mentioned as early as 27 October 1778 by Dr John Jeffries in his diary. However, on 7 January 1779 he wrote that all the sick were removed from the prisoners' hospital and that orders were given to discharge all the nurses and cooks.

175 Hamond to Commissioners for Sick and Hurt Seamen, 6 August 1781, Andrew S. Hamond, Reel 2, Sections 7, 6, PANS Micro Biography.

176 Hamond to Thomas, 13 August 1781, Andrew S. Hamond, Reel 2, Section 9:38, PANS Micro Biography. An additional lot of land was purchased for forty pounds in May 1782 from Robert Grant, Esq., formerly a member of Council and a surgeon in Halifax from 1749 to 1758, "for the use of HM Navy Hospital now being built at this Port." (Hamond to Thomas, 16 May 1782, ibid., 120).

177 Hamond to Graves, 20 August 1781, ibid., Section 7:15.

178 Hamond to Digby, 26 December 1781, ibid., 57.

179 Hamond to Thomas, 1 January 1782, ibid., Section 9:106.

180 Hamond to Andrews, 7 January 1782, ibid., Section 7:61.
Hamond informed Israel Andrews of Windsor, who had tendered for
building the naval hospital, that the contract had been awarded.

181 Hamond to Dickson, 5 November 1781, ibid., Section 9:106.

182 NSGWC, 13 February 1781.

183 Edinburgh University matriculation records indicate that John Handasyde attended lectures in the faculty of medicine during the
1777–78 term. The Examination Book of the Company of Surgeons
of London indicates that he passed an examination in surgery on
17 August 1780. He is said to have come to Halifax from London during the summer of 1781 (Joseph Peters to Samuel Peters, 13 May
1782, in Cameron, *The Papers of Loyalist Samuel Peters,* 16).

184 Hamond to Handasyde, 4 August 1781, Andrew S. Hamond, Reel 2,
Section 9:4, PANS Micro Biography.

185 Hamond to Thomas, 29 December 1781, ibid., 54. The *Stanislaus* had
been rented from its owner, Mr Winkworth Norwood, on 14 August 1781.

186 Hamond to Master Shipwright, 10 August 1781, ibid., 24.

187 Hamond to John Loader, Master Shipwright, 15 August 1781, ibid.,
32.

188 Hamond to Phips, 29 August 1781, ibid., 20.

189 Hamond to Sick and Hurt Board, 25 November 1781, ibid.,
Section 8:13.

190 Hamond to Graves, 28 October 1781, ibid., Section 7:39.

191 Innis et al., eds., *Diary of Simeon Perkins, 1780–1789* vol. 2, entry for
5 September 1781.

192 Thomas Brown to Rev. Mr Jacob Bailey, 13 September 1781, PANS
MG1, vol. 93, no. 47.

193 Hamond to Dickson, 5 November 1781, Andrew S. Hamond, Reel 2,
Section 9:106, PANS Micro Biography.

194 Halifax County Wills, PANS RG48, Book 2:273, will of Francis McLean,
Colonel of the Eighty-second Regiment and Brig. Gen. of the army
in North America. He made his will on 13 April 1781, and it was
proved on 4 May 1781.

195 Minutes of Council, 22 October 1781, PANS RG1, 189:483.

196 Halifax County Wills, book 2:287, PANS RG48, will proved 1 September 1781, Dr Francheville was buried from St Paul's on 25 August
1781.

197 *Dictionary of Canadian Biography* 5:408–9.

198 Francklin to Vandergift, PANS RG1, vol. 220, Document 61, and
     Francklin to Bulkeley, ibid., Document 62, both dated 5 November
     1781.

199 Hamond to Digby, 15 February 1782, Andrew S. Hamond, Reel 2,
     Section 7:67, PANS Micro Biography.

200 Hamond to Handasyde, 1 January 1782, ibid., Section 9:193–4.

201 Hamond to Handasyde, 14 January 1782, ibid., 57–8.

202 Digby to Stephens, New York, 9 March 1782, PANS Adm. 1/490:73.
     Halliburton had passed examinations at the Company of Surgeons
     in London on 18 May 1758, 20 March 1760, and 16 April 1761.

203 PRO Adm. 11/40:16. The ships he served on were the *Thames*,
     30 May 1758 to 30 April 1761; the *Prosperine*, 1 May 1761 to 9 April
     1762; the *Deal Castle*, 2 February 1762 to 1 February 1763; and
     the *Maidstone*, 19 April 1763 to 28 August 1766.
         He was principal surgeon of the naval hospital at Halifax from
     14 April 1782 to 31 December 1807.

204 Halliburton to Nepean, 27 November 1786, PANS CO217, 58:331.
     Halliburton mentions that he was well acquainted with a merchant in
     Halifax in 1763.

205 Halliburton to Montagu, 19 January 1773, PANS Adm. 1/484:202. The
     agreement signed on that date meant that Halliburton was to be
     paid six shillings for the cure of each man in his hospital, one shilling
     per day for victualling each man, and ten shillings for each funeral.

206 John Halliburton's Weekly Account of Sick and Wounded Seamen
     in Rhode Island Naval Hospital, 25 November 1778, PANS Adm.
     1/486:143. On that date, 142 seamen were in the hospital.

207 Memorial of John Halliburton, Halifax, March 1786, Loyalist Claims,
     Bundle 24:241–9, PANS Misc. L, AO13.

208 Petition of John Halliburton to Lords Commissioners of the Admiralty,
     9 June 1807, PANS Adm. 1/497:176.

209 Hamond to Thomas, 1 January 1782, Andrew S. Hamond, Reel 2,
     Section 9:77–8, PANS Micro Biography.)

210 Hamond to Thomas, 2 March 1782, ibid., 112. Mr Lee was paid five
     hundred pounds for work carried out during the months of Jan-
     uary and February 1782.

211 Hamond to Thomas, 1 January 1782, ibid., 80. Probably the ear-
     liest such agreement was a contract between thirty-six families in Ville
     Marie (on the Island of Montreal) and Estienne Bouchard, Master
     Surgeon, signed on 4 April 1655 (Kelly, "Health Insurance in New
     France," 535–41).

212 Hamond to Digby, 24 april 1782, Andrew S. Hamond, Reel 2, Section
     7:80, PANS Micro Biography. Hamond wrote: "As I had proceeded

before by your permission, their Plan will not be exactly followed, but attended to as far as is now practicable."

213 Hamond to Navy Board, 16 May 1782, ibid., 88.

214 Hamond to Thomson, 13 August 1782, ibid., 111.

215 Hamond to Thomas, 23 September 1782, ibid., Section 9:167.

216 Hamond to Stephens, 13 November 1782, ibid., Section 7:152.

217 Hamond to Halliburton, 15 December 1782, ibid., Section 9:200. Also Hamond to Handasyde, 1 January 1782 (ibid., 202); Hamond to Wood, 14 January 1782 (ibid., 58); Hamond to Mrs Jane Kennedy, 1 January 1782 (ibid., 203); and Digby to Stephens, 9 March 1782 (PANS Adm. 1/490:73).

218 *Pegasus: Log Book*, 135, PANS Micro Misc. s, Ships. The *Pegasus* was commanded by Prince William Henry (later William IV) and was in Halifax harbour from 5 October to 25 October 1786.

219 *Novascotian*, 29 December 1842, 410. In "Notes by an old settler," it is mentioned that the architect who planned the naval hospital was a man named Brooks. This would have been Chamberlain Brooks, a carpenter, whose will, made on 7 August 1784, was proved on 9 December 1784 (Halifax County Wills, Book 2:377, PANS RG48). Brooks's name does not appear in the Andrew S. Hamond papers.

220 Petition of Samuel Sparrow, 1782, Land Grant Petitions, PANS RG20, series A. Akins ("History of Halifax City," 213) wrote: "In the year 1765 there were two hospitals in the north suburbs, near the beach at the foot of Cornwallis Street called the Red and Green Hospitals. They were there in 1785. One stood on the site of the present North Country or Keating's market, the other stood on property now owned by the heirs of the late H.H. Cogswell." It is recorded that a property owner in Halifax by the name of McNeal was a patient in the Green Hospital *circa* 1779 (Valuation of Real Estate in the County of Halifax, PANS RG1, vol. 411). The Green Hospital appears no longer to have been used as such sometime prior to 1800, since on 22 september of that year, Richard John Uniacke, Esq., was "granted a Town lot in Halifax formerly called the Green Hospital, lately escheated" (PANS RG1, 191:53).

221 Land Grant Petitions, PANS RG20, series A.

222 Lewis Davis to Doctor Marshall, 12 January 1782, Sir Guy Carleton, Letter no. 4050, PANS Micro Biography. Lewis Davis had been a surgeon's mate in Emmerick's Chasseurs in 1779 (Raymond, "Roll of Officers of the British American," 233) and, by June 1781, was in Halifax as surgeon of the King's Rangers (King's County Deeds, 4:103, PANS RG47).

223 Examination of Mr Lewis Davis, Surgeon to the King's Rangers, 17 January 1782, Sir Guy Carleton, Letter no. 4053, PANS Micro Bi-

ography. The board consisted of John Marshall, surgeon to the hospital; George Frederick Boyd, surgeon, eighty-fourth Regiment; James Kay, Surgeon, Seventieth Regiment; George Inness, Surgeon, Eighty-second Regiment; William Lawlor, surgeon's mate to the general hospital; Peter Jaumard, surgeon's mate to the general hospital; and J.C. Helmerich, surgeon major to Regiment De Seitz.

224 Hospital Staff and Regimental Surgeons to A. Finucane, 17 January 1782, ibid., Letter no. 4057. It is interesting to note that, whereas the *Stanislaus* had been described as being able to contain four hundred persons without overcrowding (Hamond to Sick and Hurt Board, 25 November 1781, Andrew S. Hamond, Reel 2, Section 8:12, PANS Micro Biography), there were a total of 605 prisoners in Halifax, presumably on the prison ship, on 26 October 1781 (Hamond to Graves, 26 October 1781, ibid., Section 7:39).

225 Hamond to Campbell, 23 April 1782, Andrew S. Hamond, Reel 2, Section 8:18, PANS Micro Biography.

226 Minutes of Council, 21 January 1782, PANS RG1, 189:484.

227 Hamond to Campbell, 13 May 1782, Andrew S. Hamond, Reel 2, Section 8:20–1.

228 Hamond to Digby, 2 August 1782, ibid., 29.

229 Hamond to Paterson, 23 September 1782, ibid., 31.

230 Hamond to Thomas, 14 December 1782, ibid., Section 9:186. Winkworth Norwood, owner of the *Stanislaus*, was paid £1,384 for the rent of his ship from 14 May to 13 December. He had previously been paid £989 for rental for the period 14 December 1781 to 13 May 1782 (Hamond to Thomas, 14 May 1782, ibid., 119). Escape from the prison ship was very common, and the escapees were frequently given assistance by Nova Scotia residents to return to New England (Poole, *Annals of Yarmouth and Barrington*, 130–1).

231 Hamond to Digby, 15 November 1782, Andrew S. Hamond, Reel 2, Section 7:154–5, PANS Micro Biography.

232 Ontario, *Second Report of the Bureau of Archives*, 803–4.

233 Munk, *The Roll of the Royal College of Physicians of London*, 2:235. War Office to Carleton, 7 November 1781, Sir Guy Carleton, Carleton Papers, Letter no. 3860, PANS Micro Biography: "Dr Paine is to be granted the first vacancy among physicians under your command."

234 Paine, *Genealogical Notes*, 23.

235 Earl Cornwallis was a relative of Governor Edward Cornwallis, the founder of Halifax.

236 France had entered into a treaty of alliance with the Americans in February 1778, and a French fleet under Admiral d'Estaing sailed for America from Toulon in April 1778. French troops under the Marquis de Lafayette and the French fleet under Admiral François de

Grasse assisted the Americans in winning the decisive battle at Yorktown on 19 October 1781.

237 Parr to Townshend, 26 October 1782, PANS RG1, vol. 45, Document 116.

238 Parr to Townshend, 1 December 1782, ibid., Document 119. Most of these refugees arrived sometime prior to 22 November and were accompanied by part of the 82nd Regiment (Hamond to Digby, 22 November 1782, Andrew S. Hamond, Reel 2, Section 7:158, PANS Micro Biography).

239 Minutes of Council, 16 December 1782, PANS RG1, 189:493.

240 Return of Loyalists gone from New York to Nova Scotia, dated at New York, 12 October 1783, PANS RG1, vol. 369, Document 198. Nova Scotia in 1783 included the territory that later became the province of New Brunswick. Digby does not appear in the return; however, it would be expected that a portion of the 2,530 people listed for Annapolis Royal were actually settled at Digby.

241 Sydney to Parr, 7 July 1784, PANS RG1, vol. 33, Document 8.

242 Antliff, "Loyalist Claims," PANS Vertical File, vol. 312, no. 29.

243 Brown, *The King's Friends*, 290–344.

244 Leiby, *The Revolutionary War in the Hackensack Valley*, 177–8.

245 Memorial dated 19 October 1784, PANS Misc. L, AO12, 101:130.

246 Memorial of Peter Huggeford, late of New York, n.d., PANS Misc. L, AO13, bundle 64:350.

247 Memorial of the Overseers of the Poor: John Newton, Thomas Cochran, John George Pyke, and Richard John Uniacke, n.d., but circa November 1783, PANS RG1, vol. 301, Document 57.

248 —— to Parr, 23 July 1783, Sir Guy Carleton, Carleton Papers, Letter no. 8507, PANS Micro Biography.

249 Nova Scotia, *Journal*, minutes of 9 October 1783.

250 Nooth to Paine, 1 February 1783, Sir Guy Carleton, Letter no. 8026, PANS Micro Biography.

251 Campbell to Shelburne, 17 July 1782, PANS CO217, 41:9.

252 Carleton to Paterson, 3 February 1783, Sir Guy Carleton, Carleton Papers, Letter no. 6858, PANS Micro Biography.

253 War Office to Carleton, 17 June 1783, ibid., Letter no. 8059.

254 Carleton to Fitzpatrick, 27 August 1783, ibid., Letter no. 8894.

255 Donald McIntyre had been appointed surgeon to the 43rd Regiment to 13 March 1772 (*Army List*, 1777). He came to Halifax with the regiment in April 1776 when Boston was evacuated, but embarked with his regiment for New York on 19 June of the same year. On 1 March 1781, Dr McIntyre was appointed as a surgeon to a general hospital (Drew, *Roll of Commissioned Officers*, 44) and came to Halifax sometime before August 1783.

256 Office for Sick and Hurt Seamen to Commander in Chief of HM Ships and Vessels, Nova Scotia, 5 November 1783, Halifax Dockyard Records, HAL/F/2:185, Reel 4, PANS MG13.

257 Duncan to Collins, 18 Novembe 1783, ibid., HAL/F/1:23, Reel 4. It is likely that he was the same George Rutherford who signed a letter in Halifax on 29 May 1776 as surgeon on a Royal Navy ship (Rutherford to ———, 29 May 1776, PANS Adm. 1/484:622).

258 Duncan to The Principal Officers and Commissioners of HM Navy, 14 October 1785, PANS MG13, 2:362. An account of the career of Dr Duncan Clark(e) after 1783, appears in *Dictionary of Canadian Biography* 5:187–8. I have been unable to verify the *Dictionary*'s statement that "he apparently retained [the position of surgeon to the dockyard] for life." See also 259–60 for information on Dr Duncan Clarke prior to 1783.

259 Innis et al., eds., *Diary of Simeon Perkins, 1780–1789*, vol. 2, entries of 25 July, 12 October, and 16 October 1783. Hallet Collins was the father of Hon. Enos Collins, one of the wealthiest and most influential citizens of Nova Scotia in the middle years of the nineteenth century.

260 NSGWC, 16 September 1783. Rue is a small bushy herb with bitter, acrid leaves. In the eighteenth century, it was commonly used in the preparation of medicines.

261 The first mention of Dr Duncan Clark in Nova Scotia is found in Major General Eyre Massey's letter to Clinton, 20 August 1778 (Carleton Papers, Letter no. 1303). In this letter, Massey mentioned that Surgeon's Mate Clarke from the 82nd Regiment had been sent to Spanish River (later Sydney) to "take care of the working men at the colliery." Dr Clark was back in Halifax by 23 June 1783, on which date he was initiated into the St John's Lodge of Free Masonry (PANS MG20, vol. 2610, no. 1). I discovered in Special Collections at the Kellogg Library, Dalhousie University, a medical textbook printed in 1781 and bearing on its title page the signature "D. Clark, 82nd Regt." It is probable, therefore, that Clark arrived in Halifax from Great Britain with the regiment on 12 August 1778.

Two years earlier, it had been mentioned that nine men of the Nova Scotia Loyal Volunteers had died, probably from methane gas, in the "cursed coal mines" at Spanish River. Lt Col Henry Denny Denson wrote about the incident on 7 December 1776: "A surgeon of a Ship of War who saw the poor men at the Cole [*sic*] Mines [indicated] that most of them will die this Winter owing to a yellow or nervous fever occasioned by being kepted [*sic*] enveloped as they have been in sulphurous vapours" (Denson to Legge, 7 December 1776, Earl of Dartmouth 1:774–5, PANS Micro Biography).

262 Dr John Fraser, in a letter to Lieutenant Governor Wentworth
dated 31 March 1799 (PANS CO217, 70:70), stated that he had been
in Nova Scotia for twenty-one years. In land grant petitions (PANS
RG20, series A, vol. 4, 1784, no. 103), John Fraser, surgeon in the
Orange Rangers, was granted five hundred acres near the Minas
Basin on 29 March 1784. The King's Orange Rangers arrived in Hal-
ifax on 15 November 1778 (McLean to Clinton, 28 Decembe 1778,
Sir Guy Carleton, Carleton Papers, Letter no. 1634, PANS micro
Biography).

263 Innis et al., eds., *Diary of Simeon Perkins* 2:165. Perkins states that
Dr Stephen Thomas was from Lancaster, England, and was a surgeon to the King's Orange Rangers. He came to Liverpool in 1782
and resided there until 23 June 1785, when he moved his family
to Grand Manan Island to make a settlement there. From 9 March
1784 to 1 May 1785, Thomas was in England "completing his
studies in Physick, Surgery, etc." (ibid., entry of 1 May 1785).

264 General and Staff Officers by His Excellency Sir Guy Carleton's
appointment, Halifax, 1 January 1784. Signed by John Campbell,
Major General, PANS CO217, 41:43. The three mates, Gould, Gemmel, and Carter, were struck off strength on 1 March 1785 by Major
General Campbell (NAC WO1, 3:210).

265 This is undoubtedly Dr John Gamble (1755–1811). He had studied
at Edinburgh and came to New York in 1779, serving as an assistant surgeon at the general military hospital. He accompanied the re-
treating British army to Halifax, and by 1785 was practising in
Saint John. A lengthy account of his career is given by Canniff, *The
Medical Profession in Upper Canada*, 377–80.

266 Christopher Carter had been a druggist and chymist in Philadelphia
and, because of his allegiance to George III, was imprisoned in
the gaol in Philadelphia from 8 October 1775 to 8 March 1776 (Loyalist
Claims, PANS Misc. L, AO13, bundle 22. Reel 18:44). According to
his claim, he went to England after his release from prison, but returned sometime prior to 1783 to work at the general military hospital in New York. By July 1786 he was residing in Queens County,
New Brunswick, practising as a druggist and chymist (Halifax Supreme Court Records, Box 46, 1786, PANS RG39, series C).

267 Amherst to Foster, 27 February 1763, PRO WO34, 13:289 "Mr Van
Hulst, who was surgeon's mate to the 1st Battalion, Royal Americans,
having been strongly recommended to me, I have appointed him
to the Garrison of Annapolis Royal in the room of the late Mr Steele,
and he will take the first opportunity of proceeding to Nova Scotia
to attend on his duty at Annapolis."

268 Number of Inhabitants in the Province of Nova Scotia on the 1st of January 1784 as nearly as could possibly be collected from Returns of the different places where they have set down, PANS RG1, vol. 56, Document 465.

269 Parr to North, 15 January 1784, PANS RG1, 47:37.

270 These four doctors were William Faries, who studied medicine at Edinburgh during 1762–63; William Fletcher, examined by the Company of Surgeons, London, 5 July 1770; Christopher Nicolai, examined by the Company of Surgeons, 7 December 1752; and John Philipps, examined by the Company of Surgeons, London, 2 February 1758. A fifth doctor residing in Halifax, who was not practising medicine in 1775, was Rev. Thomas Wood. He studied anatomy at Edinburgh in 1743 and, on 7 May 1747, was examined by the Company of Surgeons in London.

271 Doctors who had either attended or graduated from medical schools and were practising in Nova Scotia in 1783: George Frederick Boyd, (Edinburgh, 1774–75); Duncan Clark (Edinburgh, 1777–78); James Kaye (Edinburgh, 1771–76); Donald McIntyre (Edinburgh, 1767–1770); Donald MacLean (Edinburgh, 1775–79); William Paine MD (Marischal College, Aberdeen, 1774); Fleming Pinkston (Edinburgh, 1764–67); and Robert Tucker, MD (King's College, New York, 1770).

272 Doctors who had studied at hospital medical schools and who were practising in Nova Scotia in 1783: David Landeg, St George's Hospital Medical School, London, 1772, and Edward Wyer, Guy's Hospital Medical School, London, 1776.

273 Doctors who been examined by colleges of physicians and surgeons and were practising in Nova Scotia in 1783: Peter Barnard, Company of Surgeons, London, examined 7 May 1761; Joseph N. Bond, company of Surgeons, London, examined 7 September 1775; John Gould, Company of Surgeons, London, examined 3 May 1781; J.F.T. Gschwind, College of Surgeons, Hesse Cassel, examined 1776; John Halliburton, Company of Surgeons, London, examined 18 May 1758; John Handasyde, Company of Surgeons, London, examined 17 August 1780; Joseph Hatton, Company of Surgeons, London, examined 4 April 1776; John Huggeford, Company of Surgeons, London, 2 April 1778; Daniel Kendrick, Company of Surgeons, examined 1 January 1761; David Landeg, Company of Surgeons, London, examined 2 July 1778; John Marshall, Company of Surgeons, London, examined 16 april 1778; Christopher Nicolai, Company of Surgeons, examined 7 December 1752; William Paine, Licentiate of the Royal College of Physicians, London,

1782; John Perry, Company of Surgeons, London, examined
4 February 1779; John Philipps, Company of Surgeons, London,
2 February 1758; and Fleming Pinckston, Company of Surgeons,
London, 3 November 1768.

274   During the last fifteen years of the eighteenth century and the first
part of the nineteenth, three of the most important and highly paid
positions for medical personnel in Nova Scotia were held by
Almon, Boggs, and Boyd. Dr Almon was surgeon to the Ordnance
and Artillery during the period 1784 to 1816 and also surgeon
general to the Nova Scotia Militia, Dr James Boggs served as garrison
surgeon at Halifax from 1790 to 1810 and was principal medical
officer in Nova Scotia from 1809 to 1810. John Boyd held the position
of garrison surgeon at Windsor from 1787 to 1815. The apprenticeship indenture of William J. Almon, covering the period 1 January
1771 to 14 August 1776 (see Appendix 7), indicates that he was
trained to be both a physician and a surgeon. The training that Almon
received during his apprenticeship was judged to be acceptable
by the medical faculty of St Andrew's University, Scotland. On 4 February 1792, they awarded him an MD *in absentia*.

CHAPTER FIVE

1   Abstract of the Number of Families Settled in Nova Scotia, August
1775, Earl of Dartmouth 1:349–52, PANS Micro Biography.

2   The suggestion that there would soon be a considerable emigration
from Scotland to Cape Breton was made by Lieutenant Governor
Macarmick as early as December 1792 (Macarmick to Dundas,
15 December 1792, PANS CO217, 109:1). In May 1796, the Honourable
David Mathews, President of the Council, wrote, "I have also been
informed ... that a very considerable Emigration will take place to this
Island from the Isle of Sky[e] in North Britain the moment that
Peace shall take place" (Mathews to Portland, 6 May 1796, PANS CO217,
112:55).

3   Parr to Dundas, 27 September 1791, PANS RG1, 48:58.

4   Parr to Sydney, 1 September 1784, PANS RG1, 47:55.

5   Campbell to Parr, 22 September 1784, PANS CO217, 41:151.

6   Parr to Nepean, 9 October 1784, PANS CO217, 59:208. *Canaille* is
the French word for rascals, roughs, or mobs.

7   Jades to Nepean, 11 May 1785, PANS CO217, 35:10. The passagers
on the *Sally* were kept in tents, fashioned from the ship's sails, on the
"other side of the Harbour" (Provincial Secretary to the Master of
the *Sally* Transport, 16 August 1784, PANS RG1, 221:128). By 23 Sep-

tember 1784 it was reported (ibid., 136) that they were still in tents on the eastern shore and had "no infectious disorders amongst them."

8 Minutes of the House of Assembly, 17 and 20 November 1784, PANS CO217, 58:99.

9 Nova Scotia, *Journal*, minutes of the meeting, 8 December 1784. This bill was quite likely introduced in order to deal with the "widows and children of Loyalists and soldiers and other objects of charity" as described in the Return of the Disbanded Troops and Loyalists settling in Nova Scotia mustered in the summer of 1784, (PANS RG1, 284:34–7, Document 23) which included ninety men, thirty-nine women, fifty-six children, and four servants. I have been unable to find information on the diet of the paupers in the poor house. On one occasion, however, in September 1784, John Blake delivered eleven cod, six haddock, three dozen mackerel, thirty-seven pounds of halibut, and twenty-six hake to the poor house (PANS RG5, series A, vol. 2, Document 135).

10 Nova Scotia, *Journal*, minutes of 21 December 1785.

11 Ibid., 28 June 1786.

12 Report from the Committee appointed to take into their consideration the Present State of the Poor House at Halifax, 16 June 1786, PANS RG5, series A, vol. 2, Document 33.

13 Nova Scotia, *Journal*, minutes of 15 November 1787.

14 NSGWC, 31 July 1787. High Kelly was appointed keeper of the poor house in February 1785 (Stewart to Duncan, 12 February 1785, Dockyard Records, HAL F/2:305, PANS). In April 1788 he was also appointed to the office of town clerk and, according to the NSGWC of 1 April 1788, "commenced the business of said office at the Poor House." He was still keeper of the poor house in February 1791 (*Royal Gazette and Nova Scotia Advertizer*, 1 February 1791). Hugh Kelly was also keeper of the workhouse during this period (Account of Persons Committed to the Work House of Halifax, from 1 January to 31 December 1790. Signed by Hugh Kelly, (Halifax County Court of General Sessions of the Peace, series J, vol. 4, PANS RG34–312).

15 Minutes of the House of Assembly, 23 November 1784, PANS CO217, 58:101. The master of the poor house in 1783 was Jeremiah Marshman, who had succeeded Nathaniel Russell on 1 January 1781 (Nova Scotia, *Journal*, minutes of 26 June 1781). Nicolai succeeded Mr Malachy Salter (Parr to Nicolai, 1 January 1783, PANS RG1, 169:37). Dr Nicolai was paid seventy-nine pounds for medicines and attendance at the poor house from 1 January – 30 October 1783 (Nova Scotia, *Journal*, 22 November 1783).

16 Minutes of Council, 7 July 1786, PANS CO217, 58:101.

17 Parr to Almon, 19 April 1785, PANS RG1, 170:379. Dr Almon performed the "Operation of the Trepan" on a man at the poor house in
the presence of Dr Nicolai and "the Gentlemen of the Faculty," on
28 February 1788 (Death of John Magner, PANS RG39, Series C, Box 53).
The latter records that Magner had been in a fight and had obtained a five-inch fracture in his temple bone. Trepanning is a surgical
procedure in which, to relieve pressure, a piece of bone is removed
from the skull.

18 Cameron, *The Papers of Loyalist Samuel Peters*, 70. The Loyalists received medicines and attendance gratis until 26 March 1785, when
Major General John Campbell received instructions to discontinue
the practice (Campbell to Yonge, 18 July 1785, NAC WO1, 3:224).

19 Nova Scotia, *Journal*, minutes of 20 December 1785; 16 June 1786;
and 4 December 1787.

20 Innis et al., *The Diary of Simeon Perkins 1797–1803*, 66. The Grand
Jury presented £125 to build a poor house on 14 November 1797.

21 General Sessions of the Peace, Shelburne County, PANS RG34–321,
series O, File 2.

22 General Sessions of the Peace, Shelburne County, PANS RG34–321,
series C, C. 307. By 1787, James McGrath was listed as the keeper of
the poor house and house of corrections and was paid ten pounds
per year (ibid., C. 7). Samuel Harrison was reported to be master of
the house of correction in Shelburne in 1791 (ibid., C. 309). The
house of correction and the poor house were rented from Alexander
Fraser for four pounds per year (ibid., C 20). During the three-
month period 20 January to 31 March 1786, fifteen people were sent
to the house of correction (ibid., C , 308). A fetter was a chain by
which the feet were fastened to some fixed or heavy object.

23 Parr to Sydney, 20 September 1785, PANS RG1, 47:49.

24 Rohl to Parr, 8 March 1788, PANS CO217, 61:11.

25 Parr to Nepean, 4 December 1789, PANS CO217, 62:6.

26 Memorial of the Overseers of the Poor to Parr, 18 June 1790, PANS
RG1, vol. 411, Document 13.

27 Nova Scotia, *Journal*, minutes of 6 March 1790.

28 Ibid., 11 June 1791.

29 Ibid., 27 March 1790. The only account I found of the number of persons committed to the work house during a twelve-month period
appears in Halifax County Court of General Sessions, series J, vol. 4,
PANS RG34–312, where during the period 1 January 1790 to 31 December 1790, seventeen men and twenty-five women had been committed. The average duration of a stint in the workhouse was ten
days.

30 Minutes of the House of Assembly, 21 June 1791, PANS CO217, 63:134.

31 Nova Scotia, *Journal*, minutes of meeting of 4 July 1791.

32 Ibid., 16 June 1791. The Report of the Committee to examine into the State of the Poor House indicated that on 6 March 1790 there were forty-four transient poor, including eighteen orphans in the house, and that between 6 March and 1 May 1790, eleven additional paupers were admitted. From 1 May 1790 to 17 June 1791, thirteen paupers were discharged, one ran away insane, one was sent off to Boston, six died, and three were apprenticed. This meant that, on 17 June 1791, there were thirty-one remaining in the poor house and the total included the keeper, his wife, an assistant, a cook, a nurse, a washer-woman, and fourteen orphans (PANS RG5, series A, vol. 4, Document 24).

33 Nova Scotia, *Laws*, 32 Geo. 3d, cap. 5, 1792.

34 The figures for the provincial debt and the amount spent to support the poor are found in Nova Scotia, *Journal*.

35 PANS RG5, series S, vol. 7, 31 Geo. 3d, cap. 12. An Act to raise a Revenue for the Purpose of paying off all such debts as are now due by the Province or which shall become due before the first day of July next, the Funded Debt only excepted. The act was to be in force until the whole of the principal and interest of the debt was fully paid off and discharged. Assented to by Lieutenant Governor Parr on 30 June 1791. Whereas farmers were to pay two shillings, six pence, attorneys at law, physicians, surgeons, apothecaries, merchants, and shopkeepers who were execising their profession and occupation were to pay ten shillings. According to PANS vols. 443 and 444, sixteen medical personnel paid poll tax in 1791, while twenty-two paid in 1792 and twelve in 1793. These numbers are low in comparison to the total number of medical personnel known to have practised in Nova Scotia during 1791, 1792, and 1793, according to Figure 21, the differences being due to the incompleteness in the poll tax returns for those years.

36 Nova Scotia, *Journal*, minutes of 17 June 1799.

37 Ibid., 11 July 1799.

38 Petition of the Grand Jury and the Inhabitants of Halifax, 17 June 1799, PANS RG1, vol. 287, Document 88.

39 Whitehall to Parr, 6 October 1784, PANS RG1, vol. 33, Document 11. John Parr was sworn in as governor of Nova Scotia on 9 October 1782, but upon the appointment of Sir Guy Carleton, Lord Dorchester, as governor of all the British North American colonies in April 1786, Parr's position was changed to lieutenant governor. He continued

to hold that office until he died, at Halifax, on 25 November 1791. Needless to say, Parr was not happy with his demotion (letter dated 6 June 1786, PANS CO217, 58:161).

40 Minutes of the House of Assembly, 30 November 1784, PANS CO217, 58:106. On 12 January 1784, the minutes of Council record received information that the orphans had been ill treated by the keeper of the orphan house. It appears, however, that this information was incorrect, for the committee established "to make all necessary enquiries and to give such proper orders for addressing all grievances" did not recommend that Albro be disciplined for any wrongdoing.

41 Memorial of Philipps to House, 15 November 1784, PANS RG1, vol. 301, Document 52; Minutes of the House of Assembly, 10 November 1784, PANS CO217, 58:98.

42 NSGWC, 29 July 1788.

43 Ibid., 2 December 1788.

44 Minutes of the House of Assembly, 7 June 1791, PANS CO217, 63:125.

45 Memorial of the Overseers of the Poor to Wentworth, 19 December 1795, PANS RG1, vol. 411, Document 31.

46 Ibid., Document 32. The Poor House at Halifax in account for cash received and paid for illegitimate children during the years 1798, 1799, 1800, 1801.

47 Dundas to Wentworth, 9 February 1793, PANS RG1, vol. 33, Document 65. This was the Royal Nova Scotia Regiment. The surgeon of this new regiment was Dr John Fraser, the assistant surgeon was Dr Jonathan Clarke (Return of Lodging Money due the Officers and Staff of the Royal Nova Scotia Regiment between 13 April and 12 November 1793, PANS CO217, 67:125). The surgeons appointed to the various militia regiments raised in Nova Scotia in 1793 included Dr Daniel Eaton, Colchester Corps of Militia; Dr Michael Head, 1st Regiment, Halifax Militia; Dr John F.T. Gschwind, 2nd Regiment, Halifax Militia; Dr William Fletcher, 2nd Regiment, Halifax Militia; Dr Joseph Prescott, Hants Regiment of Militia; and Dr Isaac Webster, 1st Regiment, Kings County Militia.

Dr Joseph Prescott was born in Nova Scotia in 1762, the son of Dr Jonathan Prescott. He wrote a letter dated 12 April 1852, which was printed in the *Eastern Chronicle*, 20 July 1852, page 3, column 4, in which he indicated that in the autumn of 1776, he had left Nova Scotia and entered a hospital in Albany, New York. During the course of the American war he was a hospital mate at West Point in 1778; a junior surgeon with the British army in the South in 1779; and an acting surgeon in the Maryland Regiment of Cavalry in 1782. After the war he returned to Nova Scotia, where he practised at Cornwallis, Shelburne, Lunenburg, and Halifax, where he died on 23 June

1852. Dr Isaac Webster first appears in the records of Nova Scotia in 1788, when he purchased land at Cornwallis (King's County Deeds, PANS RG47, 3:279). He was referred to as a schoolmaster in the land transaction. Dr Webster was born in Mansfield, Connecticut, in 1766, and practised in Cornwallis for over fifty years, dying there in 1851. Two of his sons, William and Frederick, practised medicine in Kentville and Yarmouth.

48 Ogilvie to Dundas, 19 May 1793, PANS CO217, 64:189.

49 Wentworth to Ogilvie, 4 August 1793, PANS RG1, vol. 50; Wentworth to Dobree, 26 May 1794, ibid., 51:119; and 22 June 1794, 51:149. According to the *Royal Gazette and Nova Scotia Advertiser*, 25 June 1793, the French prisoners were transferred from the transport ships to the Cornwallis Barracks on 23 June. They were still there on 19 November 1793, according to an advertisement that described how to deal with escaped French prisoners (ibid., 19 November 1793). The Cornwallis Barracks was shown on Captain Charles Blaskowitz's 1784 plan of the peninsula "upon which the Town of Halifax is situated" and was located near the intersection of Sackville and Brunswick streets. The Barracks was described in 1795 as consisting of sixteen rooms of twenty men each for a total capacity of 320. It had also a mess house and a kitchen (Stratton to Prince Edward, 7 March 1795, NAC RG8, series C, 1428:22).

50 Duncan to Livie, 3 September 1794, Navy Yard Papers, PANS MG13, 6:18. The *La Feliz* was in Halifax as early as December 1792, since on 18 December it was advertised for sale by order of the Admiralty (*Royal Gazette and Nova Scotia Advertiser*, 18 December 1792). A prison ship was berthed in the harbour as late as 9 December 1796 (Navy Yard Papers, 209).

51 PANS Adm. 1/492:428. Dr McEvoy was described by Halliburton (430) as being able to speak French fluently. McEvoy continued as assistant surgeon at the naval hospital until some time in 1799. In July of that year his household furniture, horse, and "sley" were advertised for sale, indicating that he was leaving the province (*Weekly Chronicle*, 6 July 1799). He was replaced in September 1799 by Dr Robert Hume, who was paid a hundred pounds per year as both dispenser and assistant surgeon (Adm. 102:256).

52 PANS Adm. 1/492:440. The naval hospital was placed on "war establishment" by Admiral Murray on 27 September 1794 (Murray to Stephens, 27 September 1794, PANS Adm. 1/492:491).

53 Ibid., 439. This is the only document that I have found describing the number and sizes of the rooms in the naval hospital. The hospital contained four wards, two with twenty patients, one with thirteen, and one with twelve; one large hall for eighteen patients; one room for

twenty-one men; four rooms for five officers each; a chamber for twenty-one men, and four garrets that held twenty-one, ten, twenty-five, and nine patients. An additional two patients were located in what was referred to as a passage.

54 Middleton, "The Yellow Fever Epidemic of 1793 in Philadelphia," 434–50.

55 Halliburton to Murray, 30 August 1794, PANS Adm. 1/492:434.

56 As early as November 1752 there had been a commodious stone house, seventy by twenty feet, and a blockhouse on "an island in the North West Arm" (*Halifax Gazette*, 18 November 1752). It is unlikely that these same buildings were on the island when James Kavanagh purchased it from John Butler Kelly for sixty-five pounds on 27 April 1784 (Halifax County Deeds, 36:168, PANS RG47). Kavanagh owned the island until 1804, when he advertised in the *Royal Gazette* of 31 May that it was for sale. He sold the island to the Commissioners for Conducting His Majestys Transport Service for a thousand pounds on 27 July 1804 (RG47, 36:214). The building on the island were described as follows: two large storage houses or prisons "which have contained 200 persons"; two cook houses; a dwelling house; a barracks for twenty-five to thirty persons; a servants' house; and a guard house. Sometime after the sale, the island was renamed Melville Island after Viscount Robert Melville, who was First Lord of the Admiralty from 1812 to 1830.

57 PANS Adm. 1/493:190.

58 State of the Royal Nova Scotia Regiment, 15 April 1796, PANS CO217, 67:81.

59 Halliburton to Duncan, 15 August 1796, Navy Yard Papers, 1794–1800, PANS MG13, 6:176.

60 Wentworth to Portland, 2 June 1797, PANS CO217, 68:124; Oxley to Wentworth, 31 May 1797, ibid., 130.

61 PANS CO217, 37:141, 144, 146; 68:209; 69:290.

62 Wentworth to Portland, 17 November 1798, PANS CO217, 69:220.

63 Fraser to Wentworth, 31 May 1799, PANS CO217, 70:70. Dr Fraser was my great, great, great, great grandfather.

64 Wentworth to Gray, 5 August 1800, PANS RG1, 53:125.

65 Bulkeley to Dundas, 3 February 1792, PANS RG1, 48:67.

66 Campbell to North, 4 February 1784, PANS CO217, 41:59.

67 Minutes of Council, 14 November 1796, PANS RG1, 213:330.

68 Mathews to Portland, 8 December 1795, PANS CO217, 112:2.

69 Minutes of Council, 9 October 1793, PANS RG1, 213:273.

70 Middleton, "The Yellow Fever Epidemic," 434–50.

71 Proclamation concerning Contagious Distempers and Quarantine, 9 October 1793, PANS RG1, 171:63.

72 Minutes of Council, 9 October 1793, PANS RG1, 190:272. According to the minutes of the Legislative Council, 8 July 1794, Peter McNab was paid twenty-five pounds for the health boat (PANS RG1, 218J:55).

73 Circular Letter, Shelburne, 1 April 1791, PANS RG34–321, C. 321.

74 Minutes of Council, 13 May 1799, PANS RG1, 214:3.

75 PANS RG1, vol. 364, Document 125. The proclamation was undated. One year earlier, on 7 June 1798, John Hill of Digby had advertised in the *Halifax Journal* that he was manufacturing and selling essence of spruce as a cure for yellow fever. Spruce beer had been used for many years as a preventive medication against epidemic fevers in Halifax, and it appears to have been the standard drink provided to inmates of the poor house (*Royal Gazette and Nova Scotia Advertiser*, 26 March 1789).

76 Statutes of Nova Scotia, 1794–1799, PANS RG5, series S, vol. 8.

77 PANS RG1, 191:12. George Henkell (ca.1751–1818), arrived in Nova Scotia in late 1797 as surgeon to the 7th Regiment of Foot, the Royal Fusiliers. By 1799, he was surgeon to the garrison at Annapolis Royal. He remained at Annapolis until his death on 8 October 1818 (*Acadian Recorder*, 31 October 1818). His obituary states that Dr Henkell spent forty years in the British army and twenty years at Annapolis Royal.

78 Dr Daniel Eaton (1769–1809), came to Onslow from Massachusetts *circa* 1790 (Onslow Township Book, marriage of 9 December 1790, PANS MG4, vol. 122), and he practised there as a physician until 1803, when he returned to the United States (Supreme Court Records, PANS RG39, series C, Box 86, 1803). He died at Salisbury, Pennsylvania, in September 1809 (*Columbian Centennial*, 9 September 1809).

79 Nova Scotia, *Journal*, minutes of 3 November 1784.

80 Memorial of John Harris to the House of Assembly, 12 November 1784, PANS RG5, series A, vol. 1b, Document 121.

81 Nova Scotia, *Journal*, minutes of 7 November 1787.

82 An extensive account of the Assembly debate which took place over the judges' affair appeared in the *Weekly Chronicle*, 21 March 1789. An informative article by Ells discussing factors leading to the affair appeared in the *Dalhousie Review* 16:475–92. The Privy Council in London subsequently advised the king that the charges brought by the House of Assembly of Nova Scotia against the two assistant judges of the Supreme Court were unfounded, and Deschamps and Brenton were acquitted (*Royal Gazette and Nova Scotia Advertizer*, 11 September 1792).

83 Halliburton to Nepean, 24 april 1790, PANS CO217, 62:266.

84 *Urban Bender vs. John Bolman*, Inferior Court of Common Pleas,

Lunenburg County, PANS RG37, vol. 1, 1784 No judgement has been found with regard to this case.

85 Ibid., vol. 2, 1786.

86 *Bolman vs. Wilkins*, 1794, Halifax Supreme Court, PANS RG39, series C. Box 70.

87 Chipman Collection, PANS MG1, vol. 184, no. 264a. Dr William Baxter (1760–1832), born in Connecticut, is recorded as being resident in Cornwallis Township as early as 1782 (King's County Deeds, PANS RG47, Reel 1279, 2:400). He practised as a physician in Cornwallis Township until he died there, on 22 November 1832 (*Nova Scotia Royal Gazette*, 12 December 1832, 3).

88 *Baxter vs. Benvie*, 1790, Halifax Supreme Court, PANS RG39, series C, Box 58; *Vanwinkle vs. Baxter*, 1791, Box 64; *Kidston vs. Baxter*, 1796, Box 75.

89 *John George Pyke vs. John Philipps Jr*, 1796, ibid., Box 75. Dr Philipps was found guilty of accosting Pyke. In the same year, Dr Lewis Davis took Alexander Woodin to court (Box 74) on a charge of "having carnal knowledge" of Davis's wife, Margaret. As a consequence of this incident, Dr Davis obtained one of the earliest divorces granted in Nova Scotia (*Davis vs. Davis*, 1796, PANS RG39, series D, vol. 1a). A second case in which a doctor brought a patient to court for non-payment involved Dr Joseph Russell and a Mr William McNiel. Dr Russell had charged McNiel twelve pounds for medicines and attendance, during the period 15 July to 27 August 1788, to cure a wound in McNiel's throat (*Russell vs. McNiel*, PANS RG39, series C, Box 53). The court asked Drs Donald McIntyre, John Halliburton, and George Gillespie to give their opinion. They responded, "We have examined a disputed bill exhibited by Mr Russell, surgeon, against Mr McNiel. From the facts stated, and which are further corroborated by Dr [Duncan] Clark, who also occasionally visited the said Mr McNiel, in company with Mr Russell, we think the charge just and reasonable."

90 Letters of William Smith, MD, British Library, Add. MSS. 19, 243, fol. 98–124. In a letter dated 3 May 1785, Dr Smith wrote: "Soon after my arrival from America I received an appointment to go to this Island, where we arrived last November." In another letter, in fol. 98, there is a statement by Squire Eleazer Davy about Dr Smith that reads, "All I know of him is from his Letters. He was at one time in great embarassment, & was obliged to hide himself from his creditors. My uncle knew him well, & had a very high opinion of his abilities, & skill in his profession." The biographical sketch of Dr Smith that appears in the *Dictionary of Canadian Biography* 5:766–7, does not refer to his activities prior to 1784, or to his published works listed in note 91 below, except for his last book which was published in 1803.

91 Affidavit of William Smith, dated 15 September 1800, PANS CO217, 118:419 indicating that his published works included *Dissertation on the Nerves* W. Owen, London, 1768, 302 pages; *A New and General System of Physic, in Theory and Practice*, London, 1769, 561 pages; *The Student's Vade Mecum*, W. Owen, London, 1770, 264 pages; *The Nature and Institution of Government*, W. Owen, London, 1771, 2 vols; *Nature Studied with a View to Preserve and Restore Health*, W. Owen, London, 1774, 210 pages; *Synopsis Medica*; *A Sure Guide to Sickness and Health*, Bew and Walter, London, 1776, 356 pages; and a *History of England*, in two volumes. It is known that he also wrote three other books: *State of the Gaols in London, Westiminister, and Borough of Southwark*, J. Bew, London, 1776, 90 pages; *Mild Punishments Sound Policy*, London, 1778, 121 pages; and *A Caveat against Emigration to America with the State of the Island of Cape Breton*, Betham and Warde, London, 1803. The British Museum has six of Dr William Smith's books. On the title of each, he refers to himself as "William Smith, MD." His *Dissertation upon the Nerves* was reviewed in *London Magazine* 37:298–301, where an anonymous reviewer referred to Smith as "the learned author [who] has discussed his subject with much ingenuity."

92 *Journal of the British House of Commons* 37:493, 503–4; 38:507. Dr Smith's address is given as Lower Brook Street in the County of Middlesex, and he is referred to as a doctor of physic. In *State of the Gaols in London*, 5, Smith wrote: "Westiminister Charity, March 25 1776. The Committee resolved that Dr Smith of Red Lion Square be desired to visit the sick in the respective gaols and prisons in London, Westminister, and the Borough of Southwark, in order to administer proper relief for which a sum of money is appropriated by the above charity." Volume 37: 505 gives a Report of the Sick, with the Expense of Medicines sent to the ten Prisons in the London area. This report indicates that, between the two dates mentioned above, Dr Smith had expended £566 while treating 1,051 prisoners. The illnesses and numbers treated are as follows: putrid, nervous and inflammatory fevers (241); diarrhoeas and dysentry (94); rheumatism (78); inflammation of the bowels (18); bilious complaints (43); asthma (57); pleurisy (68); piles (14); smallpox (28); eruptive fevers (29); consumption (21); scurvy (30); diseases of the bladder and urinary passages (12); palsy and epilepsy (8); worms (65); and cases of venereal disease and itch (159). Dr Smith had also performed surgery on fifty-four of the prisoners.

93 Mackworth to Lords of Trade, 10 July 1784, PANS CO217, 103:46.

94 Macarmick to Smith, 27 December 1791, PANS CO217, 107:343. Lieutenant Governor William Macarmick wrote: "Agreeable to your desire I now send my dispatches by the bearer and at the time I

express my sincere wish for you and Mrs Smith having a safe and speedy voyage to England. I cannot avoid transmitting testimony of the high approbation I entertain of your conduct since my arrival and particularily the just and honorable manner in which you have filled the office of Senior Puisne Judge for nearly three years and the peaceable deportment I have experienced in all description of persons in the Government during that period."

95 *Nova Scotia Royal Gazette and Weekly Chronicle*, 19 June 1798, page 3, col. 3. "The brig *Smyrna* arrived in 61 days from England. In her came passenger Mr Smith, Chief Justice of the Island of Cape Breton."

96 Fergusson, ed., *Uniacke's Sketches of Cape Breton*, 143. The 33rd Regiment had arrived at Sydney from Halifax on 22 July 1785 (DesBarres to Yonge, 27 July 1785, WO1, 3:310).

97 PANS CO217, 103:93. This hospital must have been a fair-sized building since it is recorded (ibid., 104:75) that it required 3,425 boards, 99 planks, and 5,000 shingles. It is shown in DesBarres's map of Sydney, drawn in 1786.

98 DesBarres Collection, n.d., NAC MG23 F1, series 5, 6:1063–70.

99 Perry to DesBarres, 5 March 1785, PANS CO217, 104:43.

100 Uncle to Mathews, 10 February 1786, PANS CO217, 103:132; 42:67.

101 Minutes of Some Parts of the Transactions at the Mess and among the Officers of the 33rd Regiment after their arrival at Sydney in Cape Breton extracted from the Journal of Lieutenant William Norford, PANS CO217, 104:384, entry of 30 January 1786. Major General John Campbell wrote to Sir George Yonge, secretary of state for War, on 24 November 1784 (NAC WO1, 3:147), that among the staff officers lately appointed at the garrisons in Nova Scotia were surgeons Donald McIntire (Annapolis Royal), John Irvine (Halifax), and Dr William Smith (Cape Breton); and hospital mates Joseph Pearce (Annapolis Royal), William Lawlor (Halifax), and Alexander Gordon (Cape Breton).

102 Campbell to Sydney, 22 June 1786, PANS CO217, 42:110. The Fortysecond Regiment had been in Halifax as early as 29 March 1785, according to the NSGWC of that date. The regiment embarked for Europe in August 1789, according to the Minutes of the Council of Cape Breton of 10 August 1789 (PANS RG1, 319:146).

103 DesBarres Papers, n.d., NAC MG23, series 5, 4:1010–2. In this petition Dr Smith was referred to as the "Medicinal Surgeon General," and Gordon was called an "Assistant Surgeon." The petition contained thirteen reasons why Lieutenant Governor DesBarres should "be remov'd from the Gov^t of the Island."

104 Smith to DesBarres, 5 March 1786, PANS CO217, 104:312. In this letter Smith resigned his seat on Council.

105 Ibid., 123–201. Several of the letters that passed between DesBarres and Yorke during the period 2 November 1785 to 4 March 1786 illustrate the classic power struggle between a civilian lieutenant governor and a military commanding officer on a small isolated station.

106 Minutes of the Council of Cape Breton, 27 October 1787, PANS CO217, 105:55.

107 NSGWC, 5 September 1786.

108 General Account of Provisions for the Support of 76 Convicts, dated 18 May 1789, PANS CO217, 106:34.

109 Nova Scotia, *Report of the Public Archives*, 24–7, Macarmick to Sydney, 18 March 1789.

110 Testimony from Citizens of Sydney for Dr Smith, 29 September 1791, PANS CO217, 108:347.

111 Return of the Number of Inhabitants of Cape Breton who are enrolled and liable to serve in the militia, 1 August 1790, PANS CO217, 107:273. It was estimated that, in addition, there were five hundred Jersey men who came every summer to the island. This was a substantial increase (sixty-six percent) over the 361 heads of household recorded by the Reverend Ranna Cossitt in his diary on 29 August 1788 (Rev. Ranna Cossitt, 17, PANS Micro Biography). The Reverend Mr Cossitt lists the number of families at Arichat as 170 and tabulates the number of men, women, children, and servants residing at fifteen other settlements in Cape Breton. By 1793, the number of resident inhabitants of Cape Breton Island "liable to serve in the Militia" was reduced to 423, according to PANS CO217, 109:54.

112 Minutes of the Council of Cape Breton, 8 March 1786, PANS CO217, 105:229.

113 Minutes of the Council of Cape Breton, 18 May 1791, PANS CO217, 108:165.

114 Cossitt to Secretary to the Society for the Propagation of the Gospel, 18 December 1791, PANS CO217, 108:351. The last four words in the quotation, "but to no effect," refer probably to Cossitt's difficulty in obtaining sufficient money to erect a proper church building.

115 Macarmick to Dundas, 16 September 1794, PANS CO217, 110:230. Sydney had declined in population dramatically by the year 1795, when it was reported that only 121 people resided in the town. Twenty-seven of the seventy-one houses were inhabited, with the remaining houses either uninhabited or in ruins (ibid., 111:245).

116 Anonymous letter, 18 February 1796, PANS CO217, 114:124. This was the Royal Nova Scotia Regiment.

117 Memorial of William Stafford, surgeon of HM Garrison at Cape Breton, 10 March 1798, PANS CO217, 116:80. James Miller's plan of

Sydney (Figure 23), showing the hospital of which Dr Stafford was put in charge, is taken from ibid., 111:245.

118 Ogilvie to King, 5 August 1798, PANS CO217, 115:87.

119 Smith to Ogilvie, 25 March 1799, PANS CO217, 117:62; Murray to Portland, July 1799, ibid., 123.

120 Minutes of the Council of Cape Breton, 18 May 1797, PANS CO217, 113:152. The announcement of McKinnon's suspension was made by Mathews at this meeting. Dr Smith and Mr Ball each submitted a report giving their opinion of the suspension (PANS CO217, 115:318–20, and 323–4). Mathews was replaced as president of the Council by Lieutenant General James Ogilvie six months later (Portland to Ogilvie, 12 December 1797, PANS CO217, 113:271).

121 Whitehall to Murray, 11 October 1799, PANS CO217, 117:149.

122 Despard to Portland, 23 September 1800, PANS CO217, 118:230.

123 Despard to Portland, 27 September 1800, PANS CO217, 118:232.

124 Smith to Pelham, 3 August 1801, PANS CO217, 119:178; Smith to Hobart, 4 April 1802, ibid., 120:190.

125 Because the name William Smith is so common, it has been impossible to determine when and where Dr William Smith died. It does appear that he was alive as late as 1820, since a notice placed in the *Weekly Chronicle* of 18 February 1820 stated that the property in Sydney, owned by William Smith, Esquire, Chief Justice of Cape Breton, was for sale.

126 Minutes of 12 June 1797 (first reading); 13 June 1797 (second reading); and page 250, 27 June 1797 (deferred), Nova Scotia, *Journal,* 1797, 239, 250. John Sargent (1749–1824) was a member of the Legislative Assembly for Barrington Township for the period 1793 to 1818. The minutes of the Legislative Council for the year 1797–99 (PANS RG1, vol. 218 M to O) do not mention this medical bill.

127 Nova Scotia, *Journal* 1815–20, 31.

128 Ibid., 1828, 24.

129 Clark, *A History of the Royal College of Physicians of London,* 54–5.

130 Shafer, *The American Medical Profession, 1783 to 1850,* 204.

131 Bordley and Harvey, *Two Centuries of American Medicine,* 69.

132 Shafer, *The American Medical Profession,* 206.

133 Abbott, *History of Medicine in the Province of Quebec,* 31. Persons referred to as charlatans had been practising medicine from the earliest times. These unqualified practitioners were described usually as quacks. The derivation and meaning of quackery is obscure, and there are a number of opinions concerning its origin (see Steiner, "The Conflict of Medicine with Quackery," 60). One explanation is that quackery came from the German quack-silver (mercury), for irregular practitioners used quack-silver in the treatment of syphilis. An-

other explanation is that quack is an abbreviation for quacksalver, quack being to utter loud and pretentious statements and salver being one who undertakes to perform cures by the application of ointments or cerates.

134 Quebec, Statutes, 28 Geo. 3, cap. 8, 1788.

135 Godfrey, *Medicine for Ontario*, 16.

136 Twelve newspapers were published in Nova Scotia during the period 1752–99, of which I have read 2,104 individual issues. This represents about half the issues published. Unfortunately, the remaining issues for the period have not been found.

137 Packard, *History of Medicine in the United States* 1:273.

138 Marks and Beatty, *The Story of Medicine in America*, 118.

139 Christianson, "The Emergence of Medical Communities in Massachusetts," 64.

140 The Register of Students attending medical lectures, 1768–1815 (University of Pennsylvania Archives, MSS 1575) records that Robert Clark of Halifax was attending medical lectures there during the winter of 1805–06, while William Duncan Clark attended lectures from 1810–12. These two young men were the sons of Dr Duncan Clark, who came to Halifax with the 82nd Regiment in 1778 and took up residence and practice in Halifax after the cessation of the American war. The MD that Robert Tucker was awarded in 1770 was the first earned MD granted by a medical school in the American colonies. Daniel Turner had been awarded the first honorary degree of Doctor of Medicine by Yale in 1723, according to Lane, "Daniel Turner and the First Degree of Doctor of Medicine Conferred," 367–80.

141 Medical School, in the College of New York
The Lectures to be delivered by the several Professors on Anatomy, Chemistry, Surgery, Midwifery, the Institutes of Medicine, the Practice of Physic, and on the clinical Cases of Patients in the New York Hospital, will commence in the Hall of Columbia College, in the City of New York, on the second Monday of November next.
The Lectures on Materia Medica, and on Botany, are Summer Courses, and will begin, and will continue annually, on the first Monday of July.
New York, August 28th, 1794.

142 It would be expected that a number of these men served an apprenticeship in Halifax before going to London. It is known that three of them, James Geddes, John B. Houseal, and Benjamin De St Croix, studied with Dr John Halliburton at the naval hospital, and

that George Houseal served his apprenticeship with Dr William
J. Almon. In addition to these sixteen, at least three native-born Nova
Scotians, and four others who were raised in Nova Scotia, trained
to become medical practitioners during the last twenty years of the
eighteenth century; however, the place where each received his
training is not known. They were: Jonathan W. Clark, Windsor; Gurdon Dennison, Horton; Dennis Heffernan, Halifax; John Jones,
Halifax; Joseph Prescott, Chester; Benjamin Prince, Annapolis; and
Jacob Tobias, Digby.

143 This reduction in the number of doctors in Nova Scotia was felt mainly
in the Loyalist towns of Shelburne and Digby. Of the twelve doctors who had arrived in Shelburne in 1783, four had died, and the
other eight had left the town and the province by 1799, leaving
Shelburne without a doctor for its estimated 750 residents (Rev. James
Munro visited Shelburne in 1795 and estimated that there were
only 150 families and about 750 people in the town. See Nova Scotia,
Report of the Board of Trustees, 43). Seven doctors had taken up residence in Digby after the revolution; by 1799, only one, Christian Tobias, remained. According to the Letter Book of Rev. Edward
Brudenell (PANS Micro Biography), four of the doctors, Abraham Florentine, Isaac Goodman, Fleming Pinckston, and Joseph Mervin
(or Marvin), had "gone to the States," while two others, Alexander Phillips and William Young, were said to have "left the Province."
Brudenell points out that between December 1785 and December
1787, eighty heads of households, out of 312 on the poll list of
1785, had left Digby.

144 Beekman, "The Rise of British Surgery," 549–66. Peachey, *A
Memoir of William and John Hunter*, identified forty-nine men in London
who offered private lectures in anatomy, physic, *materica medica*,
botany, chemistry, and midwifery, during the period 1700–49.

145 Lawrence, "Alexander Monro, *primus*, and the Edinburgh Manner," 193–214.

146 Gelfand, "The Paris 'Manner' of Dissection," 99–130.

147 Lawrence, "Entrepreneurs and Private Enterprise," 171–92.

148 Ransom, "The Beginnings of Hospitals in the United States,"
514–39.

149 Burnby, "A Study of the English Apothecary," 114.

150 King, *The Medical World of the Eighteenth-Century*, 233.

151 Jewson, "Medical Knowledge and the Patronage System," 369–85.

152 Porter, and Porter, *Patient's Progress: Doctors and Doctoring in 18th Century England*.

153 Ackerknecht, "From Barber-Surgeon to Modern Surgeon," 545–53.

154 Letter written by Halliburton, 21 August 1794, PANS Adm. 1/492,
folio 440.

155 State of the Royal Nova Scotia Regiment, 15 April 1796, PANS CO217, 67:81.

156 Land Grant Petitions, PANS RG20, series A, vol. 24, no. 10.

157 Drew, *Roll of Commissioned Officers* 1:114. Dr Boggs was my great, great, great, great grandfather.

158 Ibid., 37.

159 These regiments were the 4th, 6th, 7th, 16th, 20th, 21st, 24th, 47th, 57th, 65th, 66th, and the Royal Nova Scotia Regiment.

160 Stratton to Prince Edward, 27 March 1795, NAC WO1, 17:61. It is likely that the regiment using Fort Massey as its hospital was the Royal Fusiliers, or 7th Regiment, which had arrived in Halifax in 1795.

161 State of the Royal Nova Scotia Regiment, 15 April 1796, PANS CO217, 67:81. This return indicates that the regiment had a surgeon, a hospital mate, an orderly, and twenty-six patients in the regimental hospital.

162 Ibid., 125; 70:183.

163 NSGWC, 30 September 1794.

164 Ibid., 19 November 1799. The cure was described as "an excellent Remedy for a Cough, and Consumptive Complaints" by an anonymous person. It read: "Take as much pervine as will make a quart of strong tea, an equal quantity of Coltsfoot, and of Whorebound, three ounces of the root of Eleacampane, and a small quantity of Rue, put them into five points of pure water, boil them until the Liquor is reduced to one Quart, then put into it two pounds of clean heavy sugar, then boil it until it becomes so thick that when cold, it will be hard as loaf sugar, take a small piece into the Mouth and gradually melt and swallow it, often in the day or night, as the Patient shall find it convenient."

165 Ibid., 25 April 1796.

166 On 6 November 1787, Alexander Abercrombie Peters, who had been awarded an MD by the University of Aberdeen on 2 August 1787, inserted an advertisement in the NSGWC. It was unusual in that it did not mention his newly acquired medical degree; it stated simply that he "means to settle in this Town as a Medical Character. Those who see fit to honor him with their Patronage, may depend on the strictest Attention and Integrity." The *Halifax Journal* of 19 January 1788 contains an advertisement by J. Brown, surgeon and dentist. He was undoubtedly Dr Lewis Joseph Brown, who became involved in several Supreme Court cases in Halifax in 1788 (PANS RG39, series C, Box 51). One of these dealt with his being slandered by Jeremiah Marshman, who claimed that Dr Brown had absconded from town to avoid his creditors. Dr Brown's advertisement informed the public that he had removed to a house, occupied formerly by Hon. Ar-

thur Gould, on the upper side of the lower parade, where he would practise his profession.

167 Donald M'Lean could have been the surgeon by that name who married (in New York, August 1780, a daughter of Capt. Allan Mac-Donald of the 84th Regiment (NSGWC, 22 August 1780). He was stated to have been surgeon to the late 77th Regiment. The first mention of a Donald McLean, surgeon, being in Nova Scotia was on 10 November 1783 when he sold land at Shelburne (Shelburne Deeds, PANS RG47, Book 1:105). It may have been that this same Dr Donald McLean moved into Halifax and placed the advertisements shown above. A Doctor M'Lean resided in Halifax until May 1786, in which month (NSGWC, 16 May 1786) he advertised for sale a variety of elegent pieces of furniture along with a barometer and thermometer. In June 1787, a Donald McLean, surgeon, sold land at Pictou Harbour (Pictou Deeds, PANS RG47, Book 1:15) and, on 20 August 1789, Donald McLean, gentleman, sold additional land on the south side of the entrance to Pictou Harbour (Halifax Deeds, PANS RG47, vol. 28:147). On 5 May 1807, land belonging to Donald MacLean, surgeon, Eighty-second Regiment, deceased, was sold in Pictou County (Pictou Deeds, PANS RG47, Book 5:178). I have been unable to determine whether these Donald McLeans were one and the same person.

168 Dr Francis Brinley died at Shelburne in late June 1785, aged twenty-nine years, according to Shelburne records (PANS MG4, vol. 141). The advertisement in the *Royal American Gazette* of 24 January 1785 was the first mention of Dr Joseph Bond in Nova Scotia.

169 Prior to the revolution, Dr John Boyd practised in Northumberland County, Pennsylvania (Loyalist Claims, PANS Misc. L, AO13, bundle 90). By July 1783 he was a resident of Shelburne and was given Lot 5 in the South Division, Letter B, in the town (PANS RG1, vol. 372).

170 I am not absolutely sure which Dr John Philipps inserted this advertisement. Dr Philipps Sr had been in Halifax since 1758, and his son, Dr John Philipps Jr, who had trained at St George's Hospital, London, during 1778 and 1779, was established as a druggist in Halifax as early as 1789 (Nova Scotia Supreme Court Records, 1789, PANS RG39, series C, Box 56).

171 The use of electrotherapy in medicine had its beginning with the Roman physician Scribonius Largus, who lived in the first century. He described the use of the electric fish, frequently referred to as the torpedo, as follows: "For any type of gout a live black torpedo should when the pain begins, be placed under the feet. The patient must stand on a moist shore washed by the sea and he should stay

like this until his whole foot and leg up to the knee is numb. This takes away present pain and prevents pain from coming on if it has not already arisen" (see Kellaway, "The Part Played by the Electric Fish," 112–37). Instances of Europeans using electric fish in medical therapy can be found in the literature as late as the early nineteenth century. Artificially generated static electricity produced by holding an object against a rotating sphere of sulphur was accomplished first by Otto von Guericke in Magdeburg, about 1663. It is likely that physicians soon made use of static electricity in therapy. The invention of the Leyden Jar in 1745 permitted much larger electric shocks to be administered to muscles and nerves and, between 1750 and 1780, no less than twenty-six papers dealing with electrotherapy appeared in a leading French medical journal. An electric-shock machine was installed in Middlesex Hospital, London, in 1767. Within the next decade, many other hospitals followed suit. It would be expected that Dr Lewis Davis's "electric aparatus" was a variation of a static electric generator.

172 Margaret Doucet was not the first Nova Scotian woman to indicate that she was engaged in the business of offering medical therapy. Ann McGee, in a 1788 petition for a land grant (PANS RG20, series A) stated that "she had been settled in the district of Colchester upwards of 18 years and has used her knowledge of surgeonry [sic] to [help] many unfortunate travellers exposed to frost bite, who might have lost their lives." She signed the petition at Marajamish [sic] on 18 April 1788. In a second Petition (PANS RG20, series A, vol. 31), dated at Dorchester 26 October 1809, Ann McGee, who was possibly related to Barnabus McGee listed in the Return of the Township of Donegal or Pictou, dated 1 January 1770, stated that she had been granted land "in consideration of her humane exertions and relief to the crew of HM schooner *Malignant* at the time of her shipwreck." According to Wyman, "The Surgeoness: The Female Practitioner," 22–41, many women practised as surgeons in England from the sixteenth to the eighteenth century. By the early nineteenth century, however, very few women were practising as surgeons in England.

173 Benjamin Green, Esquire, was the provincial treasurer of Nova Scotia from 1768 to 1793, the year of his death. According to his brother, Francis, Benjamin was the second child of Benjamin and Margaret (Pierce) Green, who came to Halifax from Louisbourg in 1749, when the British garrison was transferred (Genealogical and Biographical Anecdotes of the Green Family ... by Francis Green, 1806, 6, PANS MG1, vol. 332D).

174 *Halifax Journal*, 9 December 1790. Dr John Chichester (ca.1765–1839) had received his medical training at St George's Hospital Medical

School, London, having attended lectures and surgery there during 1787.

175 Gullett, *A History of Dentistry in Canada*, 12.

176 *Nova Scotia Gazette and Weekly Chronicle*, 15 November 1791.

177 Ibid., 1 May 1787. There were undoubtedly many midwives in the province besides Mrs Smith. In Shelburne, for instance, James Mc-Neil was referred to in the Assessment Rolls of 1786 (PANS MG4, vol. 140) as "the midwife's husband."

178 It is noted that Dr Nicolai's name is misspelled in the advertisement. Men had been involved in midwifery since earliest times, according to Mengeit, "The Origin of the Male Midwife," 443–65. Dr Daniel Kendrick of Liverpool, Nova Scotia, professed that he was a man-midwife, according to Perkins's diary entry of 13 July 1790. In April 1796, Dr Kendrick was paid ten shillings for "delivering a woman" (Annapolis Township Book, 6 April 1796, PANS MG4). Surprisingly, this same Doctor Kendrick had been contracted by Simeon Perkins on 7 October 1790 to provide medical attention to his family for one year, for "medicines in all cases except mid-wifery and smallpox."

179 Lieutenant William Booth Diary, entry for 22 February 1789, Acadia University Archives, F1039.5, S546B6.

180 Byles Collection, PANS MG1, vol. 163. A bloodstone is a dark green subtransparent jasper with red spots and cut as a gem. It was believed by noted scientists such as Francis Bacon (1561–1626) that the bloodstone would stop nosebleed by "astriction and cooling of the spirits" (Thorndike, *Science, Medicine, and History* 1:451–4).

181 I have compiled an alphabetical list of Nova Scotians recorded as having died during the period 1749 to 1799. I estimate that these 11,503 recorded deaths represent sixty to seventy percent of the actual number of deaths that took place in Nova Scotia. Only a small fraction of deaths were recorded in newspapers, and church burial records for Halifax and rural Nova Scotia are not complete for the period.

182 The death and burial records indicate that smallpox was the cause of death for six people in Guysborough and for six in Lunenburg. People also died of smallpox in LaHave, Liverpool, and Shelburne. None of the death or burial records for Halifax for the years 1790 and 1791 indicate that anyone there died from the disease.

183 Hollingsworth, "The Demography of the British Peerage," 57. I recognize that the average age at time of death is not the same as life expectancy. The prediction of life expectancy is a statistical calculation and requires that the ages of all persons in the group being assessed are known. Also, life expectancy is calculated with respect

to a reference age; for example, it is very common to give life expectancy at birth statistics.

184 Imhof, "Methodological Problems in Modern Urban History Writing," 101–32.

185 Kunitz, "Making a Long Story Short," 269–80.

186 It is not surprising that heart disease is omitted from the causes of death in the late eighteenth century. The term did not come into general use until the late nineteenth century.

APPENDIX 2

1 King, *The Medical World of the Eighteenth Century*, 83–5.

2 Shafer, *The American Medical Profession, 1783–1850*, 25.

3 Krehl, "Mercury, the Slippery Metal." Calomel was widely used in the sixteenth century as a laxative and in the treatment of syphilis. In the nineteenth century it was recommended as a remedy for fevers, diarrhea, heart disease, worms, rheumatism, and eye disease.

4 The dried root of any of several Mexican plants of the morning-glory family, especially *exogonium purga*.

5 The dried root of the shrubby plant called *cephaelis ipecacuanha*, found in Brazil and Bolivia.

6 This was taken either orally, or as a clyster or enema. In some instances mercury was rendered into a powder and rubbed into the skin about the thighs.

APPENDIX 9

1 Accidents that were not specified.

2 Hectic fever.

3 Under one year of age.

4 These sixty-two people were American prisoners of war who, according to the *Boston Newsletter*, starved to death on a prison ship in Halifax harbour.

5 These six people were shot for desertion.

6 The type of execution was not specified, although it was probably by hanging.

Bibliography

ARCHIVAL SOURCES

ACADIA UNIVERSITY ARCHIVES, WOLFVILLE
Lieutenant William Booth Diary

ARCHIVES NATIONALES, PARIS
Colonies, C"B

EDINBURGH UNIVERSITY ARCHIVES
Matriculation Records for Students in the Faculty of Medicine
Monro, *primus*, Dr Alexander. Record Book of Scholars in Anatomy,
    1720–1749.

MASSACHUSETTS HISTORICAL SOCIETY, BOSTON
Diary of Dr John Jeffries. Jeffries Family Papers, 1686–1835. vols. 30, 31

NATIONAL ARCHIVES OF CANADA, OTTAWA
Admiralty 50   Journal of Admiral Edward Boscawen
Colonial Office 5   Military Despatches
Manuscript Group 23   DesBarres Collection
Record Group 8   British Military and Naval Papers
War Office 1   Correspondence: In-Letters

PUBLIC ARCHIVES OF NOVA SCOTIA, HALIFAX
Admiralty 1   Admiral's Despatches
Audit Office 12, 13   Loyalist Claims
Colonial Office 217   Original Correspondence, Secretary of State
             218   Letters from Secretary of State
             221   Shipping Returns

Manuscript Group	1	Papers of Families and Individuals
	3	Business Papers
	4	Church Records and Township Records
	5	Cemetery Inscriptions
	12	Great Britain, Army
	13	Great Britain, Navy
	100	Miscellaneous Manuscripts
Micro Biography		Letter Book of Chief Justice Jonathan Belcher
		Letter Book of Rev. Edward Brudenell
		Sir Guy Carleton
		George Chalmers Collection
		Rev. Ranna Cossitt
		Earl of Dartmouth
		Andrew S. Hamond
		Diary of John Salusbury at Halifax, 1749–1753
Micro Miscellaneous		A, Armies–Colonial
		L, Loyalist Claims
		s, Ships
Record Group	1	Public Records of Nova Scotia
	5	Records of the Legislative Assembly of Nova Scotia
	20	Land Grant Petitions
	22	Nova Scotia Military Records
	37	Inferior Court of Common Pleas
	39	Supreme Court
	47	Deeds
	48	Probate

Records of the Society for the Propagation of the Gospel in Foreign Parts
Vertical File. Vol. 312, no. 29. Antliff, W.B. "Loyalist Claims – A Wealth of
Information." Typescript. 1986.

PUBLIC RECORD OFFICE, KEW

Admiralty	1	Secretary's Department: In-Letters
	11	Return of Officers
	97	In-Letters
	98	Out-Letters
War Office	25	Registers
	34	Amherst Papers

ROYAL COLLEGE OF SURGEONS' LIBRARY, LONDON
Company of Surgeons' Examination Book, 1745–1800

ST GEORGE'S HOSPITAL MEDICAL SCHOOL, LONDON
Register of Pupils and House Officers, 1756–1837

ST THOMAS'S HOSPITAL MEDICAL SCHOOL, LONDON
Index to St Thomas's Pupils and Dressers, 1723–1819
Index to Pupils and Dressers, 1768–1819, for Guy's Hospital Medical
School

UNIVERSITY OF PENNSYLVANIA ARCHIVES, PHILADELPHIA
Register of Students Attending Medical Lectures, 1768–1815

PUBLISHED SOURCES

Abbott, M.E. *History of Medicine in the Province of Quebec.* Toronto: Macmillan Co., 1931.
Ackerknecht, E.H. "From Barber-Surgeon to Modern Surgeon." *Bulletin of the History of Medicine* 58 (1984): 545–53.
Akins, T.B. "History of Halifax City." In *Collections of the Nova Scotia Historical Society.* Vol. 8. Halifax: Nova Scotia Historical Society, 1895. 8.
Akins, T.B. ed. *Selections from the Public Documents of the Province of Nova Scotia.* Halifax: Charles Annand, 1869.
Anderson, Peter J. *Officers and Graduates of the University and King's College, Aberdeen.* Aberdeen: New Spaulding Club, 1893.
– ed. *Selections from the Records of Marischal College and University, 1593–1869.* Vol. 2. Aberdeen: New Spaulding Club, 1889–98.
Annals of the North British Society, Halifax, Nova Scotia, 1768–1903. Halifax: McAlpine Publishing Co., 1905.
Archibald, R.C. *Carlyle's First Love, Margaret Gordon, Lady Bannerman.* London: John Lane, 1910.
Army Lists 1758–99. An annual. London: Printed by J. Millan.
Bartlet, W.S. *The Frontier Missionary: A Memoir of the Life of the Rev. Jacob Bailey,* AM. Boston: Ide and Dutton, 1853.
Bates, G.T. "The Cornwallis Settlers who Didn't." In *Collections of the Nova Scotia Historical Society.* Vol. 38, Halifax: Nova Scotia Historical Society, 1973.
– "John Gorham, an Outline of his Activities in Nova Scotia, 1744–1751." In *Collections of the Nova Scotia Historical Society.* Vol. 30. Halifax: Nova Scotia Historical Society, 1954.
Baugh, D.A. *British Naval Administration in the Age of Walpole.* Princeton: Princeton University Press, 1965.
Beekman, F. "The Rise of British Surgery in the Eighteenth-Century." *Annals of Medical History* 9, n.s. (1937): 549–66.
Bell, W.P. *The Foreign Protestants and the Settlement of Nova Scotia.* Toronto: University of Toronto Press, 1961.
Bordley, J., and A.M. Harvey. *Two Centuries of American Medicine.* Philadelphia: Saunders, 1976.

Bowers, J.Z., and E.F. Purcell, eds. *Advances in American Medicine: Essays at the Bicentennial*. Vol. 1. New York: Macy Foundation, 1976.

Brebner, J.B. *The Neutral Yankees of Nova Scotia: A Marginal Colony during the Revolutionary Years*. New York: Columbia University Press, 1937. Reprint. Toronto: McClelland and Stewart, 1969.

Brown, W. *The King's Friends; The Composition and Motives of the American Loyalist Claimants*. Providence, RI: Brown University Press, 1965.

Burnby, J.G.L. "A Study of the English Apothecary from 1660 to 1760." *Medical History*. Supplement 3 (1983).

Burrage, W.L. *A History of the Massachusetts Medical Society: with Brief Biographies of the Founders and Officers, 1781–1922*. Norwood, Massachusetts: Plimpton Press, 1923.

Bynum, W.F. "Health, Disease, and Medical Care." In *The Ferment of Knowledge*. Edited by G.S. Rousseau and R. Porter, Cambridge: Cambridge University Press, 1980.

Bynum, W.F., and V. Nutton, eds. *Theories of Fever from Antiquity to the Enlightenment*. London: Wellcome Historical Medical Institute, 1981.

Cameron, K.W. *The Papers of Loyalist Samuel Peters*. Hartford: Trancendental Books, 1978.

Campbell, D.A. "Pioneers of Medicine in Nova Scotia." *Maritime Medical News* 16 (1904): 195–210, 243–53, 519–27; 17 (1905): 8–17.

Canniff, W. *The Medical Profession in Upper Canada, 1783–1850*. Toronto: Briggs, 1894. Reprint. Toronto: Clarke Irwin for the Hannah Institute for the History of Medicine, 1980.

Cartwright, F.F. *Disease and History*. London: Hart-Davis, 1972.

Chaplin, A. *Medicine in England during the Reign of George III*. London: Kimpton, 1919.

Chichester, H.M., and G. Burges-Short. *The Records and Badges of Every Regiment and Corps in the British Army*. London: Gale and Polden Ltd, 1900.

Christianson, E.H. "The Emergence of Medical Communities in Massachusetts, 1700–1794, The Demographic Factors." *Bulletin of the History of Medicine* 54 (1980): 64–77.

Clark, A.H. *Acadia, the Geography of Early Nova Scotia to 1760*. Madison: University of Wisconsin Press, 1968.

Clark G. *A History of the Royal College of Physicians of London*. 3 vols. Oxford: Clarendon Press, 1964.

Clark, W.B., and W.J. Morgan, eds. *Naval Documents of the American Revolution*. Vols 2–6. Washington: US Government Printing Office, 1966 (vol. 2), 1968 (vol. 3), 1969 (vol. 4), 1970 (vol. 5), 1972 (vol. 6).

Clark-Kennedy, A.E. *Stephen Hales: an Eighteenth Century Biography*. Cambridge: Cambridge University Press, 1929.

Columbia University. *Columbia University Alumni Register, 1745–1931*. New York: Columbia University Press, 1931.

Comrie, J.D. *History of Scottish Medicine to 1860.* London: Wellcome Historical Medical Museum, 1927.

Cooter, R., ed. *Studies in the History of Alternative Medicine.* New York: St Martin's Press, 1988.

Cope, Z. *The History of the Royal College of Surgeons of England.* London: Blond, 1959.

Cunningham, A. "Thomas Sydenham: Epidemics, Experiment and the 'Good Old Cause.'" In *The Medical Revolution of the Seventeenth Century.* Edited by R. French and A. Wear. Cambridge: Cambridge University Press, 1989.

Davies, K.G., ed. *Documents of the American Revolution, 1770–1783.* Colonial Office series. Dublin: Irish University Press, 1976.

"Documents Related to Cape Breton, 1788–1789." In *Annual Report of the Public Archives of Nova Scotia.* Halifax: Public Archives of Nova Scotia, 1950.

Donnison, J. *Midwives and Medical Men: A History of Inter-Professional Rivalries.* London: Heineman Foundation, 1977.

Doughty, A.G., ed. *An Historical Journal of the Campaigns in North America for the Years 1757, 1758, 1759, and 1760 by Captain John Knox.* 3 vols. Toronto: The Champlain Society, 1914–16.

Drake, G.H. "The Wet Nurse in France in the 18th Century." *Bulletin of the History of Medicine* 8 (1940): 934–48.

Drew, R. *Roll of Commissioned Officers in the Medical Services of the British Army, 1660–1960.* 2 vols. London: Wellcome Historical Medical Institute, 1968.

Duncanson, J.V. *Falmouth. A New England Township in Nova Scotia, 1760–1965.* Windsor, Ontario, 1965. Private printing.

Ellis, R.L. *A Genealogical Register of Edmund Rice Descendants.* Rutland, Vermont: C.E. Tuttle & Co., 1970.

Ells, Margaret. "Nova Scotian, Sparks of Liberty." *Dalhousie Review* 16 (1937): 475–92.

Fildes, V.A. *Wet Nursing. A History from Antiquity to the Present.* New York: Blackwell, 1988.

Force, P., comp. *American Archives.* 4th ser., vols. 3–6. Containing a Documentary History of the English Colonies in North America from the King's Message to Parliament, of March 7, 1774 to the Declaration of Independence by the United States. Washington: M.S. Clarke, 1840 (vol. 3), 1843 (vol. 4), 1844 (vol. 5), and 1846 (vol. 6).

French, R., and A. Wear, eds. *The Medical Revolution of the Seventeenth Century* Cambridge: Cambridge University Press, 1989.

Garrison, F.H. *An Introduction to the History of Medicine.* Philadelphia: Saunders, 1914.

Gelfand, T. "The Paris 'Manner' of Dissection: Student Anatomical Dissection in Early Eighteenth-Century Paris." *Bulletin of the History of Medicine* 46 (1972): 99–130.

Glass, D.V., and D.E.C. Eversley, eds. *Population in History: Essays in Historical Demography.* Chicago: Aldine Publishing Co., 1965.

Godfrey, C.M. *Medicine for Ontario, A History.* Belleville: Mika, 1979.

Gordon, M.B. *Aesculapius Comes to the Colonies; The Story of the Early Days of Medicine in the Thirteen Original Colonies.* Ventnor, NJ: Ventnor, 1949.

Gordon, William Augustus. "Journal Kept by Gordon, one of the Officers engaged in the Siege of Louisbourg under Boscawen and Amherst." In *Collections of the Nova Scotia Historical Society.* Vol. 5. Halifax: Nova Scotia Historical Society, 1887.

Granshaw, L., and R. Porter, eds. *The Hospital and History.* London and New York: Routledge, 1989.

Gullett, D.W. *A History of Dentistry in Canada.* Toronto: University of Toronto Press, 1971.

Haliburton, T.C. *An Historical and Statistical Account of Nova Scotia.* 2 vols. Halifax: Joseph Howe, 1829.

Hannaway, C.C. "Veterinary Medicine and Rural Health Care in Pre-Revolutionary France." *Bulletin of the History of Medicine* 51 (1977): 431–47.

Harris, E.D. *An Account of Some of the Descendants of Capt. Thomas Brattle.* Boston: Clapp and Son, 1867.

Heagerty, J.J. *Four Centuries of Medical History in Canada, and a Sketch of the Medical History of Newfoundland.* Vol. 1. Toronto: MacMillan, 1928.

Hessische Truppen im Amerikanischen Unabhängigkeitskrieg (Hetrina). Vol. 2. Marburg: Archivschule, 1974.

Hoad, L.M. *Surgeons and Surgery in Île Royale.* Publication no. 6. National Historic Parks and Sites Branch. Ottawa: Supply and Services Canada, 1976.

Hofstadter, R. *America at 1750, A Social Portrait.* New York: Random House, 1971.

Hollingsworth, T.H. "The Demography of the British Peerage." *Population Studies.* Supplement to vol. 18, no. 2 (1964): 57.

Hopkins, D.R. *Princes and Peasants: Smallpox in History.* Chicago: University of Chicago Press, 1983.

Howie, W.B. "Finance and Supply in an Eighteenth-Century Hospital, 1747–1830." *Medical History* 7 (1963): 126–46.

Imhof, A. "Methodological Problems in Modern Urban History Writing: Graphical Representation of Urban Mortality, 1750–1850." In *Problems and Methods in the History of Medicine.* Edited by R. Porter and A. Wear. London: Croom Helm, 1987.

Innis, H.A., D.C. Harvey, and C.B. Fergusson, eds. *The Diary of Simeon Perkins.* 4 vols. Toronto: The Champlain Society, 1948–67.

Jeffries, J.T.L. *Jeffries of Massachusetts, 1658–1914.* N.p., 1914.

Jewson, N. "Medical Knowledge and the Patronage System in 18th Century England." *Sociology* 8 (1974): 369–85.

Jones, E.A. *The Loyalists of Massachusetts, Their Memorials, Petitions, and Claims.* London: Saint Catherine Press, 1930.

Journal of the Commissioners for Trade and Plantations. Vols. 8 and 9, 1741–53. London: HM Stationery Office, 1931 (vol. 8), 1932 (vol. 9).

Kellaway, P. "The Part Played by the Electric Fish in the Early History of Bioelectricity and Electrotherapy." *Bulletin of the History of Medicine* 20 (1946): 535–41.

Kelly, A.D. "Health Insurance in New France." *Bulletin of the History of Medicine* 28 (1954).

King, L.S. *The Medical World of the Eighteenth Century.* Huntington, New York: Krieger Publishing Co., 1958.

Knap, Nathaniel. *The Diary of Nathaniel Knap of Newbury in the Province of Massachusetts Bay in New England written at the Second Siege of Louisbourg in 1758.* Publication no. 2. Proceedings of Colonial Wars. Boston: Society of Colonial Wars, 1895.

Knowles, J.H. *Hospitals, Doctors, and the Public Interest.* Cambridge: Harvard University Press, 1965.

Krehl, W.A. "Mercury, the Slippery Metal." *Nutrition Today* 7 (1972): 4–15.

Kunitz, S.J. "Making a Long Story Short: A Note of Men's Height and Mortality in England from the 1st through the 19th Centuries." *Medical History* 31 (1987): 269–80.

Lane, J.E. "Daniel Turner and the First Degree of Doctor of Medicine conferred in the English Colonies in North America by Yale College in 1723." *Annals of Medical History* 2 (1919): 367–80.

Laufe, L.E. *Obstetric Forceps.* New York: Harper and Row, 1968.

Lawrence, C. "Alexander Monro, *primus*, and the Edinburgh Manner of Anatomy." *Bulletin of the History of Medicine* 62 (1988): 193–214.

Lawrence, Charles. "Journal, and letters, being a day-by-day account of the founding of Lunenburg, by the Officer in Command of the Project." Bulletin no. 10. Public Archives of Nova Scotia. Halifax: Public Archives of Nova Scotia, 1953.

Lawrence, S.C. "Entrepreneurs and Private Enterprise: The Development of Medical Lecturing in London, 1775–1820." *Bulletin of the History of Medicine* 62 (1988): 171–92.

LeFanu, W.R. "The Lost Half-Century of English Medicine, 1700–1750." *Bulletin of the History of Medicine* 46 (1972): 319–48.

Leiby, A.C. *The Revolutionary War in the Hackensack Valley.* New Brunswick, NJ: Rutgers University Press, 1962.

Levine, I.E. *Conqueror of Smallpox, Dr Edward Jenner.* New York: Messner, 1960.

Lind, J. *A Treatise of the Scurvy in Three Parts Containing an Inquiry into the Nature, Causes, and Cure of that Disease, together with a Critical and Chronological View of what has been published on the Subject.* Edinburgh: Sands, Murray, and Cochran, 1753.

Lonie, I.M. "Fever Pathology in the 16th Century: Tradition and Innovation." In *Theories of Fever from Antiquity to the Enlightenment*. Supplement 1. Edited by W.F. Bynum and V. Nutton. London: Wellcome Historical Medical Institute, 1981.

"Louisbourg Soldiers." *The New England Historical and Genealogical Register*. vol. 24. Boston: New England Historic Genealogical Society, 1870.

MacKay, R. "Poor Relief and Medicine in Nova Scotia, 1749–1783." In *Collections of the Nova Scotia Historical Society*. Vol. 24. Halifax: Nova Scotia Historical Society, 1938.

MacLennan, J.S. *Louisbourg, from its Foundation to its Fall, 1713–1758*. London: Macmillan and C., 1918. Reprint. Sydney: Fortress Press, 1969.

Marble, A.E. "He Usefully Exercised the Medical Profession: The Career of Michael Head in Eighteenth-Century Nova Scotia." *Nova Scotia Historical Review* 8, no. 2 (1988): 40–56.

– "The History of Medicine in Nova Scotia, 1783–1854." *Collections of the Nova Scotia Historical Society*. Vol. 41. Halifax: Nova Scotia Historical Society, 1982.

Marks, G., and W.K. Beatty. *The Story of Medicine in America*. New York: Scribner's, 1973.

Martin, J. "Sauvages's Nosology: Medical Enlightenment in Montpellier." In *The Medical Enlightenment of the Eighteenth Century*. Edited by A. Cunningham and R. French. Cambridge: Cambridge University Press, 1990.

McDonald, Captain Alexander. "Letter Book of Captain Alexander McDonald." In *Collections of the New York Historical Society*. Vol. 15. New York: New York Historical Society, 1882.

McKeown, T. "A Sociological Approach to the History of Medicine." *Medical History* 14 (1970): 342–51.

Shortt, S.E.D., ed. *Medicine in Canadian Society*. Montreal: McGill-Queen's University Press, 1981.

Medvei, V.C., and J.L. Thornton, eds. *The Royal Hospital of Saint Bartholomew, 1123–1973*. London: Cowell, 1974.

Mengeit, W.F. "The Origin of the Male Midwife." *Annals of Medical History* 4, n.s. (1932): 453–65.

Middleton, W.S. "The Yellow Fever Epidemic of 1793 in Philadelphia." *Annals of Medical History* 10 (1928): 434–50.

Miller, G. *The Adoption of Inoculation for Smallpox in England and France*. Philadelphia: University of Pennsylvania Press, 1957.

Milner, W.C. "Records of Chignecto." In *Collections of the Nova Scotia Historical Society*. Vol. 15. Halifax: Nova Scotia Historical Society, 1911.

Munk, W. *The Roll of the Royal College of Physicians of London*. Vol. 2, 1701–1800. London: Royal College of Physicians, 1878.

Munro, Rev. James. "MSS History and Description and State of the Southern and Western Townships of Nova Scotia in 1795." *Annual Report of the Public Archives of Nova Scotia*. Halifax: Public Archives of Nova Scotia, 1946.

Murdoch, B. *A History of Nova Scotia, or Acadie.* 3 vols. Halifax: Barnes, 1865–67.

Northcliffe Collection. The papers of General Robert Monckton. Ottawa: King's Printer, 1926.

Nova Scotia Calendar or, an Almanack. Halifax: Printed by A. Henry, 1778.

Nova Scotia. House of Assembly. *Journal of the House of Assembly.* 1758–1799. Halifax: King's Printer.

– *Nova Scotia Laws, 1758–1804.* The Statutes at Large Passed in The Second General Assemblies held in His Majesty's Province of Nova Scotia. Halifax: R.J. Uniacke, 1805.

– Public Archives of Nova Scotia. *Report of the Board of Trustees of the Public Archives of Nova Scotia for 1946.* Halifax: Public Archives of Nova Scotia, n.d.

– *Report of The Public Archives of Nova Scotia.* Halifax: Public Archives of Nova Scotia, 1950.

Ontario. Bureau of Archives. *Second Report of the Bureau of Archives of The Province of Ontario, Part 2.* Proceedings of the Loyalist Commissioners, St John, 1786. Vol. 11. Printed by Order of The Legislative Assembly of Ontario, 1904.

Osler, W. *The Evolution of Modern Medicine.* New York: Arno Press, 1972.

Packard, F.R. *History of Medicine in the United States.* New York: Hafner Publishing Co., 1963.

Paine, N. *Genealogical Notes on the Paine Family of Worcester, Massachusetts.* Albany, 1878. Privately printed.

Patterson, G. *A History of Pictou County, Nova Scotia.* Montreal: Dawson Bros, 1877.

Peachey, G.C. *A Memoir of William and John Hunter.* Plymouth: Brendon Press, 1924.

Piers, H. *The Evolution of the Halifax Fortress, 1749–1928.* Publication no. 7. Public Archives of Nova Scotia. Halifax: Public Archives of Nova Scotia, 1947.

– "The Fortieth Regiment Raised at Annapolis Royal in 1717; and Five Regiments subsequently Raised in Nova Scotia." In *Collections of the Nova Scotia Historical Society.* Vol. 21. Halifax: Nova Scotia Historical Society, 1927.

Poole, E.D. *Annals of Yarmouth and Barrington, Nova Scotia, in the Revolutionary War.* Yarmouth: Lawson, 1899.

Porter, D., and R. Porter. *Patients's Rights: Doctors and Doctoring in 18th Century England.* Stanford: Stanford University Press, 1989.

Porter, R. "The Gift Relation: Philanthropy and Provincial Hospitals in Eighteenth-Century England." In *The Hospital and History.* Edited by L. Granshaw and R. Porter. London and New York: Routledge, 1989.

– "Before the Fringe: 'Quackery' and the Eighteenth-Century Medical Market." In *Studies in the History of Alternative Medicine.* Edited by R. Cooter. New York: St Martin's Press, 1988.

– *A Social History of Madness*. London: Weidenfeld and Nicolson, 1987.

Porter, R., and A. Wear, eds. *Problems and Methods in the History of Medicine.* London: Croom Helm, 1987.

Potter, J. "The Growth of Population in America, 1700–1800." In *Population in History: Essays in Historical Demography.* Edited by D.V. Glass and D.E.C. Eversley. Chicago: Aldine Publishing Co., 1965.

Punch, T.M. "The Irish Catholics, Halifax's First Minority Group." *Nova Scotia Historical Quarterly* 10, no. 1 (1980): 23–40.

Quebec. Legislative Council. Statutes of the Quebec Legislative Council.

Ransom, J.F. "The Beginnings of Hospitals in the United States." *Bulletin of the History of Medicine* 13 (1943): 514–39.

Raymond, W.O. "Colonel Alexander McNutt and the Pre-Loyalist Settlements of Nova Scotia." In *Transactions of the Royal Society of Canada.* 3d ser., section 2. Ottawa: Royal Society of Canada, 1911.

– "Roll of Officers of the British American or Loyalist Corps, 1775–1783." *Collections of the New Brunswick Historical Society.* Vol. 2, no. 5. St John, NB: Barnes and Co., 1904.

Razzell, P. *The Conquest of Smallpox: The Impact of Inoculation on Smallpox Mortality in Eighteenth-Century Britain.* Sussex: Caliban Books, 1977.

Reiser, S.J. *Medicine and the Reign of Technology.* New York: Cambridge University Press, 1878.

Risse, G.B. "Typhus Fever in the 18th Century Hospitals: New Approaches to Medical Treatment." *Bulletin of the History of Medicine* 59 (1985): 176–95.

Rodger, N.A.M. *The Wooden World, An Anatomy of the Georgian Navy.* London: Collins, 1986.

Rousseau, G.S., and R. Porter, eds. *The Ferment of Knowledge.* Cambridge: Cambridge University Press, 1980.

Scott, H.E., ed. *The Journal of the Reverend Jonathan Scott.* Boston: New England Historic Genealogical Society, 1980.

Shafer, H.B. *The American Medical Profession, 1783 to 1850.* New York: AMS Press, 1936.

Smith, D.C. "Concept of Typhus in Mid-Eighteenth-Century Britain." In *Theories of Fever from Antiquity to the Enlightenment.* Supplement 1. Edited by W.F. Bynum and V. Nutton. London: Wellcome Historical Medical Institute, 1981.

Smith, Dr William. *State of the Gaols in London, Westminster, and Borough of Southwark.* London: J. Bew, 1776.

Spencer, H.R. *The History of British Midwifery from 1650 to 1800.* London: Bale, 1927.

Stark, J.H. *The Loyalists of Massachusetts and the Other Side of the American Revolution.* Boston: Clarke Co., 1907.

Steel's Original and Correct List of the Royal Navy. An annual. London: Printed for D. Steel, 1781–99.

Steiner, W.R. "The Conflict of Medicine with Quackery." *Annals of Medical History* 6 (1924): 60–70.

Stubbing, C.H. "Dockyard Memoranda, 1894." *Collections of the Nova Scotia Historical Society.* Vol. 13. Halifax: Nova Scotia Historical Society, 1908.

Thacher, J. *American Medical Biography*, New York: Da Capo Press, 1967.

Thomas, John. "Diary of John Thomas." In *Collections of the Nova Scotia Historical Society.* Vol. 1. Halifax: Nova Scotia Historical Society, 1879.

Thorndyke, L. "The Attitude of Francis Bacon and Descartes towards Magic and Occult Science." In *Science, Medicine, and History.* Vol. 1. Edited by E.A. Underwood. New York: Arno Press, 1975.

Traux, R. *Joseph Lister, Father of Modern Surgery.* London: Harrap & Co., 1947.

"Trials for Treason, 1776–1777." In *Collections of the Nova Scotia Historical Society.* Vol. 1. Halifax: Nova Scotia Historical Society, 1879.

Tunis. B. "Dr James Latham (c.1734–1799): Pioneer Inoculator in Canada." *Canadian Bulletin of Medical History* 1, no. 1 (1984): 1–12.

Tutty, Rev. William. "Letters and Other Papers relating to the Early History of the Church of England in Nova Scotia." In *Collections of the Nova Scotia Historical Society.* Vol. 7. Halifax: Nova Scotia Historical Society, 1891.

Underwood, E.A., ed. *Science, Medicine, and History.* New York: Arno Press, 1975.

Fergusson, C.B., ed. *Uniacke's Sketches of Cape Breton.* Halifax: Public Archives of Nova Scotia, 1958.

Upton, L.F.S. *Micmacs and Colonists: Indian-White Relations in the Maritimes, 1713–1867.* Vancouver: University of British Columbia Press, 1979.

Vernon, C.W. *Bicentennial Sketches and Early Days of the Church in Nova Scotia.* Halifax: Chronicle Printing Co., 1910.

von Eelking, M. *The German Allied Troops in the North American War of Independence, 1776–1783.* Baltimore: Baltimore Genealogical Publishing Co., 1969.

von Riedesel, Baroness. *Baroness von Riedesel and the American Revolution, Journal and Correspondence of a Tour of Duty, 1776–1783.* Chapel Hill: University of North Carolina Press for the Institute of Early American History and Culture at Williamsburg, Virginia, 1965.

Walford, R.I. *The 120-Year Diet.* New York: Simon and Shuster, 1986.

Webster, J.C., ed. *Journal of William Amherst in America, 1758–1760.* London: Butler and Tanner, 1927.

Willard, Abijah. "Journal of Abijah Willard of Lancaster, Massachusetts, 1755." *Collections of the New Brunswick Historical Society.* No. 13. St John, NB: Barnes and Co., 1930.

Williams, R. See MacKay, R.

Wilson, John. *A Genuine Narrative of the Transactions in Nova Scotia since the Settlement, June 1749 till August the 5th 1751.* London: A. Henderson, 1751.

Winslow, John. "Journal of John Winslow of the Provincial Troops while engaged in the Siege of Fort Beauséjour." In *Collections of the Nova Scotia Historical Society*. Vol. 4. Halifax: Nova Scotia Historical Society, 1885.

– "Journal of Colonel John Winslow of the Provincial Troops while Engaged in Removing the Acadian French Inhabitants from Grand Pré, and the Neighbouring Settlements; in the Autumn of the Year 1755." In *Collections of the Nova Scotia Historical Society*. Vol. 3. Halifax: Nova Scotia Historical Society, 1883.

Wrigley, E.A., and R.S. Schofield. *The Population History of England, 1541–1871*. Cambridge, MA: Harvard University Press, 1981.

Wyman, A.L. "The Surgeoness: The Female Practitioner of Surgery, 1400–1800." *Medical History* 28 (1984): 22–41.

Young, J.H. *The Toadstool Millionaires. A Social History of Patent Medicines before Federal Regulation*. Princeton: Princeton University Press, 1961.

Index

Abercrombie, Dr Alexander, physician, surgeon, and apothecary's mate, 17, 29, 42–4, 52, 55, 56, 59, 62, 70, 85, 86, 193, 214, 244n.26, 260n.191; chief surgeon to the hospital, 46

Abernethy, John, surgeon at St Bartholomew's, 175

Acadians, 13, 46, 47, 66, 68, 70; expulsion, evacuation, and deportation of, 37, 49, 247n.57, 261n.209; and smallpox epidemic at Quebec in 1757, 9

Accoucheur, 92. *See also* Man-midwife

Act, legislative, 136; in England, the first concerning medical matters, 167; in Nova Scotia, concerning the disabled and infirm, 79, 80, 88, 93, 152, 202; concerning the poor, 80, 82, 93, 152; concerning the workhouse, 75, 76, 93; for punishing rogues, 89; for registering marriages, births, and deaths, 234n.67; for regulating the militia,

108; to prevent the spread of contagious distempers, 67, 200. *See also* Bill, Medical Act, Stamp Act, Sugar and Molasses Act, Townshend Act

Adair, Robert, inspector of regimental infirmaries in the British army, 119, 120

Adair, William, director of the military hospital in Halifax, 59, 61, 214

Adams, Charles, surgeon at Annapolis Royal, 204

Adelheit, William, surgeon and practitioner of physic, 261n.204

Advertisements, 61, 78, 92, 96, 104, 105, 122, 123, 124, 125, 126, 133, 141, 161, 172, 179, 180, 182, 183, 184; first, by a medical practitioner in Canada, 38, 39; related to medicine and dentistry, 38; for veterinary services, 126

Ainslie, Thomas, surgeon at Halifax, 261n.204

Aix-la-Chapelle, Treaty of, 222n.3

Akins, Thomas Beamish, historian, 25, 234n.68

Albemarle Street: now known as Market Street, 77, 127

Allotment Book for Halifax, 22

Almon, Dr William John, physician and surgeon at Halifax, 101, 144, 148, 170, 185, 204, 206, 212–14, 220n.4, 300n.17; visiting physician to the sick at the poor house, 150, 214; surgeon's mate with the Royal Artillery, 206; surgeon to the Ordnance and Artillery, 298n.274

Alms house, 64, 87

Amherst, Major General Jeffery, 58, 61, 65

Amherst, Colonel William, 58

Amputation. *See* Surgical procedures

Anaesthetics: including alcohol, opium, and nitrous oxide, 221n.8

Anatomy: teaching of, in the eighteenth century, 174

Anderson, Andrew, physician and surgeon of New York, 212, 213

Andrews, Israel, of Windsor, 290n.180

Anne, 27, 30, 33, 236n.84

Annapolis, Township of, 68, 70, 102, 205; population in 1762, 70; relief of the poor in, 81

Annapolis Royal, 18, 19, 23, 37, 38, 47, 51, 58, 81, 121, 137, 143, 158, 159, 206, 210; English garrison at, 16

Anwyl, Rev. William, 234n.66

Apothecaries, in Nova Scotia: number of, from 1749–53, 35; from 1750–1800, 173

Apothecary, drug, and medicine stores: at Halifax, 38, 61, 96, 179, 181, 288n.166, 314n.170; at Lunenburg, 161; at Shelburne, 179, 180; at Windsor, 123

Apprenticeship, 4, 79, 81, 90, 144, 152; of orphans, 240n.124

Arbuthnot, Lieutenant Governor Mariot, 108, 111, 112, 115, 117, 118, 276n.44; commander of the Naval Yard at Halifax, 276n.44

Argyle Highlanders (the 74th Regiment), 119, 122

Argyle Street, 59, 77

Argyle, Township of, 158

Army hospital. See Military hospital

Arichat, 222n.1

Art Gallery of Nova Scotia, 60, 78

Artillery, train of, 58, 246n.52

Asia, 156

Autopsy. See Surgical procedures

Ayer, Abijah, 277n.46

Baie Verte, 47

Bailey, Rev. Jacob, 108, 129

Ball, Ingram, chief justice of Cape Breton, 165

Balsams: Fryar's, 125; Turlington's, 179–81

Baltimore, 193, 224n.10

Barbers, 4, 15, 168

Barclay, Major Thomas, 151

Barkley, Capt. Andrew, 115

Barnard, Peter. See Bernard, Peter

Barracks, 84

Barrington, Lord, 119, 120

Barrington Street, 46, 77

Barrington, Township of, 66, 68–70, 118, 158, 167; population in 1762, 70

Barry, Dr Edward: his book *A Treatise on a Consumption of the Lungs*, 271n.146

Bartelo, Francis, 236n.86

Bastide, Colonel John, military engineer, 257n.154

Batt, Major Thomas, 282n.99

Baugh, D.A., naval historian, 245n.33

Baxter, John, surgeon at Halifax, 30, 38, 59, 264n.31; agent to the Hospital for Sick and Wounded Seamen, 55; assistant surgeon at the naval hospital, 54; surgeon in attendance at Grand Battery Hospital at Louisbourg, 67

Baxter, William, physician and surgeon at Cornwallis, 14, 142, 159, 161

Beath, John, travelling dentist, advertising repair of natural and artificial teeth, 184

Beaufort, 19, 193, 224n.10

Beauséjour, Fort: capture of, 37, 46

Bedlam. *See* Hospital: of St Mary of Bethlehem

Belcher, Benjamin, 151

Belcher, Chief Justice Jonathan, 61, 66–8, 73, 77, 81, 82; appointed lieutenant governor, 255n.142

Belchiss, Mr, surgeon's mate, 17, 226n.24

Bell, Winthrop, historian, 234n.68

Bender, Urban, 161

Bennett, Rev. Joseph, 261n.201; and smallpox in his family, 274n.15

Bent, Jesse, 277n.46

Bernard, Peter, apothecary, physician, and surgeon at Halifax, 119, 139, 297n.273

Berton, Peter, surgeon, 204, 206

Best, William, merchant, 49, 51, 265n.41

Betts, Azor, surgeon at Digby and Saint John, 204, 206, 209, 210; of the Queen's Rangers, 204

Bevan, Mr, apothecary and chymist, 16, 17

Bicêtre, Paris asylum for men, 272n.158

Bigot, François, intendant of New France: and Medical Act, 168

Bill: for the Maintenance and Support of Transient Poor, Maimed and Disabled Seamen and Soldiers, and other Distressed People, 148; poor, 152; to Regulate the Practice of Physick and Surgery, 167. *See also* Act

Binney, Jonathan, 77, 130

Birch Point: location of smallpox house, 129

Bishop, John, 112

Bishop Street, 32, 77, 81, 214, 216

Black hole, 98, 75, 275n.27

Black, Joseph, professor at Glasgow, 175

Black people, 156; their servitude in America in the eighteenth century, 224n.10

Black scurvy. *See* Diseases and illnesses

Blake, Charles, surgeon at Montreal, 169

Blaskowitz, Charles: his plan of the Naval Yard, 133, 134

Blistering, 196

Blooding (also bleeding, and blood-letting), 4, 41, 141, 195–7

Bloodstone, 185, 316n.180

Blowers Street, 59, 77, 110, 178, 214

Bode, Charles, surgeon at Shelburne, 204, 206

Boerhaave, Dr Hermann, professor of medicine at Leiden, 4, 7, 15, 28, 195; on fever, 4, 195

Boggs, James, physician and surgeon at Halifax, 143, 144, 178, 204, 206, 209, 210; portrait of, 100; principal medical officer in Nova Scotia, 298n.274; surgeon to garrison at Halifax, 178

Bohme, Frederick Ludovic, surgeon at Clements, 142; silhouette of, 72

Bolman, John, surgeon, apothecary, and dentist at Lunenburg, 142, 159–61; accusations and charges against, 161; health officer for LaHave, Chester, and Lunenburg, 159

Bolus: defined, 197; kinds

of, 40, 41, 197, 198, 199

Bond, Joseph N., surgeon at Shelburne and Yarmouth, 101, 137, 179, 204, 206, 297n.273; portrait of, 100

Booth, Lt William, 163, 185; his watercolour of Sydney, 163

Borias, 58

Boscawen, Vice Admiral Edward, 45, 48, 58, 61; naval commander at the Siege of Louisbourg, 49, 58

Boston, 51, 84, 102, 104, 107; artificers and labourers from, 24; cartel from, 228n.165; civilians from, moved to Halifax, 109; evacuation of, 110; newspapers, 25, 27, 31, 118; Tea Party, 102

Bourn, William, 263n.13

Bowman, James, hospital mate at Halifax, 119

Boyd, George Frederick, surgeon at Windsor, 112, 142, 170, 281n.82; surgeon to the 2nd Battalion, Royal Highland Emigrants, 112

Boyd, John, surgeon at Windsor, 144, 180, 204, 206, 209, 210

Boyleston, Zabdiel, physician in Boston: first to carry out an inoculation in North America, 8

Bragg's Regiment (the 28th), 57

Brattle, William, physician at Boston, 109, 110, 209, 210; attorney general of Massachusetts Bay Colony, 36; portrait of, 36

Breast pipe, 180

Brebner, J.B., historian, 233n.61

Brehm, Phillip, overseer of the poor, 87

Brenton, James, judge of the Supreme Court, 160

Brewhouse: at the workhouse, 75

Brewse, John, engineer. *See* Bruce, John.

Breynton, Rev. John, 70, 74, 90, 103, 139; administrator of the orphan house, 46; promotes inoculation, 103

Bridekirk, W., 207

Bridewell, 74, 146. *See also* House of Correction, Workhouse

Brinley, Francis, surgeon at Shelburne, 179, 204, 206; of the New York Volunteers, 204

Bromfield, William, surgeon at St George's Hospital, 174

Brookes, Richard: his book *The General Practice of Physic*, 171n.146

Brooks, Chamberlain, architect of the Naval Hospital, 292n.219

Brown, Daniel, surgeon's mate at Halifax, 193

Brown, J., surgeon and dentist at Halifax, 313n.166

Brown, John, surgeon at Shelburne, 204, 206

Brown, Lewis Joseph, surgeon and dentist at Halifax, 313n.166

Brown, Thomas, owner of smallpox house in Liverpool, 129

Brown, Thomas: advertised Sal Salutis in Halifax, 122

Browne, Peter, hospital mate at New York

General Hospital and
Halifax, 143, 204, 206,
209, 210
Bruce, Lt Col James,
officer commanding
the forces in Nova
Scotia, 73
Bruce, John, engineer, 19,
20
Brudenell, Rev. Edward:
his *Letter Book*,
312n.143
Brunswick Troops, 120,
122, 284n.136
Bruscourt, Georginus,
doctor of physic and
surgeon at Halifax, 193
Buchan, William: his book
Domestic Medicine, 8
Bulkeley, J.M. Freke,
Secretary of Council,
156
Bulkeley, Richard, provincial secretary, 77, 91,
106; member of a com-
mittee to report on the
orphan house, 91; and
smallpox, 106
Bullein, Nathaniel,
surgeon 204, 209, 210
Burbidge, John, overseer
of the poor 265n.33
Burgoyne, General,
117
Burns, William, surgeon at
Shelburne, 157, 204,
206; inoculating at
Shelburne, 157
Butler, Lt Col John,
commanding officer of
the Halifax Militia,
275n.22
Buttler, John, distiller, 91,
128; lawsuit brought
against by John Grant,
surgeon, 40, 41; and
orphan house, 91
Byles, Rev. Mather, 110,
185
Bynum, William, xvi

Cahill, Matthew, surgeon

of the 20th Regiment,
204, 206
Calef, John, surgeon at
Saint John, 204, 206,
209, 210; silhouette of,
72
Calendar: Gregorian
supercedes Julian, 11
Callendar, Alexander,
227n.35
Callendar's Division, 31
Calomel, 103, 196
Cambridge, University of,
15, 177
Camp fever. *See* Fever
Camp followers, 3, 35, 73,
74, 88, 97, 98, 109,
112, 146, 185, 186, 188
Campbell, Archibald,
surgeon's mate at Hal-
ifax, 193
Campbell, Colonel, 118
Campbell, Dr D.A., xv
Campbell, John. *See*
Loudon, Lord
Campbell, Maj. Gen. John,
129, 135, 139, 140, 156
Campbell, Governor
William, 73, 88, 93
Canard, 222n.1
Cancer. *See* Cures,
Diseases and illnesses
Cape Breton, 55, 147, 162,
164
Cape Forchu, 66
Cape Sable, 261n.206
Cape Sable Island, 165
Capitation tax. *See* Poll tax
Captail Reed's Company,
204
Carbolic acid: used as an
antiseptic, 221n.7
Careening Yard, in
Halifax, 96, 133, 140;
surgeon at, 140
Carleton, Sir Guy, 136,
140, 142
Carlyle, Thomas, 163
Carnegie, David, surgeon
at Halifax, 193
Carr, Robert, apothecary's
mate at Halifax, 17. *See
also* Kerr, Robert

Carter, Christopher, hos-
pital mate at Halifax,
143; druggist and chem-
ist in Philadelphia and
Queen's County, New
Brunswick, 296n.266
Cast, Phillip Geoffrey,
surgeon, Shirley's
Regiment, 47, 49
Cathartics. *See* Drugs,
medications, and treat-
ments
Catherwood, Ann,
midwife at Halifax, 42,
61, 62, 91, 255n.140
Catherwood, William,
surgeon's mate of the
45th Regiment, 24
Catholics: Irish, 102
Census. *See* Halifax
Chaplin, Arnold, 97
Charity school: established
in Halifax, 154
Charlatans: practising in
Lower Canada, 168,
169, 171
Charlestown, North
Carolina, 137
Charlton, 93, 193, 224n.10
Chatham, 110
Chebucto, 14, 18, 19,
22, 23, 74; renamed
Halifax, 226n.26
Chebucto Harbour, 14,
18, 19, 23
Cheselden, William,
surgeon in London, 5,
124, 174; and Barber-
Surgeons, 4
Chester, 70, 158, 159, 204,
206; population of in
1762, 70
Chester, Simeon, 277n.46
Chichester, John, surgeon
at Halifax, 170; adver-
tises a course of lectures
in chemistry in
Halifax, 183
Chignecto, 46, 47, 49, 51,
56, 222n.1
Childbirth, 91, 92, 217
Child mortality, 147
Children 30, 67, 73,

79–81, 83, 95, 108, 109, 112, 119, 120, 138, 139, 141, 151, 154, 156, 158; illegitimate, in poor house, 154; of poor, in orphan house, 68; with Cornwallis in 1749, 14; Children's hospital. *See* Hospital
Chipman, John, 161
Chloroform: introduced as an anaesthetic, 221n.8
Chymists, in Nova Scotia: number of, 35, 173
Citadel Hill, 115
Citrus juices, 271n.146
Claims: for loss of property and income by Loyalist doctors, 209
Clapham, William, 242n.3
Clapham's Rangers, 242n.3
Clark, A.H., historian, 222
Clark, Duncan, surgeon at Halifax, 140, 142, 170, 221n.10; appointed surgeon to the Careening Yard, 140; picture of, 36; sent to Spanish River, 295n.261
Clarke, Jonathan W., surgeon in Windsor, assistant surgeon of the Royal Nova Scotia Regiment, 178
Clark, Parker, physician at Fort Cumbeland, 116, 282n.102
Clark, Robert, son of Duncan Clark, surgeon, 311n.140
Clark, William Duncan, son of Duncan Clark, surgeon, 311n.140
Clements Township, 142, 205, 207
Cleveland, Hon. John, Secretary of the Admiralty, 55
Clinton, Sir Henry, commander in chief of

British forces, 118, 119, 131, 138, 140
Clysters, 197
Cobequid, 68, 130, 160, 222n.1
Cochran, John, surgeon at Halifax, 261n.204; portrait of, 12
Coffin, William, apothecary in Boston, 109
College of Physicians, London, 176
College of Surgeons, Hesse-Cassell, 170
Collier, Admiral Sir George, 111, 113–16; his *Journal*, 113
Collier, John, 227n.35
Collier's Division, 31
Collins, Hallet: two of his children die of measles, 141
Collins, Robert, mason 127
Columbia College, New York: first medical school to advertise in a Nova Scotia newspaper, 172
Colville, Admiral Alexander, 58, 65, 67
Commeus, Windilinus, surgeon on the *Murdoch*, 239n.113
Company of Barber-Surgeons, 168, 174, 220n.3
Company of Surgeons, 4, 15, 124, 168, 170, 174, 176, 287n.153
Concord, Massachusetts, 101, 102
Connecticut, Colony of, 66, 141, 168; and regulating the practice of medicine, 168
Connor, John, 34
Consumption. *See* Cures, Diseases and illnesses
Contagious distempers. *See* Diseases and illnesses

Continental Congress, 102, 125
Convicts, 151, 157, 164
Conway Township, 138, 204, 206, 211
Cooper, Sir Astley, surgeon at Guy's Hospital, 175
Cope, Sir Zachery, historian of the Royal College of Surgeons of England, 124
Cork, Ireland, 51
Cornwall, Daniel, surgeon at Country Harbour, 204
Cornwallis Barracks, 154; description and location of, 303n.49
Cornwallis, General Earl: defeat of, at Yorktown, 136
Cornwallis, Governor Edward, 14, 18, 19, 22–7, 31, 33, 44, 46, 116, 220n.1
Cornwallis, Township of, 70, 93, 121, 129, 142, 150, 158, 189; arrival of New England families, 66; population in 1762, 70
Cornwallis Island, 52, 53. *See also* McNab's Island
Corporal punishment, 75
Cossitt, Rev. Ranna, rector of St George's Anglican Church at Sydney, 164, 165; his *Diary*, 309n.111
Country Harbour, 34, 158, 204, 205
Court of St James, 88
Cowpox, 6
Crafts, Edward, surgeon at Halifax, 30
Crawford, John, hospital mate at Halifax, 119
Creighton, James: granted military hospital lots, 178
Criminals, 149

Cuffey, Barbara, midwife at Liverpool, 269n.117
Cullen, Walter, surgeon's mate at Halifax and Fort Cumberland, 116, 140, 142
Cullen, Dr William, professor at Edinburgh and Glasgow, 5, 15, 29, 175, 196
Culloden, battle of, 223n.8
Culpeper, Nicholas: his book *The English Physician enlarged with three hundred, sixty, and nine medicines, made of English herbs*, 171n.146
Cumberland, Township of, 68, 70, 108, 137; and Militia Bill, 108; population in 1762, 70
Cupping, 196
Cures, 122; for cancer, 183; for consumptive weaknesses, 123; for cough, advertised, 141, 178; for gout, 125, 314n.171; for hydrophobia, advertised, 178; for mad-dog bite, 141; for scurvy, 254n.135; for venereal disease, advertised, 122, 178; for wens, 183; for yellow fever, 123, 305n.75

D'Anville, Mons: his map of Nova Scotia, 227n.34
Dartmouth, 38, 42, 51, 60, 96, 145, 155, 156, 158, 206, 210, 214, 216, 237n.91; building on, 27; Indian attack on, 30; arrival of Maroons, 156; Maroon hospital, 156; tent hospital, 155; population in July 1752, 38
Dartmouth College: establishes a Faculty of Medicine, 171

Dartmouth, Earl of, 106, 107, 109
Dartmouth, Lord, 91, 95
Davidson, Andrew: and smallpox in Horton Township, 112
Davidson, Hugh, treasurer of the colony, 26, 27
Davies, Lt Thomas, of the Royal Artillery, 52, 53; his watercolour of Halifax, 53
Davis, Lewis, surgeon of the King's Rangers, 133, 135, 142, 182, 306n.89; his electric apparatus advertised for sale, 182, 314n.171; surgeon's mate in Emmerick's Chasseurs, 292n.222
Day, Henrietta, 270n.143
Day, John, surgeon at the naval hospital, 48, 93–7, 233n.61; his advertisement for drugs and medicine, 61; agent victualler of the army, 270n.142; appointed as a surgeon's assistant in Nova Scotia, 48; his drugstore on Hollis Street, 61; elected to House of Assembly, 93; inserts first election advertisement in a Halifax newspaper, 95; picture of, 12
Day and Scott, merchants in Halifax, 270n.142
Debt, provincial, 85–8, 94, 97, 98, 146, 153
Death: causes of, among Nova Scotians from 1749–99, 147, 188, 189, 217, 218; mean and median ages of Nova Scotians at time of, 186; rate, among Nova Scotians from 1749–84, 147, 187

Deaths, in Halifax, 49, 56; in Nova Scotia, number of, 103, 186
Deglen, Johann C., surgeon on the *Gale*, 38, 70
de Grasse, Admiral François, 293n.236
de Haen, Dr Anton: and introduction of the thermometer as a diagnostic aid in 1758, 124
De Heister, Lieutenant General, commander of Hessian Regiment, 111
de Labertouche, Anna, 38
DeLancey's Brigade, 205
de Layfayette, Marquis, commander of French troops during American Revolution, 293n.236
de la Roche, Rev. Peter: and outbreak of smallpox in Lunenburg in 1775, 105, 106
Dennison, Gurdon, physician in Horton, 159, 160; representative for Horton in House of Assembly, 159
Denson, Lt Col Henry Denny, 249n.74; elected to House of Assembly, 270n.138
Dentistry, 137, 184; advertisements by dentists, 184, 313n.166; anodyne water for teeth, 96; artificial teeth, 184; chewsticks, 184; extraction of teeth, 161; toothbrushes, 182; tooth powders, 180, 182; transplanting teeth, 184. *See also* von Riedesel, Baroness
de Rodohan, Alexandre, surgeon of the *Gale*, 31, 243n.6; and Acadians, 246n.55, 47
DesBarres, Lieutenant

Governor J.F.W., 162, 163, 164
Deschamps, Isaac, judge of the Supreme Court, 106, 160
de Seitz, Lt Col Fritz Carl Erdman, commander of the Hessian Regiment, 120. *See also* Hessians
Deserters, 22
Despard, Major General John, 165
d'Estaing, Admiral, 293n.236
De St Croix, Benjamin, surgeon, 172
Devices, medical and surgical. *See* Supplies
Dick, 27
Dickson, Cochran, surgeon at Halifax, 193
Dickson, James, surgeon and agent for sick and hurt seamen at Halifax, 110, 111, 113, 114, 130, 214, 215; principal surgeon at the naval hospital, 129, 130; surgeon to the sick prisoners of war, 129
Digby, 137, 138, 150, 158, 204–6, 208–11; number of Loyalists who settled there, 137
Digby, Rear Admiral Robert, 128, 130
Dimsdale, Thomas, physician, 8
Diseases and illnesses: apoplexy, 217; asthma, 217; black scurvy, 156; cancer, 217; cholera, 217; constipation of the bowels, 123; consumption, 123, 190, 217; contagious distempers, 200; convulsions, 217; dropsy, 217; dry grips, 123; dysentry, 56, 218; fits,

217; flux, 67; gangrene, 29; gout, 84, 125, 126, 190, 217; jaundice, 28, 29, 118, 123, 196; King's Evil, 123; leprosy, 123; lung disease, 217; malaria, 125; measles, 141, 217; of horses, 126; palsy, 217; paralysis, 217; pleurisy, 217; putrid sore throat, 156; quinsy, 217; rheumatism, 123, 196; scurvy, 56, 67, 123, 126, 254n.135; stealoma encysted tumor, 183; steckfluss, 217; stone in the bladder, 217; strangury heat, 123; stroke, 217; syphilis, 6, 310n.133, 317n.3; ulcers, 123; ulcerated legs, 123; venereal disease, 44, 45, 178; wens, 183; worms, 217; yaws, 123. *See also* Cures, Fever; yellow fever, 123, 156, 217. *See also* Cures, Fever, Smallpox
Dispenser, 52, 84, 131, 155
Distemper, 67, 103
Diuretics, kinds of, 196, 197
Doane, Mrs Elizabeth, midwife at Barrington, 67, 70, 118
Doctor of Cobequid. *See* Harris, John
Doctor Rare, 125, 126
Doggett, John, 129
Dolhonde, John, surgeon at Halifax, 261n.204
Dundon, Dr Patrick, of the 52nd Regiment, 107
Dorchester, Lord, 169
Dragoons, 17th Light, 109
Draper, William, surgeon at Halifax, 29
Drops, 40; kinds of, 122, 125, 179, 180, 182, 198

Druggists, in Nova Scotia: number of, from 1749–53, 35; from 1750–1800, 173
Drugstores. *See* Apothecary, drug, and medicine stores
Drugs, medications, and treatments: alcohol, 182; alum, 180, 182, 197; anisette, 197; anodyne draught, 41, 196; antimony, 197, 198; arsenic, 196; astringent electuary, 41, 197; balsam, 125; barberry bush, 196; bark, 182, 197; barley water, 103; Bateman's Golden and Plain Scurvy Grass, 125; benedictine, 197; bleeding, 196, 197; blistering, 196; bloodstone, 185; calomel, 103, 196; cathartic, 196; camphor, 181, 197; camphorated spirits of wine, 41, 197; Carolina Pinkroot, 181; castor oil, 179, 181, 198; cephalic mixture, 197; chloride of mercury, 196; coltsfoot, 182, 313n.164; cooling clysters, 41; corn salve, 180; cream of tartar, 124; Darby's carminative, 181, 182; detergent decoction, 41, 198; digestive, 41; elecampane, 313n.164; electuary, 198; enema, 40, 197; fermentation, 41, 198; flower of sulphur, 123; foxglove, 197; frankincense, 126; Galenicals, 125; gargarsm, 41, 198; garlic, 141; Godfrey's General Cordial, 125, 180; hartshorn shavings, 41, 180, 181, 185, 198; herbs and

roots, 118; Hoff-
mann's Anodyne, 196;
ipecac, 196, 197, 198;
iron, 196; isinglass, 41,
179–82, 198; jalap,
103, 196; Jesuit's Bark,
181; lavender, 180,
182, 185; laxatives, 196,
197; linseed, infusions
of, 141; liquorice, 40,
141, 182, 185; loz-
enges, 182; magnesia
alba, 123; marshmal-
low, 141; mercury, 196;
mithridate, 141; mor-
phine, 196; musk, 196;
mustard, 199; nos-
trums, 125; ointment
for the itch, 180;
opium, 196, 198; pecto-
ral lozenges, 182; pep-
permint, 182; pewter,
scrapings of, 141; pop-
pies, syrup of, 141; pur-
gative mixture of
calomel and jalap, 196;
purging, 195, 199;
quinine, 197; rhubarb,
181, 199; rue, leaves
of, 141; Russian Pearl
Ash, 181; saffron, 181,
198; Sal Salutis, 123,
125, 199; Salt Petre,
181, 182; sarsaparilla,
141; Spanish liquorice,
40, 180, 199; spirits of
hartshorn, 199; spruce
beer, 305n.75;
static electricity,
314n.171; Steer's Opo-
deldoc, 181, 182; Sto-
rey's Worm Destroying
Cakes, 181;
Stoughton's Bitters, 180,
181; tamarinds, 180,
181; tannin, 197; tarr,
vomit of, 103;
turpentine, 179, 196,
199; verdigris, 181,
182; Ward's Medicines,
96; whorehound,
313n.164; wine, 197. See

also Balsams, Bolus,
Diuretics, Drops, Elix-
irs, Emetics, Essences,
Mixtures, Nostrums,
Oils, Patent medi-
cines, Pills, Plasters,
Poultice, Powders
Drummond, George, sur-
geon at Shelburne,
185, 204, 206, 209, 210;
of the New York Gen-
eral Hospital, 204
Duckworth, John, surgeon
at Halifax, 30
Duke of Cumberland's
Regiment, 156, 205
Duke of Hamilton's
Regiment (the 82nd),
119, 122, 140, 142
Duncan, Henry, 207
Dundon, Dr Patrick,
surgeon at Halifax,
107
Dunmore, 119
Durell, Admiral Phillip,
Commander in Chief
of the Fleet in America,
64
Duties: collected on
spirituous liquors, 76,
77, 82, 84, 85, 94,
264n.21
Duty Fund, 82
Duty: on articles from the
United States, 151
Dysentery. See Diseases
and illnesses

Earl of Halifax, George
Montagu-Dunk:
appointed president of
the Board of Trade
and Plantations.
Eastern Battery, 135
Eaton, Daniel, physician
and surgeon at
Onslow, 159; member
of the House of As-
sembly, 159; surgeon of
the Colchester Militia,
302n.47
Eddington, Maine, 116

Eddy, Captain Jonathan,
116
Edinburgh Infirmary, 5, 6
Edinburgh University, 5,
175, 196; medical
faculty established, 175
Edmund, Johann
Edmund Heinrich,
surgeon on the Pearl,
38
Electrotherapy, 314n.171.
See also Torpedo
Elixirs: defined, 198;
kinds of, 40, 125, 133,
180, 181, 198
Ellis, Edward, surgeon at
Newport,
Emetics: defined, 197,
198; kinds of, 40, 196,
197, 198
Emigrants: lists of, 224
Emigration, Scottish, 147
Emmerick's Chasseurs,
292n.222
Enactment concerning
medical matters, 167;
first by the English
Parliament, 167
Engineers, Corps of, 58
Enniskillens (the 27th
Regiment), 276n.44
Epidemic: of 1749–50
misdated, 25; in Nova
Scotia, 28, 55, 56, 61,
105, 112, 141
Erad, Johann Berghard,
surgeon on the Pearl
and at Lunenburg, 31,
38, 65
Essences: kinds of, 125,
180, 182
Executions, 217

Fair Lady, 18, 193, 224n.10
Fallon, Eleanor, midwife
of Halifax, 91
Falmouth, Township of,
67, 70, 81, 118, 160;
arrival of New England
families, 66; popula-
tion in 1762, 70; relief
of the poor in, 81

Falt, Joseph, surgeon at Petite Rivière, 137, 161, 204, 206

Families: with Cornwallis in 1749, 224n.10

Fane, John, seventh earl of Westmoreland, 225

Faries, William, surgeon's mate at Halifax, 107, 108, 129, 274n.13; of 65th Regiment, 107; assistant surgeon at the naval hospital, 105, 107

Farish, Henry Greggs, surgeon at Yarmouth, 172

Farquhar, John, surgeon's mate at Halifax, 17

Farrington, John, chymist and surgeon at Halifax, 193

Fencible, definition of, 273n.8

Fenton, John, appointed to be a governor of the orphan house, 91

Fever, 28, 32, 54, 55, 56, 119, 136, 155–7, 190, 195, 196, 217; bilious, 28, 123; camp, 28; contagious, 54; epidemical, 61; hectic, 123, 217; hospital, 28; infectious, 155, 201; inflammatory, 28, 29, 48; intermittent, 59; jail, 28, 135; low nervous, 29; malignant, 29, 135, 136, 155, 200; nervous, 185, 295n.261; putrid, 28, 135, 158, 217; scarlet, 156; spotted, 56, 217; typhus, 28, 29; yellow, 118, 119, 121, 125, 157–9, 196. See also Boerhaave, Dr Hermann, Cures, Fevers

Fillis, John, overseer of the poor, 265n.33

Fish, electric, 314n.171

Fisher, James, surgeon to the garrison at Quebec, 168, 169, 171

Fitzpatrick, Thomas, keeper of the gaol and workhouse, 88, 269n.105

Flanders, 28, 29; hospitals in, 16, 28; military campaigns in, 224n.26

Fleming, Elizabeth, midwife at Halifax, 92

Fletcher, Dr Richard, 170

Fletcher, William, surgeon at Halifax, 107, 297n.270, 302n.47

Florentine, Abraham, surgeon at Digby, 204, 206, 209, 211

Foot, Zachariah, 117

Forceps: secretely used by Chamberlen family of physicians, 92

Forts: Beauséjour, 37, 46, 47, 57, 130; Cornwallis, 76, 77; Cumberland, 57, 114, 116, 130; Edward, 112; Horseman's 46, 77; Lawrence, 38, 47; Lee, 138; Massey, 172, 178, 216; William Henry, 57

Foster, Robert, 277n.46

Foye, William, 255n.145

France, 26; declares war on Great Britain in 1793, 154

Francheville, George, surgeon at Halifax, 31, 130

Francklin, Lieutenant Governor Michael, 77, 84, 87, 88, 130

Fraser, John, surgeon at Windsor, 142, 156, 214, 215, 302n.47

Freeholders: committee of, 57; of Halifax, 89

Friendship, 164

Fuller's Regiment (the 29th), 222n.4

Fumigation: procedures

used at the Edinburgh Infirmary, 5

Fury, William, 133

Gale, 30, 33, 42, 238n.109

Galen, 287n.157

Galenicals, 125

Galland, John, 227n.35

Gamble, John, hospital mate in Halifax, 143, 296n.264, 296n.265

Gangrene. See Diseases and illnesses

Gaol, 94, 119, 120, 149, 162, 163, 202, 240n.126; building for, 263n.14; location of in Halifax, 75, 88; provincial, 149

Gardiner, Sylvester, physician at Boston, 109, 209, 211; portrait of, 36

Garnier, Mr, apothecary general to the army, 16, 17

Gates, Horatio, 19

Geddes, James, surgeon, 172

Gemmel, John. See Gamble, John

General military hospital. See Military hospital

Gentleman's Magazine and Historical Chronicle, 24, 55

George III, 81, 88, 97, 98, 109, 150

George Street, 60

George's Island, 18, 41, 51, 67, 110, 112–15, 122, 135, 137, 157, 214–16, 285n.143; naval hospital on, 113, 121; quarantine hospital on, 110, 112, 113

Germain, Lord George, 110, 112, 115, 117–19, 127

German Auxillary Forces, 204

Germans, 27, 34, 102

Germany, 30, 239n.113

Gerrish, Joseph, 254n.133
Gibbons, Richard, over-
  seer of the poor,
  265n.33, 268n.105
Gillespie, George, surgeon
  at Halifax, 170,
  306n.89
Gisiquash, Claude, 34
Glasgow, 118, 147, 175
Glazier, Beamsley,
  228n.44
Goldthwaite, assistant
  surgeon at Halifax, 110
Goldthwaite, Michael B.,
  hospital mate at hospi-
  tal in New York,
  279n.65
Goodman, Isaac, surgeon
  at Digby, 138, 204,
  206, 209, 211
Gordon, Alexander,
  surgeon at Sydney,
  163; surgeon's mate to
  the 33rd Regiment,
  163; silhouette of, 72
Gordon, William Augus-
  tus: his *Journal*,
  253n.122
Goreham's Corps, 109
Gorham, John, 242n.3
Gorham, Lt Col Joseph,
  commander of the
  Royal Fencible Ameri-
  cans, 103
Gorham, Major, 239n.115
Gorham, William, 127
Gorham's Point, 254n.133
Gorham's Rangers, 242n.3
Gould, John, hospital
  mate at Halifax, 143,
  204, 206, 209, 211,
  296n.264, 297n.273
Grace, James, 34
Grafton Street, 77, 178
Grand Battery Hospital, at
  Louisbourg, 65
Grand Pré, 38, 47, 49,
  222n.1
Grant: to Nova Scotia, 62,
  63; hospital expenses
  omitted from, 64
Grant, John, surgeon, 17,

31, 38, 39, 41, 44, 45,
  57, 193; and orphan
  house, 42; assistant
  surgeon of the naval
  hospital, 54; lawsuits
  against patients, 39, 40,
  41; man-midwife at
  Halifax, 44, 92
Grant, Robert, surgeon at
  Halifax, 17, 39, 45, 48,
  52, 54, 93, 193, 215; advertising medicines for
  sale, 38; his grocery, dry
  goods, and medicine
  store in Granville Street,
  40, 41; principal sur-
  geon at naval hospital,
  52; surgeon and agent
  to the sick and wounded
  at Halifax, 45, 55;
  sworn in as member of
  Council, 93
Grant, William, surgeon at
  Halifax, 193
Granville, Township of,
  66, 70, 81, 117, 121,
  138, 172, 205, 207;
  population in 1762,
  70; relief of the poor in,
  81
Granville Street, 45, 59,
  177
Graves, Rear Admiral
  Samuel, 128
Greaves, George, surgeon
  to the naval hospital,
  84, 104, 215; advertises
  patent medicines, 105;
  inoculation hospital in
  his house, 104
Greaves, William, surgeon
  at Halifax, 172
Green, the Honourable
  Benjamin, 82, 86, 93,
  94, 183; administrator
  of the government, 86;
  provincial treasurer, 82,
  88
Gregory, Dr James,
  physician, 5
Grenville, George, Lord of
  the Treasury, 225

Griffith, Fenton, surgeon's
  mate at Halifax, 77,
  193
Gschwind, John Frederick
  Traugott, surgeon at
  Halifax, 127, 142, 159,
  170, 289n.171,
  302n.47; appointed
  health officer for
  Halifax, 159;
Guards: two companies
  arrive in Halifax, 111
Gut of Canso, 158
Guysborough, 157, 186,
  205, 208
Guy's Hospital, London, 6,
  170, 172

Hales, Stephen, clergy-
  man, 16
Haliburton, Thomas
  Chandler, historian,
  223n.7
Halifax, 22, 23, 48, 51, 57,
  59, 73, 102, 103, 109,
  117, 226n.33, 268n.93;
  assessment on inhabi-
  tants for the poor, 85,
  87, 88; Britain's major
  naval base in North
  America, 3; census of
  1752, 33; cost of
  establishing the settlement, 31; intended
  attack on, by the
  French, 249n.76; North
  Suburbs, 31, 104, 105,
  120, 133, 241n.131;
  number of houses, 24,
  68; number of Loyalists
  who settled there, 137;
  number of persons in,
  24, 25, 52, 102,
  234n.72, 241n.131; oli-
  garchy in, 96; plan for
  fortifying, 20; plan
  showing forts, batter-
  ies, etc., 50; proposed
  attack by New England
  rebels on, 107; rendez-
  vous of fleets and
  armies at, 37, 70; small-

pox in, 55, 107; South
Suburbs, 23, 241n.131;
unemployment in, 73;
view of, by Moses Har-
ris, 21; worst storm
ever experienced in,
268n.93
Hall, John Sr, of Granville,
117
Hall, John Jr, 117
Halliburton, John,
surgeon at Halifax,
131, 133, 140, 142, 155,
160, 177, 178, 209,
211, 215, 220n.6,
291n.205; surgeon of
the naval hospital, 131,
215; appointed to care
for the sick and
wounded naval prison-
ers, 155; appointed to
HM Council, 160; pic-
ture of, 100
Halliburton, John Jr,
surgeon at Halifax,
172
Hamilton, Lt Col Otto,
commander of HM
Troops in Nova Scotia,
267n.65
Hamond, Lieutenant
Governor Sir Andrew
Snape, 121, 122,
127–31, 135, 136
Hancock, 118
Handasyde, James,
surgeon at Halifax, 17,
193
Handasyde, John, surgeon
at Halifax, 129, 131,
215, 290n.183;
appointed assistant
surgeon and surgeon at
naval hospital, 129,
130, 215
Hangings: in Halifax, 217
Harbin, Augustus, assis-
tant surgeon at Hali-
fax, 193
Hardy, Sir Charles, 52, 56,
58
Harris, John, physician at

Pictou and Truro, 130,
159, 160; member of
the House of Assembly
for Truro, 130, 160; re-
ferred to as the Doctor
of Cobequid, 130
Harris, Jonathan, 82, 83,
87, 88
Harris, Matthew, 130
Harris, Moses: his plan of
Halifax, 19, 21, 24, 25,
32
Harris, Mrs, midwife in
Falmouth, 118
Harrison, Samuel, master
of the House of Cor-
rection at Shelburne,
300n.22
Hartshorn, Ebenezer,
surgeon at Annapolis,
70
Harvard University, 136;
establishes a Faculty of
Medicine, 171
Harvey, Dr William: on
midwifery, 92
Hatton, Joseph, surgeon
at Country Harbour,
205, 297n.273
Hawkins, Mr, master of
Surgeons' Hall, 17
Hay, Alexander, surgeon's
mate in Halifax, 31, 193
Hay, Charles, captain of
the Port of Halifax, 41
Hay, Patrick, surgeon at
Halifax, 193
Hay, Thomas, Lord
Dupplin, 225n.19
Hays, Lewis, 27
Head, Dr —, surgeon at
Halifax, 48
Head, Michael, surgeon
and druggist at Wind-
sor, Lunenburg, and
Halifax, xvi, 48, 49,
123, 181, 249n.74,
281n.85, 302n.47;
drugstores on Granville
and Hollis Streets,
181; and inoculations,
106

Head, Samuel, surgeon at
Halifax, 172
Heagerty, Dr J.J.: his
description of attempt
to introduce smallpox
into Halifax, 57
Health boat, in Halifax
Harbour, 157
Health officers: first
appointed in Nova
Scotia, 158, 159
Heffernan, Dennis,
surgeon at Halifax and
Liverpool, 312n.142
Helmerich, Johan
Christian, surgeon at
Halifax, 127, 214
Henkell, George, surgeon
and health officer at
Annapolis, 159
Henry, Anthony, King's
Printer, 122, 158;
advertises patent medi-
cines, 122
Hessian Hospital, 127,
214, 216
Hessians, 101, 111, 120,
122, 127, 138, 142; de
Heister Regiment of,
111; de Seitz Regiment
of, 120
Highlanders, 117
Hill, John, of Digby,
manufacturer of Es-
sence of Spruce,
305n.75
Hill, Trotter, surgeon at
Halifax, of the 59th
Regiment, 92
Hillsborough, Lord, 88
Hinshelwood, Mr, 82
Hippocrates, 1
Hoar, Frike Dilks, 77
Hoffman, John, justice of
the peace for Halifax
County, 238n.101
Hofstadter, R., historian, 9
Holburne, Admiral, 37,
51, 52, 55, 58; and
siege of Louisbourg, 55
Holland, George, surgeon
at Halifax, 137, 205

Hollingsworth, T.H.: his study of life expectancy, 187

Hollis Street, 61

Hoose, John, surgeon at Shelburne, 137, 157, 205, 207

Hopson, Governor Peregrine Thomas, 18, 32–4, 38, 42, 46, 228n.38; commander of the 29th Regiment, 223n.4; lieutenant governor of Louisbourg, 223n.4; governor of Nova Scotia, 33

Hopson's Regiment (the 40th), 18, 24, 51, 57, 236n.86, 278n.52

Horseman, Lt Col John, 246n.40

Horses: medicines for, 126, 182

Horton, Township of, 66, 70, 81, 112, 118, 121, 158, 159, 206, 210; population in 1762, 70; relief of the poor in, 81

Hospital, civilian, in Halifax, 25, 32, 44, 46, 52, 57, 64, 67, 85, 116, 149, 214, 216; administration and operation of, 42, 57; condition of, 57; grant for the operation of, 1753–63, 63; location of, 25, 77; expenses of, 32, 42, 62; number of patients, 32, 42; medicines requested for, 26; surgeons, assistant surgeons, apothecaries, and midwife on staff of, 42, 235n.79; to be used as an alms house, 87

Hospital fever. See Fever

Hospital for Hurt and Sick Seamen, 48, 52, 215, 216; location, 45, 215

Hospital Street, 45, 46, 75, 77

Hospitals: children's, 145; first private, 104–6; for the Maroons, 156, 214, 216; French, at Louisbourg, 61; Green, on Cornwallis Street, 216; in Fort Edward, 112; in poor house, 82, 214, 216; in Sydney, 163, 165, 308n.97; prison, in Halifax, 101, 127, 133, 215, 216; prison, on Kavanagh's Island, 155, 178, 216; quarantine, 113, 214, 215; rebel, 119, 127; Red, 133, 216; regimental, 178, 215, 216; tent, at Dartmouth, 155. See also the following hospitals by name: for Hurt and Sick Seamen, Grand Battery, Hessian, Hotel Dieu, Middlesex, Military, Naval, New England, Ships: hospital

Hospitals: in Halifax and environs, 1749–99, 214–16

Hotel Dieu Hospital, Paris: death rate among patients, 26

Hotham, Commodore William, 111

Households: heads of, in Nova Scotia, 223n.7

House of Assembly: established, 76

House of Commons, 31, 98, 162

House of Correction, 46, 75, 79, 83, 93, 94, 153. See also Workhouse, Bridewell

House of Lords, 162

House of Representatives, 57

Houseal, John B., surgeon, 172

How, Edward, 236n.86

Howe, Colonel, of the 58th Regiment, 61

Howe, Joseph, 96

Howe, General Sir William, 104, 107–10, 112, 113, 115, 117–19, 185, 211

Huggeford, John, surgeon at Shelburne, 205, 207, 209, 211, 297n.273

Huggeford, Peter, surgeon at Digby, 138, 150, 205, 207, 209, 211

Hughes, Lieutenant Governor Richard, 119

Hume, Robert, assistant surgeon and dispenser at Halifax, 221n.10

Humors (blood, phlegm, choler, and melancholy), 287n.157

Hunter, John, English surgeon and teacher, 4, 15, 174

Hunter, Dr William, teacher of anatomy, 174, 175

Hunter, 253n.106

Huxham, Dr John: his book An Essay on Fevers, To which is now added a Dissertation on the Malignant Ulcerous Sore Throat, 271n.146

Idiots, 79, 80, 93, 97. See also Lunacy; Lunatics

Ile St Jean, 163

Imhof, A.E.: his study of urban mortality, 187, 188, 190

Indians, 18, 24, 30, 33, 34, 38, 46, 47, 66, 86, 154, 236n.86; attack on Dartmouth by, 232n.56; bounty placed on, 233n.56; at Louisbourg, 55; population of, 13, 70; of Shubenacadie, 33; and smallpox epidemic at Quebec, 9; surgeon to care for, 86

Ingonish, 222n.1
Inman, John, surgeon at Halifax, 17, 193
Inness, Dr George, surgeon, 82nd Regiment, 293n.223
Inoculation, 7, 8, 56, 70, 71, 103–5, 117, 157, 158, 184; advertisement concerning, 105; first administered in Canada, 71; first administered in Great Britain, 7; first administered in North America, 8; first administered in Nova Scotia, 71; hospital for, in Liverpool, 112; two methods of inoculating described, 118. See also Breynton, Rev. John, de la Roche, Rev. Peter, Dimsdale, Thomas, Greaves, George
Insane, the, 5, 86, 93, 97
Insanity, 98
Insurance: medical, established during construction of naval hospital, 131; in New France, 291n.211
Ipswich, Massachusetts, 116
Ireland, 27, 107, 151
Irish Town, 126
Irvine, John, surgeon at Halifax, 308n.101
Irwin, Josiah, 17
Irwin, Thomas, surgeon at Annapolis Royal and Halifax, 178; assistant inspector of hospitals in Nova Scotia, 178
Island of St John. See Ile St Jean

Jacot, Hector, surgeon on the Gale, 239n.113
Jades, C.N.G.: contracted yellow fever from convicts on Sally, 148, 157
Jager Corps, 205, 208
Jail, 85. See also Gaol

Jail fever. See Fever
Jamaica, 156
Jaumard, Peter, surgeon's mate to the hospital in Halifax, 293n.223
Jaundice. See Diseases and illnesses
Jeffries, Dr John, physician and surgeon at Halifax, 109, 110, 112, 117, 119, 209, 211, 214; and inoculation, 118, 119; surgeon to quarantine hospital on George's Island, 110; first native-born American to be awarded an MD by the University of Aberdeen, 279n.59; portrait of, 36; purveyor of the general military hospital in Halifax, 113, 119; surgeon to the military hospital in Halifax, 112, 214
Jenner, Dr Edward, 8
Jenny, 271n.154
Jews: burying ground of, 76
Jones, John, surgeon at Halifax, 312n.142
Jones, Matthew, surgeon, 17, 27–9, 44, 59, 193, 214
Joppe, Ludovic, of the 60th Regiment, surgeon at Guysborough, 205
Judges: impeachment of, 160
Justices of the peace, 74, 79, 83, 153, 201, 202

Karr, David Thomas: surgeon for the sick and wounded prisoners of war at Louisbourg, 251n.99
Kast, Phillip Geoffrey. See Cast, Phillip Geoffrey
Kavanagh's Island: prison hospital on, 155, 178, 216; renamed Melville

Island, 304n.56
Kay(e), James, surgeon at Halifax, 119, 140, 142, 297n.271
Kelly, Hugh, 299n.14
Kelly, John Butler: sells Island in North West Arm to James Kavanagh, 304n.56
Kendrick, Daniel, surgeon and man-midwife at Liverpool, 156, 157, 205, 207, 297n.273
Kennedy, Jane, matron and head nurse at the naval hospital, 133
Kennedy, Robert, assistant surgeon at naval hospital, 254n.134
Kennedy's Regiment (the 43rd), 57–9, 205, 278n.52
Kent, John, 40, 41
Kerr, Robert, apothecary's mate at Halifax, 29, 193. See also Carr, Robert
Kilby, Christopher, agent for the settlement of Halifax, 16, 26
Killam, Amasa, 227n.46
Killo, Robert, overseer of the poor, 280n.79
King's American Regiment, 204
King's College, New York: establishes the first Faculty of Medicine in the American colonies, 170–2
King's Evil, 123
Kingslaugh, John, 68
King's Naval Hospital. See Naval hospital
King's Naval Yard, 59
King's Orange Rangers, 120, 133, 142, 182
King's Own Regiment (the 4th), 154, 183
Kinsman, Robert, 121
Klett, Johann Ulrich, surgeon at Halifax and Lunenburg, 30, 38

Knap, Nathaniel, carpenter, 59, 65; and hospital for the sick at Louisbourg, 59

Kneeland, William, 39, 40, 197

Knowles, J.H., 26

Knox, Captain John, 56, 59, 84

Kunitz, S.J.: his study on life expectancy, 187

LaHave, 158, 159

Lake Champlain, 57

Lancet, 182; used to convey infection of the smallpox, 118

Landeg, David, surgeon at Shelburne, 205, 207, 297n.272, 297n.273

Largus, Scribonius, Roman physician, 314n.171

Lascelles, William, surgeon at Halifax, 193

Lascelles, Colonel Peregrine, 73

Lascelles's Regiment (the 47th), 27, 30, 33, 42, 47, 51, 57, 73, 74, 236n.86

Latham, Dr James: Canada's pioneer inoculator, 71

Lavoisier, Antoine Laurent, 14

Lawlor, Dr William Digby, hospital mate at Halifax, 119, 293n.223

Lawrence, Lieutenant Governor Charles, 35, 38, 41, 45–47, 51, 54, 57, 61, 62, 64, 68, 75, 76, 93, 108, 145, 243n.19; and civilian hospital, 62; his proclamation concerning lands vacated by the Acadians, 66; and transfer of settlers to Lunenburg, 38

Lawrence, John: physician and surgeon at Granville, 205, 207

Lawrencetown, 51

Lawsuits: for non-payment of medical fees, 39, 40, 162, 195, 306n.89

Lazaretto, 32

LeClerc, Dr Daniel: his book A Natural and Medicinal History of Worms, Bred in the Bodies of Men and other Animals, 271n.146

Lee, William: and building of new naval hospital, 131

LeFanu, Dr William, 5, 15

Legge, Governor Francis, 90, 91, 93, 95, 102, 103, 106, 107, 108, 109

Legislation: medical, first mentioned in Nova Scotia House of Assembly, 167

Leprosy. See Diseases and illnesses

LeRoy, Louis, surgeon on the Speedwell, 239n.113

Levison-Gower, Granville, first marquis of Stafford, 225

Lexington: skirmish at, 101, 102

Leyden, University of, 15, 174, 195

Life expectancy, 187

Lind, Dr James: his book A Treatise of the Scurvy, 271n.146

Liquor, Spirituous, 74, 76, 77, 82, 84, 94

Lister, Dr Joseph, 221n.7

Lithotomy. See Surgical procedures

Liverpool, England, 24

Liverpool, Township of, 66, 70, 81, 118, 120, 129, 130, 141, 142, 150, 157, 205, 208; hospitals in, 112; population

in 1762, 70; relief of the poor in, 81; and smallpox, 112, 129

Loader, John, master shipwright, 129, 131

Lockman, Leonard, surgeon at Halifax and Lunenburg, 16, 17, 27, 38, 45, 65, 193, 214; surgeon and agent for the Hospital for Sick and Hurt Seamen, 45; surgeon on the hospital ship Roehampton, 224n.11

London: Hospital, 6; smallpox hospital, 8

London, City of, 39, 55, 58, 96, 98, 122, 148; and examining persons in medicine, 168

London Gazette, 13, 22

London Magazine or Gentleman's Monthly Intelligencer, 30

Lords of Trade, 16, 19, 22, 24–6, 32–5, 42, 57, 62, 64, 67, 68, 76, 84, 89, 91, 93, 145, 162

Loring, Benjamin, surgeon at Shelburne, 205, 207

Loudon, Lord, fourth earl of Loudon, 37, 52, 54, 55, 56, 57, 59

Louisbourg, 3, 13, 22, 24, 31, 33, 37, 49, 52, 53–5, 58, 59, 61, 64–7, 69, 73, 84, 93, 222n.1; English garrison at, 13, 18, 22; hospitals at, 59, 65, 67; and smallpox outbreak, 49

Louthian, Thomas, surgeon's mate at Halifax, 193

Lower Canada, 168–71

Loyal American Regiment, 205

Loyal Nova Scotia Volunteers: formation of, 106, 108

Loyalist: claim commission and claims, 137, 209; physicians and surgeons who came to Nova Scotia in 1783, 137, 209
Loyalists, in Nova Scotia, 107, 109, 136, 137, 143, 144, 151, 165, 171, 186, 209, 300n.18
Lunacy: trade in, 98
Lunatics, 79, 80, 89, 93, 97, 98, 126. *See also* Idiots, Lunacy
Lunenburg 34, 37, 38, 42, 46, 51, 65, 69, 70, 84, 91, 92, 104, 122, 142, 157–60, 186, 205; hospital at, 65; number of families in 1762, 70; referred to as Merlegash, Merleguash, and Merlequash, 34, 42; return of settlers there from 1753–58, 241n.140; smallpox epidemic in, 105
Lutgens, Johannes Matthew, surgeon on the *Gale*, 31
Lyons, Major ———, town major, 113

Macarmick, Lieutenant Governor William, 164
McColme, Dr John, physician and surgeon at Halifax, 261n.204
McCormick, John, assistant surgeon to the naval hospital, 251n.95
McDonald, Captain Alexander, 117, 118, 179, 272n.7; his *Letter Book*, 275n.27
McEvoy, John, assistant surgeon and dispenser at Halifax, 155
McGee, Ann, surgeoness at Merigomish, 315n.172
McGrath, James, listed as keeper of the poor house and House of Correction at Shelburne, 300n.22
Machias: pirates from, 102
McIntyre, Donald, surgeon at Halifax, 140, 143, 147, 178, 205, 207, 214, 297n.271
MacKay, Relief. *See* Williams, Relief, 48
McKeown, Thomas, xvi
McKinnon, Hon. William: suspended from the Council of Cape Breton, 165
Mackintosh, Catherine: autopsy on, 48
Mackworth, Sir Herbert, 162
McLean, Donald, of New York, 118
McLean, Donald, surgeon, 179, 205, 207, 297n.271, 314n.167; advertisement to sell drugs and medicine, 179
McLean, Brig. Gen. Francis, 119–22, 127, 130; officer commanding the British army at Halifax, 122
McLean, Colonel, 118
Maclean's Corps, 109
MacLennan, J.S., historian, 222
McLeod, Murdock, surgeon at Country Harbour, 205, 207, 209, 211
McMonagle, John H., surgeon, 172
McNab's Island, 52
MacNeil, Mrs, midwife at Shelburne, 185
McNutt, Colonel Alexander, 68, 69
McPherson, John, surgeon at Manchester, 205, 207
Mad-dog bite: prescription for, 178; recipe for, 141
Malaria, 125
Manchester, 159, 205
Man-midwife: Daniel Kendrick, 316n.178; John Grant, 44, 92; Henry Meriton, 39, 92; Christopher Nicolai, 71; John Phillipps, 65, 92
March, Jacob, surgeon's mate, Shirley's Regiment, 47; at Louisbourg, 246n.52
Marines, 65, 109, 114, 116, 117
Marischal College, 136, 176, 177
Maroons, 145, 155, 156; hospital for, 145
Marsh, Francis, captain of the 65th Regiment, 272n.3
Marshall, John, surgeon at Halifax, 119, 120, 127, 129, 133, 136, 139, 140, 214, 215, 221n.10, 297n.273; surgeon to general military hospital, 120, 129, 214
Marshall, Josiah, 76
Marshman, Jeremiah, 399n.15
Martha, 165
Martial law: proclaimed in Nova Scotia, 107
Marvin, Joseph, surgeon's mate at Digby, 205, 207
Maryland Volunteers, 165
Mascarene, Paul, lieutenant governor at Annapolis Royal, 18
Massachusetts Bay, Colony of, 66; grants right to regulate medical practice, 168; vote against Acadians landing at Boston, 262n.209
Massey, Major General Eyre, 107, 112–17,

119, 121; duel with
Admiral Sir George
Collier, 115
Mather, Rev. Cotton: and
inoculation, 8
Mathews, Hon. David,
president of HM Coun-
cil, Cape Breton, 165
Mauger's Beach, 157
Maxwell, William, sent
277n.46
Measles, 6, 141
Medical Act, of Lower
Canada, 169
Supplies: medical and surgical. See Breast pipe,
Truss, Electrotherapy,
Lancet, Nipple glasses,
Syringes, Thermometer
Medications: and treat-
ments administered by
surgeons in Halifax,
195. See also Drugs,
medications, and treat-
ments
Medicine: and drugs,
advertised for sale, 96,
122, 123, 179, 180;
chests, 24, 131, 180,
181; English, 14; regu-
lation of price of, 39;
for the hospitals at Hal-
ifax and Louisbourg,
65; for the settlers to go
to Nova Scotia, 17;
patent, advertised, 122,
123, 179, 180; stores,
advertisment of, 38, 61,
96, 123, 161, 179, 180
Medlicot, Ann, midwife at
Halifax, 193
Melville Island. See
Kavanagh's Island
Melville, Viscount Robert,
First Lord of the
Admiralty, 304n.56
Mercury, H.M., 270n.142
Meres, James S., 132, 133
Meriton, Henry, apothe-
cary and surgeon at
Halifax, 38, 92, 193; ad-
vertisement of ser-

vices, 38, 39; his school
on Sackville Street, 40;
man-midwife at Halifax,
39, 92
Merlegash. See Lunenburg
Merry, William, surgeon
and apothecary at Hal-
ifax, 17, 38–40, 46, 193,
197; lawsuit against
William Kneeland, 39,
40
Merry Jacks, 224n.10
Messervy, Colonel, 61
Methane gas: causing
deaths in coal mines at
Spanish River, 295n.261
Micmacs, (also Micmaks
and Mick Mack): lan-
guage of, 121; popula-
tion of, 222n.2; treaty
with those in eastern
part of the province,
33
Microscope, 15
Middlesex Hospital,
London, 6
Middleton, Mr, surgeon
general to the army
abroad, 16, 17
Midwife, 34, 91, 92, 118,
145, 146, 184; and
midwives, 17, 32, 46, 83,
91, 118, 137; at
Barrington, 66, 118; at
Halifax, 62, 91, 92,
118, 184, 193, 194; at
Horton, 118; at Liver-
pool, 269n.117; at
Lunenburg, 91,
269n.117; at Shelburne,
185; provincial, 42, 61,
62
Midwifery, 62, 92, 169,
170
Military hospital, 83, 84,
110, 112, 119, 120,
121, 139, 145, 146, 178,
210, 214, 216; closed
in 1797, 178; directions
to substitute regimen-
tal hospitals for general
hospital, 120, 140;

location of, 77; plans
for, 59; referred to as
the general military
hospital, 61
Militia, 108, 164, 227n.35;
and smallpox, 106
Miller, James: his plan of
Sydney drawn in 1795,
165, 166
Minutemen, 101
Mixtures, 57; attenuating,
41, 197; cephalic, 40,
197; hysteric, 40, 198
Monckton, Lt Col Robert,
47, 59
Monk, James, 231n.48,
263n.13
Monro, Dr Alexander,
primus, 15, 174, 175,
220n.5
Mons, 239n.113
Montague, Lord Charles,
commanding officer of
the Duke of Cumber-
land's Regiment, 156
Montague, Admiral John,
84
Montague, Lady Mary
Wortley: her son inoc-
ulated in Constanti-
nople, 7
Montcalm, 57
Montreal, 71, 107, 168,
169, 209
Moreau, Rev. J.B., of Halifax and Lunenburg,
33, 84
Morehead, Mr ———:
recommends to over-
seers of poor in Liver-
pool concerning
smallpox, 129
Morehead, Mr ———,
assistant surgeon at
Halifax, 110
Morgagni, Giovanni-
Battista, founder of
modern pathology, 5
Morgan, Dr John: his
book A Discourse upon
the Institution of Medical
Schools in America, 96

Morris, Charles, 76, 77; member of a committee to report on the orphan house, 91
Mortality, 51, 92, 147, 188, 234n.68; infant, in Nova Scotia, 147, 189; in Halifax, 25, 28; in orphan house, 69; on four foreign-Protestant ships arriving in Halifax in 1751, 30; on the five foreign-Protestant ships arriving in Halifax in 1752, 33; on trans-Atlantic crossings in the eighteenth century, 225n.18. *See also* Death
Morton, Dr William: demonstrated use of ether in 1846, 221n.8
Moser, Maria, midwife at Lunenburg, 269n.117
Moses Harris: his plan of Halifax, 21
Murder, 217
Murdoch, 30, 239n.111
Muriatic acid, 5
Murray, Rear Admiral George, 155
Murray, Brig. Gen. John: replaced as president of Council for Cape Breton, 165
Murray, Colonel, of the 15th Regiment, 61

Namur, 58
Nancy, 27, 30
National Gallery of Canada, 53
Naval hospital, 48, 52, 54, 55, 58, 59, 64, 65, 67, 83, 84, 108, 111, 113–15, 122, 127, 128, 130, 131, 133, 140, 142, 145, 155, 177, 211, 215, 216; assistant surgeons sent out from London for, 254n.134; at Louisbourg,

257n.154; descriptions of, 122, 127, 128, 303n.53; drawing of, by J.S. Meres, 132; establishment of, 57, 131, 133; location of, 113, 121, 122, 216; number of seamen in hospital from 1757–61, 54
Navigation Acts, 102
Navy Yard, 134; set on fire, 102
Needham, Lieutenant, 113
Negroes: arrived in Halifax from St Augustine, 151
Nepean, Evan, Secretary of State, 148, 151, 160
Neptune, 256n.153
Nesbitt, William, overseer of the poor, 254n.133
New Brunswick, province of, established, 137
New Brunswick, New Jersey, 33
Newcomb, Simon, 277n.46
New Dublin, Township of, 69
Newell, Dr Thomas, physician and surgeon in England, 172
New England, 18, 55, 59, 66, 107, 115; emigration to Nova Scotia from, 22, 66, 237n.98; first hospital established in, 26; planters, and land vacated by Acadians, 66
New England Provincial Troops, 47, 49, 51, 111
New England Hospital. *See* Hospital
Newfoundland, 103, 104
New Jersey, 121, 168, 210; first colony to adopt a law requiring physicians to be examined, 168
New Jerusalem, Maine, 106

Newport, Rhode Island, 131
Newport, Township of, 68, 70, 81, 94; number of families and people there in 1762, 70; relief of the poor in, 81
"New Settlers," 160
Newton, Henry, 77
Newton, Hibbert, overseer of the poor, 64, 87
Newton, Sir Isaac, 14
New York, 25, 52, 110, 111, 113, 118, 131, 135, 137, 138, 140, 150, 151, 159, 168, 179, 207, 209–11; and Act to Regulate the Practice of Physick and Surgery, 168; hospitals at, 131, 140, 142, 204; poor house there,
New York Volunteers 139
Nicolai, Christopher Adam, surgeon on *Murdoch*, 31, 38, 71, 150, 184, 214, 297n.270; advertises that he will perform inoculation, 71; appointed physician at the poor house, 150, 214; advertises his services as a man-midwife, 71, 184; dispensing apothecary and surgeon to the poor
Nipple glasses, 182
Nooth, Dr J.M., superintendent general of hospitals for the forces in North America, 139, 140
North Carolina Volunteers, 205
Northern Ireland, 68, 69
Northern University: infamous for physical diplomas, 43
Norwood, Lieutenant William, of the 33rd Regiment: his *Journal*, 308n.101

Nostrums, 14
Nourse, Edward, surgeon at St Bartholomew's Hospital, 174
Nova Scotia: estimated population of, in 1762, 70
Nova Scotia Historical Society, Collections of, xv, xvi
Nurses, 118, 185; at George Greaves's inoculation hospital, 105; at general or public hospital, 42, 45, 57; at naval hospital, 54, 133; at the poor house, 89; at the prison hospital, 289n.174
Nye, Cornelius, surgeon's mate, Shirley's Regiment, 47, 49

Oakum: description of, 263n.13; picking of, 75, 89
Oats, Samuel, referred to as doctor at Cape Forchu, 66, 70
Oath of Allegiance, 46,108
Ogden, Jonathan, hospital mate at Halifax, 143, 205, 207; of the New York General Hospital, 205
Ogilvie, Lt Gen. James, 154; replaces Hon. David Mathews as president of Cape Breton Council 310n.120
Ohme, Johann C., surgeon of the Sally, 240
Oils (also Oyls), kinds of, 40, 179–81
"Old Settlers," 160
Oliver, Lieutenant Governor, 279n.60
Oliver, Dr Peter, physician in Boston and in England, 109, 209, 211

Onslow, Township of, 68, 70, 81, 108; reaction to the Militia Bill and tax to support the militia, 108; population in 1762, 70
Orphan house, 32, 33, 42, 43, 46, 49, 68, 81, 85, 86, 89, 90, 91, 108, 120, 130, 145, 149, 154, 214, 216; and children of poor, 68; building and lot placed for auction, 149; closed in 1784, 154; condition of, 69, 90, 91; costs and expenses of, 68, 90; doctors appointed to attend, 85, 86; grant for, 63; keepers of, 68, 130, 154; location of, 77
Orphans, 68, 148, 149; apprenticeship of, 79, 240n.124; binding out of, 79, 81, 90; from New York 139; mortality among, in orphan house, 69; number in orphan house, 240n.125; number sent to orphan house from the Gale, 33; placement of, as servants, 265n.44
Oswald, Mr, commissioner of Trade and Plantations, 26
Overseers of the poor, 64, 77, 79–83, 87–9, 124, 139, 149, 151–4, 157, 254n.133, 265n.33, 268n.105, 280n.79
Oxford University, 15, 177
Oxley, John, surgeon of the 96th Regiment, 156, 214

Paine, Charles, surgeon at Halifax, 193
Paine, Dr William, physician at Halifax and

Passamaquoddy, 136, 139, 142, 170, 209, 211, 214; director of all hospitals for the British army in Halifax, 139; portrait of, 72
Papists, 230n.48
Paracelsus, 287n.157
Paris, Treaty of, 37, 73
Parr, Governor John, 139, 147, 148, 151, 152, 154, 160; demoted to lieutenant governor, 301n.39
Passamaquoddy, New Brunswick, 136, 211
Patent medicines 122, 124, 179–80. See also Balsams, Drops, Drugs, mediations, and treatments, Elixirs, Oils, Pills, Powders, Salts, Syrups, and Tinctures
Paterson, Major General, commander of HM Forces in Nova Scotia, 136, 140
Paupers, 149, 152, 154
Peace treaty: of 1752, 33; with Claude Gisiquash, 34
Pearce, Joseph, hospital mate in Annapolis Royal, 308n.101
Pearl, 30, 33
Pegasus, 132, 133
Pembroke, 58
Penal Laws: prohibiting Roman Catholics from owning land, 22, 229n.48
Penobscot, Maine, 122
Pepperell, Sir William, 223; ordered to raise a regiment to assist in taking Fort Beauséjour, 47
Pepperell's Regiment (the 51st), 222n.4
Pereau (also Pero), 246n.56
Perkins, Nathaniel, physi-

cian in Boston, 109, 210, 211

Perkins, Simeon, 118, 123, 129, 141, 156, 157, 208; his *Diary*, 118, 141, 156

Perkins, Dr William Lee, physician in Boston and England, 109, 210, 211

Perry, John, surgeon and practitioner of physic at Shelburne, 157, 205, 207, 298n.273

Peters, Dr Alexander A., physician and surgeon at Halifax, 170, 172; advertises his practice in a Halifax newspaper, 313n.166

Petitcodiac, 47

Petite Rivière, 204

Petition: of Cumberland County residents to General George Washington, 108, 277n.46; of residents to George III concerning Governor Legge's policies, 109

Petty larceny, 74, 75

Pharmacopoeia, used in Flanders, 16

Philadelphia, 26, 95, 102, 130, 155, 157, 159, 196

Philipps, George, surgeon at Halifax, 170, 172

Philipps, John, surgeon at Halifax, 86, 91, 96, 108, 120, 135, 154, 159, 160, 170, 172, 180, 214, 215, 254n.134, advertisement to sell an assortment of medicines, 96, 180; appointed surgeon of the Loyal Nova Scotia Volunteers, 108; assistant surgeon and surgeon at the naval hospital, 113, 215; elected to the House of Assembly, 93; involvement with

orphan house, 86, 91, 214; and smallpox, 105; surgeon at the naval hospital, 215

Philipps, John Jr, surgeon at Halifax, 170, 172, 314n.170

Philipps, William, surgeon at Halifax, 172

Philipps's Regiment (the 40th), 24

Phillipps, Lieutenant John, surgeon at Lunenburg, 38, 65, 70, 84; man-midwife at Lunenburg, 92; appointed surgeon for all Independent Companies of Rangers, 31

Phillips, Alexander Josiah, practitioner of physic at Digby, 205, 207

Philosophical Society of Edinburgh, 15

Phlebotomy, 4

Physicians: Chamberlen family of. *See* Forceps

Pictou, 130, 147, 158, 160

Pills, kinds of, 40, 41, 96, 122, 125, 179–82, 196, 199

Pinckston, Fleming, doctor of physic at Digby, 170, 205, 207, 298n.273

Pinel, Dr Philippe, pioneer in the treatment of the mentally ill, 98

Pisiquid (also Piziquid), 51, 58, 66, 222n.1

Pitt, Harry, surgeon at Halifax, 193

Pitt, William, first earl of Chatham, 225

Plan: for the Town of Halifax by John Bruce, 20; for the Town of Halifax by Moses Harris, 21; of the Naval Yard by Charles Blaskowitz, 134

Plasters: kinds of, 40, 125, 179, 180, 196, 197, 199

Pleurisy, 135, 196

Plymouth, England, 224n.10

Plymouth, New England, 26

Point Edward: workhouse and sawmill there, 163

Point Pleasant, 22

Police, 149

Poll tax, 146, 153

Poor, 103, 151, 268n.93; employment for, 89; relief and support of, 73, 80–3, 85, 87, 88, 89, 145; tax, on citizens of Halifax, 80, 87, 88; transient, 3, 98, 146, 148–53. *See also* Act, Bill, Overseers of the poor

Poor bill. *See* Act, Bill, Poor, transient

Poor house, 3, 26, 77, 85, 87, 89, 98, 112, 126, 139, 145–50, 152, 177, 299n.9; as part of workhouse, 83, 85; hospital in, 83, 142, 214, 216; illegitimate children in, 154; keepers of, 126, 299n.114, 299n.115; list of persons there in 1773, 88, 89; records pertaining to, 1779–80, 126, 127

Poor relief. *See* Poor

Popery: suppression of, 229n.48

Porter, Roy, medical historian, 5, 6, 98, 177

Portland, Lord, 165

Port Medway, 157

Port Mouton, 206

Port Roseway: number of Loyalists who settled there, 137

Portsmouth, England, 224n.10

Pott, Percival, surgeon at St Bartholomew's, 174
Poultice, 183, 199
Powders: kinds of, 40, 124, 179–81, 196
Power, Thomas, 231
Prebble, Major Jedidiah, 49
Prescott, Jonathan, surgeon at Halifax and Chester, 31, 40
Prescott, Joseph, physician and surgeon at Cornwallis, Lunenburg, and Halifax, 302n.47; portrait of, 100
Preston, 207
Price, Arthur, surgeon of the 47th Regiment, 30, 51
Prince, Benjamin, physician at Annapolis and Truro, 312n.142
Prince Carl Regiment, 205
Prince Edward's Regiment, 165
Prince George, 271n.154
Prince, John, physician at Salem, Massachusetts, 107, 109, 142, 210, 211; merchant and trader in Halifax, 108
Prince of Wales Regiment, 205
Prince Street, 78
Pringle, Sir John, physician to military hospitals: his observations concerning fever, 28; and sanitation in military camps, 29
Pringle, William, surgeon's mate, 107
Prins, David, surgeon on the *Pearl*, 239n.113
Prison hospital. See Hospital
Prison ships. See Ships
Prisoners, 30, 32, 48, 49, 65, 119, 120, 129, 130, 136, 154, 155, 186; and smallpox, 117; from

St Domingo 155; from St Pierre and Miquelon, 154, 155; health of, 32, 118; naval, housed in *La Feliz*, 155; rebel, 117, 119, 121
Proclamation: concerning quarantine for yellow fever, 157; ending victualling of original settlers, 234n.72; to the Settlers to Assemble in order to Draw Lots, 228n.41; to Prevent Desertion from the Settlement of Halifax, 19
Proctor, Colonel Charles, 95
Protestants, foreign, in Nova Scotia, 30–4, 37, 38, 66, 220n.1
Public hospital. See Hospital, civilian
Purging, 195, 199
Pye, Captain, chief commander of the squadron at Halifax, 45

Quackery: definitions of, 310n.133; golden age of, 15
Quacks, 177
Quarantine: hospital, 113, 214, 215; of foreign Protestants in Halifax Harbour in 1752, 33; proclaimed by Council in January 1754, 41, 42. See also Proclamation
Quebec: 3, 71, 93, 168, 169; bill to prevent persons from practising medicine, surgery, and midwifery, 168, 169; fall of, 65; smallpox epidemics in, 9
Queen Street, 77
Queen's Rangers, 204
Quin, Mr ———, surgeon's mate of the 84th Regiment, 275n.27

Rangers, Independent Companies of, 31, 58
Ransom, John, author, 176
Ratio: of persons in Nova Scotia to the number of practising doctors, 171
Rebels, 106–9, 115, 116, 120, 122, 129–31, 138; sympathy with, from Cumberland County, 108
Red hospital. See Hospital
Redman, Dr John, 198
Reeves (or Reeve), Thomas, surgeon and apothecary at Halifax, 17, 85, 112, 116, 120, 19, 214; appointed to care for the sick in the workhouse, 85; surgeon's mate at the hospital, 42
Regiments: number designation of, 226n.29; in Nova Scotia, movements of, 18, 19, 24, 27, 30, 33, 47, 51, 56–8, 59, 61, 69, 73, 74, 79, 80, 84, 102, 107, 112, 116, 117, 118, 119, 122, 138, 140, 142, 154, 156, 163, 164, 179, 183, 204, 205, 207, 216, 223n.8, 224n.4, 236n.86, 250n.88, 250n.90, 254n.126, 266n.65, 267n.65, 275n.27, 276n.44, 277n.45, 278n.52, 308n.101. See also the following regiments by name: Argyle Highlanders, Bragg's, Duke of Cumberland's, Duke of Hamilton's, Enniskillens, Fuller's, Hopson's, Kennedy's, King's Own, Lascelles's, Pepperell's, Royal Fusiliers, Royal Highland Emigrant, Royal,

Royal Regiment of Artillery, Shirley's, Waldeck, Warburton's
Representative government, 96
Rheumatism, 123, 196
Rhode Island, Colony of, 66, 131, 137, 138
Rice, Jesse, physician at Yarmouth, 123, 142
Robertson, William, surgeon of the 42nd Regiment, 164
Robinson, Sir Thomas, late governor of Barbados, 225
Roehampton, 17, 23, 193
Rohl, Andrew, Loyalist admitted to the poor house, 151
Roman Catholics, 23; discrimination against, 22, 229n.48
Roots, 22; Carolina Pinkroot, 181; elecampane, 313n.164; marshmallow, 141
Rosine, 126
Rotterdam, 28, 30
Rous, Captain John, 45, 48, 49
Rowlands, Dr David, surgeon at Halifax, 172
Royal College of Physicians of London, 136, 170, 176, 177, 220n.3
Royal College of Surgeons of London, 124
Royal Fencible Americans, 102, 103, 142
Royal Fusiliers (7th Regiment), 156, 216
Royal Highland Emigrant Regiment (the 84th), 102, 112, 116, 117, 142, 179
Royal Navy, 49, 101, 131; disposition of HM ships under command of Lord Colville in 1760, 67; first fleet to arrive in Halifax, 48

Royal Nova Scotia Regiment, 154, 155, 178
Regimental Hospital. See Hospital
Royal Regiment (the 1st), 56–8
Royal Regiment of Artillery, 51, 52, 109, 204, 206
Rum: sold by unlicensed retailers, 94, 146
Rush, Dr Benjamin, of Philadelphia, 196
Russell, Joseph, doctor and surgeon at Halifax, 205, 207; lawsuit against patient for non-payment for medicines, 306n.89
Russell, Nathaniel, 126
Rust (also Rush), Thomas, doctor and surgeon at Halifax, 193
Rutherford, Dr George, surgeon at Halifax, 140

Sacheverell, Joshua, surgeon at Halifax, 24, 193
Sackville, 51, 108; Street, 40; Township of, 108
Saint John, 137, 138, 204, 206, 210; number of Loyalists who settled there, 137
Salem, Massachusetts, 107, 108
Sally, 33, 147, 148, 151, 157
Salter, Malachy Sr, 126, 228n.166
Salter, Malachy, surgeon at Halifax, 214; his drug and medicine store on Granville Street, 288n.166
Salts: Glauber's, 40, 198; of copper, 199; Scarborough's, 40
Salusbury, John: his Diary, 19, 23, 27, 30

Salve, 126
Sarah, 24
Saratoga, battle of, 117
Sargent, John, member of the House of Assembly: introduces first bill to regulate the practice of medicine in Nova Scotia, 167
Saunders, Admiral Charles, 65
Sauvage, F.B. de C.: on typhus, 29
Saxony, 240n.127
Scalpings, 30, 34, 217, 233n.56, 236n.86, 238n.105
Scarlet fever. See Fever
Scatari Island, 256n.153
Schmitt, Johann Michael: his family Bible, and entries describing deaths from smallpox, 253n.109
Schools, 40, 240n.124
School of Anatomy and Surgery, Great Windmill Street, 174
Schwartz, William, overseer of the poor, 265n.33
Scott, Ann, midwife, 118
Scott, Captain George, 47
Scott, John, assistant surgeon at the naval hospital, 114
Scott, Joseph, 263n.13
Scurvy. See Cures, Diseases and illnesses
Sears, Richard, physician at Horton, 66, 70
Seaton, Robert, 4th Regiment: his wens cured by Benjamin Green, 183
Seidler (also Scidler and Scidleir), Andrew, surgeon at Clements, 137, 205
Servants, 74, 79, 118, 203, 230n.48; with the Cornwallis passengers, 22

Settlers: living on transports in Halifax Harbour, 18; quitting the settlement of Halifax, 18, 19, 23; unable to pay for medical services, 32; transferred from transports to George's Island, 18
Seven Years' War, 73, 185
Sharman, Ambrose, of 59th Regiment, surgeon's mate at Halifax, 267n.65
Sharp, Samuel, surgeon at Guy's Hospital, 174
Shaw, Dr Peter: his book *A New Practice of Physic*, 271n.146
Shelburne, 150, 151, 156–7, 172, 185, 204–11; establishment of a poor house and workhouse in, 150
Sherman, John, surgeon's mate at Halifax, 17
Ship fever. *See* Fever, 28
Ships: emigrant, 27–30, 33, 42; hospital, 17, 23, 25, 51, 56, 109, 110–12, 193, 214, 216, 225n.23; of war, 14, 49, 58, 136, 249n.76; passenger lists of, 22, 23, 224n.10, 236n.84, 238n.107, 238n.109, 239n.110, 239n.111; prison, 129, 130, 131, 133, 135, 136, 155, 290n.185, 293n.224, 293n.230; transport, 18, 19, 156,193, 194; with illness on board, 28, 32, 33, 42, 58, 135, 148, 155, 236n.86, 284n.130
Ships, miscellaneous, 22, 23, 24, 30, 42, 51, 95, 110, 113, 118, 119, 132, 133, 147, 151, 157, 162, 164, 207, 249n.76, 253n.106, 256n.153,

270n.142, 271n.154, 308n.95, 315n.172
Shipton, Sam, 228
Shipwrecks, 164, 165
Shirley, Governor John, 46, 47, 51, 66
Shirley's Regiment (the 50th), 33, 47, 222n.4
Short, Richard: his engravings, 60, 77, 78
Shubenacadie, 68
Shubenacadie Indians. *See* Indians
Shuldham, Rear Admiral Molyneux, 109, 110, 111
Sick and Hurt Board: commissioners of, 127
Sieger (also Seege), John Christian, physician and surgeon at Halifax, 137, 205, 208
Sierra Leone, 156
Silver, James, surgeon of Marines and at Fort Cumberland, 116
Simpson, James, surgeon in London, 172
Simpson, Dr James, 221n.8
Skene, William, surgeon of the 40th Regiment, 24, 51
Skener, Johannes (also Skinner, John), surgeon at Digby, 137, 205
Skye, Isle of, 298n.2
Slater, William, merchant, 133
Slocombe, George, surgeon at Halifax, 24, 30
Small, Lt Col John, commander of the Second Battalion of the 84th Regiment, 102
Smallpox, 3, 6, 35, 37, 57, 58, 59, 61, 67, 71, 96, 101, 103–8, 110, 112, 117, 118, 121, 125, 129, 130, 157–9, 184, 186, 190, 200, 201,

217; among infants in Halifax, 129; and inoculation against, 105, 118, 157; deaths from, August-December 1775, 104; description of, at Lunenburg, 105, 106; epidemics of, 48, 55, 56; house, at Liverpool, 129, 157; outbreaks of, 104, 105, 117; precautions against infection with, 104
Smellie, Dr William, man-midwife in London, 39, 92
Smith, Edward, surgeon at Liverpool, 205, 208
Smith, Isaac, 74
Smith, William, a governor of the orphan house, 91
Smith, William, physician and surgeon in London and Sydney, 162–5, 307n.92
Smith, William Howard, overseer of the poor, 268n.105
Society for the Propagation of the Gospel, 84, 121
Society of Apothecaries, 176, 220n.3
Solomon, John, wheelwright, 51
Sorcery and witchcraft, 167
South Barracks, 127
South Carolina, 137, 147; regiment, 204, 205
South Suburbs. *See* Halifax
Southwark, borough of London, 162
Sparrow, Samuel, 133
Speedwell, 30, 238n.107
Sphinx, 14
Spithead, England, 14, 55, 111
Sprainger, Katherine, 246n.6

Spring Garden Road, 214, 216

Spruce beer: part of orphans' diet in the orphan house, 240n.124; preventive medication against epidemic fevers, 305n.75; standard drink provided to inmates at poor house, 305n.75

Spry, Captain Richard, 51

Stafford, William, surgeon at Sydney, 164, 165

Stamp Act, 102

Stapleton, ———, physician with the Yorkshire settlers, 97, 271n.154

Starvation, 118, 217

Static electricity: used in medical therapy, 315n.171

St Augustine: negroes from, 151

St Bartholomew's Hospital, London, 5, 175

St Christopher's, Island of, 96

St Domingo: French prisoners from, 155

Steele, John, lieutenant and surgeon at Halifax and Annapolis, 17, 70, 194; elected to House of Assembly, 93; surgeon's mate at the hospital, 42

Steer's Opodeldoc, 181, 182

St George's Anglican Church, Sydney, 164

St George's Hospital, London, 6, 170, 172, 174

Stickells, John F.T., surgeon at Liverpool and Guysborough, 137, 205, 208

Stills, 31, 40, 128

Stimulents: kinds of, used to rebuild the body, 196

St John's Anglican Church, Lunenburg, 105

Story, Mark, 17

St Paul's Anglican Church, Halifax, 30, 33, 49, 103; burial records, 24, 28

St Peters, Cape Breton Island, 222n.1

St Pierre and Miquelon, 154

St Thomas's Hospital, London, 6, 39, 174

Sugar and Molasses Act, 102

Sullivan, Bartholomew, doctor at Shelburne and merchant at Halifax, 109, 205, 208

Supplies: medical and surgical. See Breast pipe, Truss, Electrotherapy, Lancet, Nipple glasses, Syringes, Thermometer

Surgeoness, 315n.172

Surgeons, in Nova Scotia: dispute between, 57; number of, from 1749–53, 35, from 1753–63, 71, from 1763–74, 97; civilian, naval, and military, number of, from 1750–1800, 173; pay received by, in Halifax, 42; quitting settlement of Halifax, 23

Surgeon's instruments, 52; for sale, 179, 182

Surgeons' Hall, London: examinations at, 16

Surgery, antiseptic, 221n.7

Surgical procedures: amputation, 4; autopsy, 48; lithotomy, 4, 124; trepanning, 300n.17

Sutton, Mr: and air pipes for transports, 16, 225n.18

Sweet, Benoni, bonesetter at Falmouth, 67, 70

Switzerland: passengers from, 30

Sydenham, Dr Thomas, 7, 14, 15

Sydney, Cape Breton, 156, 162–5; arrival of first settlers, 162; described, 163; hospital in, 163, 165; plan of, by James Miller, 165, 166; regiments there, 156, 163; watercolour of, by Lt William Booth, 163

Syphilis. See Diseases and illnesses

Syringes, 182

Syrup: of poppies, 141; Velmo's vegetable, 96

Tait, David, 163

Tarleton's Legion, 205

Tattray, Maria, midwife at Lunenburg, 269n.117

Templeman, Dr ———, travelling dentist, 184

Textbooks, medical: advertised, 271n.146

Thermometer: advertised in a Halifax newspaper in 1780, 124

Thomas, George, naval storekeeper at Halifax, 127

Thomas, John, surgeon's mate, Shirley's Regiment, 47, 49; portrait of, 12

Thomas, Stephen, surgeon at Liverpool, 142, 296n.263; picture of, 72

Thomson, Alexander, purveyor of the naval hospital, 131

Throckmorton, Robert, pupil surgeon at Halifax, 194

Tinctures: colic, 40, 197; compound Senna, 125; description of, 199; Greenough's, 182

Tobias, Christian, physician at Digby, 205, 210; only doctor remaining in Digby in 1799, 312n.143

Tobias, Jacob, physician at Digby, 312n.142

Tonge, William, 96

Tonics: kinds of, used to rebuild the body, 196

Torpedo (or electric fish), 314n.171

Torrington's Bay, 227n.34

Townsend, George: sells patent medicines, 122

Townshend Act, 102

Townshend, Maria, 223

Townshend, Lord, 223

Transient poor. See Poor

Transport ships. See Ships

Treatments. See Drugs, medications, and treatments

Trepanning. See Surgical procedures

Triggs, Darius, 225n.145

Triggs, Mrs Dorcas, midwife at Halifax, 62

Tritten, Richard, overseer of the poor, 88, 124

Truro, Township of, 68, 70, 81, 108, 130, 150, 160; and reaction to the Militia Bill and the tax to pay for the militia, 108; population in 1762, 70

Truss, elastic: advertised in Halifax, 180

Tucker, Dr Robert, physician and surgeon at Annapolis Royal, 170, 176, 205, 210, 211; awarded first MD granted by King's College, New York, 170, 171, 176

Tumor, stealoma encysted, 183

Tunis, Barbara, 71

Turner, Edward, 17

Tutty, Rev. William, 230n.48

Two Brothers, 109, 110

Tyler, John, surgeon's mate, 47, 49, 51

Typhus. See Fever

Uniacke, Richard John, 116, 148, 161; charged with treason

University: of Aberdeen, 170, 172, 176, 177; of Edinburgh, 170, 176; of Glasgow, 5, 175, 176; of Pennsylvania, establishes a Faculty of Medicine, 171; of St Andrews, 170, 176, 177

Upton, L.F.S., historian, 222

Urquhart, William, surgeon at Halifax, 31, 48

Utrecht, Treaty of, 13

Van Buren, James, physician at Granville, 138, 205, 210, 211

Van Buskirk, Abraham, surgeon at Shelburne, 205, 208, 210

Van Hulst, Abraham, surgeon at Annapolis Royal, 143, 296n.267

Vaudreuil, Monsieur, governor of Three Rivers, 249n.76

Veale, Dr Richard, physician and surgeon at Halifax and Louisbourg, 30, 45, 51, 69

Venereal disease. See Cures, Diseases and illnesses

Ventilators, on ships, 16, 27; description of, 225n.17

Victualling list: for May and June 1750, 25, 31

Vienna, 124

Viets, Rev. Roger: and efforts to obtain medical assistance for the people of Digby, 150

Vincent, Rev. Robert, 261n.201

Vinegar: ship washed down with, 96

Virginia, 47, 207

Von Haller, Dr Albrecht, 14

Von Riedesel, Baroness: her tooth pulled by a surgeon in Halifax, 288n.170

Von Specht, Lieutenant Colonel, 120

Wade, Captain, ———, aide-de-camp to Major General Massey, 115

Waldeck Regiment, 142

Walker, Hugh: in charge of the House of Correction at Shelburne, 150

Wallace, John, surgeon's mate at Halifax, 194

War Office, 140

Warburton's Regiment (the 45th), 19, 24, 30, 33, 47, 51, 57, 59, 69, 79, 80, 84, 222n.4, 232n.54

Washington, George, 102, 106, 108, 111, 112, 138; comments on proposed invasion of Nova Scotia, 103, 106, 108

Webb, Godfrey, surgeon at Halifax, 59, 215; assistant surgeon and surgeon at the naval hospital, 54, 55, 215

Webster, Isaac, physician and surgeon at Cornwallis, 189, 303n.47

Wenman, Mrs Ann, matron of the orphan house, 32, 46

Wenman, Richard, 45, 46, 75–77, 107, 130; overseer of the poor, 265n.33
Wens. *See* Cures, Diseases and illnesses
Wentworth, Lieutenant Governor John, 154, 156–8
Westminister, 162
Westminister Hospital, London, 6
Wet nurses: advertisements of, 124; cost of, 90; at orphan house, 90
Wethered, Samuel, 116
Weymouth, 205, 207
Whipping: of inmates, 150
Whipping post, common, 263n14; in workhouse, 76, 150; public, 75
White, Charles, surgeon at Halifax, 83, 110, 215, 279n.68; in charge of naval hospital at Halifax, 83, 215
White, Francis, overseer of the poor, 87
White (also Whyte), Robert, surgeon at Halifax, 24, 194
White servitude: in eighteenth-century America, 9, 224n.10
Whitehall, 31, 51, 62, 63, 115, 118, 146, 151, 154
Whitehaven Harbour, Guysborough County, 225n.21
Whitehead, on Whitehaven Harbour, 225n.21
Whitworth, Sir Charles, 162
Whitworth, Miles, surgeon, Shirley's Regiment, 47, 49
Wildman, John, surgeon at Halifax, 29, 194
Wilkins, Lewis Morris, 161

William IV: in Halifax in 1786, 292n.218
William and Ann, 207
Williams, Elizabeth, midwife at Halifax, 194
Williams, Relief, author, 48; her article on poor relief and medicine in Nova Scotia, xv
Williams, Richard, storekeeper of the Halifax Careening Yard, 272n.4
Willis, John, chymist and surgeon at Halifax, 194
Willoughby, Samuel, physician at Cornwallis, 66,70, 93; and member of House of Assembly, 93, 94
Wilmington, 193, 224n.10
Wilmot, Dr, physician general of the army, 16, 17
Wilmot, Governor Montague, 84, 89, 116
Wilmot Township, 66
Wilson, John, 238n.105
Wilson, Thomas, surgeon at Halifax, 17, 194
Winchelsea, 193, 224n.10
Windsor, Town of, 48, 102, 106, 116, 142, 150, 158, 160, 172, 180, 181, 204, 205, 209–11; hospital there, 112
Winslow, George, surgeon at Halifax, 31
Winslow, Col John, 47–9
Witchcraft. *See* Sorcery and witchcraft
Women, 30, 73, 74, 79, 83, 89, 109, 112, 118, 126, 151, 167; and children, of the army, 73, 74
Wood, Richard, surgeon's mate at the naval hospital, 133
Wood, Rev. Thomas, vicar of St Paul's Church,

physician and surgeon, 33, 121, 285n.141, 297n.270; silhouette of, 12
Woodbury, Jonathan, physician at Granville and Wilmot, 66, 70
Woodin, John, 88, 112, 126; keeper of the workhouse, 88
Workhouse, at Halifax, 3, 74, 75, 77, 80, 82, 83, 85, 86, 87–9, 93–5, 97, 98, 116, 150, 152; funding of, 75, 76; keepers of, 45, 46, 75–7, 82, 83, 87, 88, 107, 126, 130, 299n.14; location of, 45, 75, 76, 77; surgeon appointed to, 85. *See also* Bridewell, House of Correction, Shelburne
Workhouse, at Point Edward, 163
Wurtemberg (also Wertemberg), 239n.113
Wyer, Edward, surgeon at Halifax, 120, 124, 127, 142, 170, 214, 285n.139; performed first recorded lithotomy in Halifax, 124; surgeon to the poor house, 120, 214

Yarmouth, Township of, 66–70, 81, 104, 123, 142, 150, 179, 204, 206; population in 1762, 70
Yellow fever. *See* Cures, Fever
Yonge, Sir George, secretary of state for War, 308n.101
Yorke, Colonel John, 164
Yorkshire: immigrants to Nova Scotia from, 97; passenger lists of boats from, 271n.154

Yorktown, Virginia: de-
feat of the British
forces at, 136
Young, Colonel, of the
60th Regiment, 61
Young, William, Loyalist
surgeon at Digby, 205

Zouberchuler, Mr
Sebastian, of Lunen-
burg, 269n.117